Automation and Emerging Technology in Clinical Microbiology

Editor

CAREY-ANN D. BURNHAM

CLINICS IN LABORATORY MEDICINE

www.labmed.theclinics.com

September 2013 • Volume 33 • Number 3

ELSEVIER

1600 John F. Kennedy Boulevard ● Suite 1800 ● Philadelphia, Pennsylvania, 19103-2899

http://www.theclinics.com

CLINICS IN LABORATORY MEDICINE Volume 33, Number 3
September 2013 ISSN 0272-2712, ISBN-13: 978-0-323-18860-9

Editor: Patrick Manley

Reprints. For copies of 100 or more, of articles in this publication, please contact the Commercial Reprints Department, Elsevier Inc., 360 Park Avenue South, New York, New York 10010-1710. Tel. (212) 633-3813, Fax: (212) 462-1935, E-mail: reprints@elsevier.com.

Clinics in Laboratory Medicine (ISSN 0272-2712) is published quarterly by Elsevier Inc., 360 Park Avenue South, New York, NY 10010-1710. Months of issue are March, June, September, and December. Business and Editorial offices: 1600 John F. Kennedy Blvd., Suite 1800, Philadelphia, PA 19103-2899. Periodicals postage paid at NewYork, NY and additional mailing offices. Subscription prices are $240.00 per year (US individuals), $382.00 per year (US institutions), $129.00 per year (US students), $291.00 per year (Canadian individuals), $483.00 per year (Canadian institutions), $177.00 per year (Canadian students), $370.00 per year (foreign individuals), $483.00 per year (foreign institutions), $177.00 (foreign students). Foreign air speed delivery is included in all Clinics subscription prices. All prices are subject to change without notice. POSTMASTER: Send address changes to *Clinics in Laboratory Medicine*, Elsevier Health Sciences Division, Subscription Customer Service, 3251 Riverport Lane, Maryland Heights, MO 63043. **Customer Service: 1-800-654-2452 (US). From outside of the US and Canada, call 1-314-447-8871. Fax: 1-314-447-8029. E-mail: journalscustomerservice-usa@elsevier.com (for print support) or journalsonlinesupport-usa@elsevier.com (for online support).**

Clinics in Laboratory Medicine is covered in *EMBASE/Exerpta Medica, MEDLINE/PubMed (Index Medicus), Cinahl, Current Contents/Clinical Medicine, BIOSIS and ISI/BIOMED.*

Printed and bound by CPI Group (UK) Ltd, Croydon, CR0 4YY
Transferred to Digital Printing, 2013

Contributors

EDITOR

CAREY-ANN D. BURNHAM, PhD, D(ABMM)
Assistant Professor of Pathology and Immunology, Division of Laboratory and Genomic Medicine, Department of Pathology and Immunology, Washington University School of Medicine, Washington University in St Louis, St Louis, Missouri

AUTHORS

NIAZ BANAEI, MD
Assistant Professor, Departments of Pathology and Medicine, Stanford University School of Medicine, Stanford, California; Clinical Microbiology Laboratory, Stanford University Medical Center, Palo Alto, California

RICHARD S. BULLER, PhD, D(ABMM)
Research Assistant Professor of Pediatrics, Department of Pediatrics, Washington University School of Medicine, St Louis, Missouri

CAREY-ANN D. BURNHAM, PhD, D(ABMM)
Assistant Professor of Pathology and Immunology, Division of Laboratory and Genomic Medicine, Department of Pathology and Immunology, Washington University School of Medicine, Washington University in St Louis, St Louis, Missouri

SUSAN M. BUTLER-WU, PhD
Department of Laboratory Medicine, University of Washington Medical Center, Seattle, Washington

KAREN C. CARROLL, MD, F(CAP), F(AAM), F(IDSA)
Division of Microbiology, Department of Pathology, School of Medicine, The Johns Hopkins University, and The Johns Hopkins Hospital, Baltimore, Maryland

MARI L. DEMARCO, PhD
Clinical Assistant Professor, Department of Pathology and Laboratory Medicine, University of British Columbia, St. Paul's Hospital, Vancouver, Canada

TANIS C. DINGLE, PhD
Department of Laboratory Medicine, University of Washington Medical Center, Seattle, Washington

CHRISTOPHER D. DOERN, PhD
Department of Pathology, Children's Medical Center Dallas, University of Texas Southwestern Medical Center, Dallas, Texas

SHERRY A. DUNBAR, PhD
Luminex Corporation, Austin, Texas

BRADLEY A. FORD, MD, PhD
Clinical Assistant Professor of Pathology, Associate Director of Clinical Microbiology, Department of Pathology, University of Iowa Hospitals and Clinics, Iowa City, Iowa

GEORGE KALLSTROM, PhD
Medical Director, Clinical Microbiology; Department of Microbiology, Tripler Army Medical Center, Honolulu, Hawaii

BENJAMIN C. KIRKUP, PhD
Deputy Director, Department of Wound Infections, Walter Reed Army Institute of Research, Silver Spring, Maryland

ROBERT F. LUO, MD, MPH
Clinical Instructor, Department of Pathology, Stanford University School of Medicine, Stanford, California; Clinical Microbiology Laboratory, Stanford University Medical Center, Palo Alto, California

DUNCAN MACCANNELL, PhD
Science Officer, National Center for Emerging and Zoonotic Infectious Diseases, Centers for Disease Control and Prevention, Atlanta, Georgia

STEVEN MAHLEN, PhD
Director, Bacterial Diseases Branch, Walter Reed Army Institute of Research, Silver Spring, Maryland

ELIZABETH M. MARLOWE, PhD
Southern California Permanente Medical Group, Regional Reference Laboratories, North Hollywood, California

ERIN MCELVANIA TEKIPPE, PhD
Division of Laboratory and Genomic Medicine, Department of Pathology and Immunology, Washington University School of Medicine, Washington University in St Louis, St Louis, Missouri

SUSAN M. NOVAK, PhD
Southern California Permanente Medical Group, Regional Reference Laboratories, North Hollywood, California

MORGAN A. PENCE, PhD
Division of Laboratory and Genomic Medicine, Department of Pathology and Immunology, Washington University School of Medicine, Washington University in St Louis, St Louis, Missouri

BOBBI S. PRITT, MD
Associate Professor of Pathology and Laboratory Medicine, Director of Clinical Parasitology, Division of Clinical Microbiology, Department of Laboratory Medicine and Pathology, Mayo Clinic, Rochester, Minnesota

STEFAN RIEDEL, MD, PhD, D(ABMM), F(CAP), F(ASCP)
Division of Microbiology, Department of Pathology, School of Medicine, The Johns Hopkins University, and Johns Hopkins Bayview Medical Center, Baltimore, Maryland

AUDREY N. SCHUETZ, MD, MPH
Assistant Professor of Pathology and Laboratory Medicine, Weill Cornell Medical College, New York-Presbyterian Hospital, New York, New York

YI-WEI TANG, MD, PhD
Clinical Microbiology Service, Department of Laboratory Medicine, Memorial
Sloan-Kettering Cancer Center, New York, New York

SHAWN VASOO, MBBS, MRCP
Instructor of Pathology and Laboratory Medicine, Division of Clinical Microbiology,
Department of Laboratory Medicine and Pathology, Mayo Clinic, Rochester, Minnesota

HONGWEI ZHANG, MD, PhD
Luminex Corporation, Austin, Texas

Contents

Sepsis, severe sepsis, and septic shock cause significant morbidity and mortality worldwide. Rapid diagnosis and therapeutic interventions are desirable to improve the overall mortality in patients with sepsis. However, gold standard laboratory diagnostic methods for sepsis, pose a significant challenge to rapid diagnosis of sepsis by physicians and laboratories. This article discusses the usefulness and potential of biomarkers and molecular test methods for a more rapid clinical and laboratory diagnosis of sepsis. Because new technologies are quickly emerging, physicians and laboratories must appreciate the key factors and characteristics that affect the clinical usefulness and diagnostic accuracy of these test methodologies.

Over the past several years a wide variety of molecular assays for the detection of respiratory viruses has reached the market. The tests described herein range from kits containing primers and probes detecting specific groups of viruses, to self-contained systems requiring specialized instruments that extract nucleic acids and perform the polymerase chain reaction with little operator input. Some of the tests target just the viruses involved in large yearly epidemics such as influenza, or specific groups of viruses such as the adenoviruses or parainfluenza viruses; others can detect most of the known respiratory viruses and some bacterial agents.

Molecular parasitology represents an emerging field in microbiology diagnostics. Although most assays use nonstandardized, laboratory-developed methods, a few commercial systems have recently become available and are slowly being introduced into larger laboratories. In addition, a few methodologies show promise for use in field settings in which parasitic infections are endemic. This article reviews the available techniques and their applications to major parasitic diseases such as malaria, leishmaniasis, and trichomoniasis.

The biomarkers galactomannan and 1,3-β-D-glucan have been well studied over the past years and are gaining a role in the diagnosis of invasive fungal infections. Although not as well studied until recently, molecular methods for the diagnosis of invasive fungal infection are also being evaluated. Outcomes data for molecular testing are expanding, but have not yet provided enough evidence for inclusion of molecular diagnostics in formal clinical guidelines. Lack of standardization and validation of the various molecular assays and platforms has hindered their widespread acceptance in the evaluation of invasive fungal infections, although the future is promising.

Gastroenteritis persists as a worldwide problem, responsible for approximately 2 million deaths annually. Traditional diagnostic methods used in the clinical microbiology laboratory include a myriad of tests, such as culture, microscopy, and immunodiagnostics, which can be labor intensive and suffer from long turnaround times and, in some cases, poor and Yi-Wei Tang sensitivity. This article reviews recent advances in genomic and proteomic technologies that have been applied to the detection and identification of gastrointestinal pathogens. These methods simplify and speed up the detection of pathogenic microorganisms, and their implementation in the clinical microbiology laboratory has potential to revolutionize the diagnosis of gastroenteritis.

Tuberculosis (TB) continues to be a public health emergency, compounded by the lack of adequate diagnostic testing in many regions of the world. New advances in the molecular detection of *Mycobacterium tuberculosis*, including faster and simpler nucleic acid amplification tests, have resulted in rapid and cost-effective methods to diagnose TB and test for drug resistance. Ongoing research on biomarkers for TB infection may lead to new tests for blood, urine, breath, and sputum. Sustained investment in the development and dissemination of diagnostic tests for TB is critical for increasing TB case finding, placing patients on appropriate treatment, and reducing transmission.

Imagine a clinical microbiology laboratory where a patient's specimens are placed on a conveyor belt and sent on an automation line for processing and plating. Technologists need only log onto a computer to visualize the images of a culture and send to a mass spectrometer for identification. Once a pathogen is identified, the system knows to send the colony for susceptibility testing. This is the future of the clinical microbiology laboratory. This article outlines the operational and staffing challenges facing clinical microbiology laboratories and the evolution of automation that is shaping the way laboratory medicine will be practiced in the future.

> Matrix-assisted laser desorption/ionization time-of-flight mass spectrometry (MALDI-TOF MS) is a rapid, reliable, and high-throughput diagnostic tool for the identification of microorganisms. The technology is unique in clinical microbiology, allowing laboratories to definitively identify bacterial and fungal isolates within minutes. The rapid turnaround time and minimal cost for consumables per specimen compared with conventional identification methods have resulted in MALDI-TOF MS being increasingly used in clinical laboratories worldwide. This article summarizes the current literature on MALDI-TOF MS for microbial identification and provides a preview of the method's potential future applications in clinical microbiology.

> The routine use of matrix-assisted laser desorption/ionization time-of-flight mass spectrometry (MALDI-TOF MS) has revolutionized microorganism identification in the clinical microbiology laboratory. Building from these now common microorganism identification strategies, this review explores future clinical applications of MALDI-TOF MS. This includes practical approaches for laboratorians interested in implementing direct identification processing methods for MALDI-TOF detection of microbes in bloodstream infection (BSI) and urinary tract infection (UTI), as well as, post-analytical approaches for classifying MALDI-TOF spectral data to detect characteristics other and species-level identification (e.g. strain-level classification, typing, and resistance mechanisms).

> Over the course of the past several decades, rapid advancements in molecular technologies have revolutionized the practice of public health microbiology, and have fundamentally changed the nature, accuracy, and timeliness of laboratory data for outbreak investigation and response. Whole-genome sequencing, in particular, is becoming an increasingly feasible and cost-effective approach for near real-time high-resolution strain typing, genomic characterization, and comparative analyses. This review discusses the current state of the art in bacterial strain typing for outbreak investigation and infectious disease surveillance, and the impact of emerging genomic technologies on the field of public health microbiology.

> The detection of blood stream infections is one of the most important functions of the clinical microbiology laboratory. Sepsis is a clinical emergency, and mortality increases if commencement of appropriate antimicrobial therapy is delayed. Automated blood culture systems are the most sensitive approach for detection of the causative agent of sepsis. Several

Preface

Automation and Emerging Technology in Clinical Microbiology

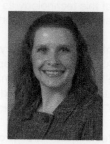

Carey-Ann D. Burnham, PhD, D(ABMM)
Editor

This is an exciting time in the field of Clinical Microbiology and the "state of the art" is evolving at a rapid pace. This can be attributed to new technology, rapid development and evolution of antimicrobial resistance, and the discovery of new pathogens. In addition, advances in modern medicine, such as solid organ and stem cell transplantation, have resulted in an explosion of infections with agents that historically have been considered to be of low virulence. This issue of *Clinics in Laboratory Medicine* highlights some of the recent advances in diagnostic microbiology, including high-throughput sequencing methods, matrix-assisted laser desorption ionization-time-of-flight mass spectrometry (MALDI-TOF MS) for organism identification, molecular diagnostics, and the use of biomarkers in the diagnosis of infectious diseases.

This monograph includes articles devoted to contemporary approaches to a number of different types of infection. For example, in the diagnostic virology laboratory, viral culture is becoming almost obsolete; in the article by Dr Buller, advances in molecular diagnostics for respiratory viruses and some of the advantages and limitations of these methods are discussed. In Drs Vassoo and Pritt's article, advances in diagnostic parasitology beyond the traditional "ova and parasite" exam are explored. Next, Drs Dunbar, Zhang, and Tang present novel and advanced techniques for diagnosis of gastrointestinal pathogens.

An area of great interest in medicine is the development and validation of diagnostic biomarkers—noninvasive assays that can predict the presence of a particular disease state accurately. Biomarkers can be especially helpful for diagnosing infections due to slowly growing organisms and high-acuity clinical syndromes or confirming a disease state when an organism is isolated that can both colonize and cause infection. In clinical microbiology, there are a number of circumstances where biomarkers would have diagnostic utility. These have been investigated in detail for the diagnosis of sepsis (reviewed in the first article by Drs Riedel and Carroll) and invasive fungal infections (addressed in the article by Dr Schuetz). While these biomarkers are enticing diagnostic tools, to date, most of them fall short for use in the definitive diagnosis of an infectious disease.

Traditionally, the clinical microbiology laboratory has been considered a somewhat "low-tech" area, void of the automation that is becoming commonplace in Chemistry and Hematology laboratories. However, this is rapidly changing with the advancement of microbiology total laboratory automation systems. Widespread use of automation in microbiology will be an enormous change; a description of this technology as well as considerations for cost justification and implementation are detailed in the article by Drs Novak and Marlowe.

Another "chemistry" concept that is poised to supplant traditional phenotypic microbial identification methodology is MALDI-TOF MS. MALDI-TOF MS is a rapid, accurate, and inexpensive identification method that to date has been used primarily for bacterial identification; MALDI-TOF MS for organism identification is reviewed by Drs Dingle and Butler-Wu, and advanced uses of MALDI-TOF MS in microbiology are described by Drs DeMarco and Ford in their article.

So-called "next generation sequencing" (NGS) techniques are producing sequencing data at a rapid pace while the cost of this analysis has been steadily decreasing. However, the role that NGS will play in diagnostic microbiology is still unclear. In the article by Drs Kirkup, Mahlen, and Kallstrom, some of the challenges of integrating this methodology into clinical practice, including bioinformatics and regulatory issues, are described. I think it will be very interesting to see how this technology evolves and is used in the microbiology lab in the future.

All of this exciting new technology is coupled with challenges for the Microbiology laboratory. For example, with the shift toward molecular diagnostics, laboratories will have to be aware of the impact that the constant evolution of organisms will have on the analytical performance characteristics of these assays. There will be an ongoing need to train the workforce in new techniques, the challenge of choosing the technology that is the most appropriate for the patient population that is served by the laboratory, as well as choosing methods that fit the size, clinical needs, and budget of the hospital. In addition, laboratories will have to consider the impact of "active" compared to "passive" reporting of results, and effective communication with the end-user on the utility and performance characteristics of new methods. Some of these challenges are detailed in Dr Doern's article on integration of new technology into clinical practices. In addition to the direct challenges to the diagnostic laboratory, public health considerations are emerging as a result of the shift away from culture-based techniques—strain typing and outbreak investigation may prove difficult in the absence of isolates of microorganisms. A review of the advances in strain typing techniques is found in the article by Dr McCannell.

I have very much enjoyed working on this monograph, and I would like to thank the contributors for all of their efforts in preparing interesting submissions. I hope you will enjoy reading it.

Carey-Ann D. Burnham, PhD, D(ABMM)
Assistant Professor of Pathology and Immunology
Division of Laboratory and Genomic Medicine
Department of Pathology and Immunology
Washington University School of Medicine, Washington University in St Louis
660 South Euclid Avenue, Campus Box 8118
St Louis, MO 63110, USA

E-mail address:
cburnham@path.wustl.edu

Laboratory Detection of Sepsis
Biomarkers and Molecular Approaches

Stefan Riedel, MD, PhD, D(ABMM)[a],*, Karen C. Carroll, MD[b]

KEYWORDS

- Biomarkers • Procalcitonin • C-reactive protein • Molecular diagnostics
- Nucleic acid amplification testing • Sepsis • Bacteremia

KEY POINTS

- Sepsis, severe sepsis, and septic shock are significant medical problems worldwide; sepsis is the 10th leading cause of death in the United States.
- Although numerous biomarkers are available no single assay has consistently emerged for use as a single marker with high diagnostic accuracy for the prediction and outcome assessment of sepsis.
- The best evidence in support of usefulness and diagnostic and prognostic performance in the management of patients with sepsis exists for the following biomarkers: C-reactive protein, procalcitonin, adrenomedullin, and a few select interleukins (IL-6 and IL-8).
- Although blood cultures are still considered the gold standard in clinical practice for the detection of sepsis, molecular technologies provide more rapid organism identification from positive blood cultures in patients with bacteremia/sepsis. Direct whole-blood assays are not yet sensitive enough to replace existing culture amplification.
- Diagnostic approaches for early sepsis diagnosis using biomarkers, together with rapid organism identification by molecular technologies, will likely lead to a reduction of turnaround time for test results and subsequent improvements of therapeutic interventions and patient care outcomes.

S. Riedel has received research funding from Cubist Pharmaceuticals, Lexington, MA; Siemens Healthcare Diagnostics, Tarrytown, NY; Meridian Bioscience, Cincinnati, OH; Becton, Dickinson and Co, Sparks, MD; and Quidel, Inc, San Diego, CA.
K.C. Carroll has received research funding from BioFire, Inc, Salt Lake City, UT; Nanosphere, Inc, Northbrook, IL; and AdvanDx, Inc, Woburn, MA. She is also on the scientific advisory boards for Quidel, Inc, San Diego, CA, and NanoMR, Inc, Albuquerque, NM.

[a] Division of Microbiology, Department of Pathology, School of Medicine, The Johns Hopkins University, and Johns Hopkins Bayview Medical Center, 4940 Eastern Avenue, A Building, Room 102-B, Baltimore, MD 21224, USA; [b] Division of Microbiology, Department of Pathology, School of Medicine, The Johns Hopkins University, and The Johns Hopkins Hospital, Meyer B1-193, 600 North Wolfe Street, Baltimore, MD 21287, USA
* Corresponding author.
E-mail address: sriedel2@jhmi.edu

Clin Lab Med 33 (2013) 413–437
http://dx.doi.org/10.1016/j.cll.2013.03.006
0272-2712/13/$ – see front matter © 2013 Elsevier Inc. All rights reserved.

INTRODUCTION

Sepsis, severe sepsis, and septic shock are the increasingly severe stages of the systemic inflammatory host response to bloodstream infections. The host response to infection is commonly known as systemic inflammatory response syndrome (SIRS). Uniformly accepted definitions of these three conditions were first established in 1992 by an expert panel from the American College of Chest Physicians and the Society of Critical Care Medicine.[1] In the years to follow, and as a result of these consensus definitions, numerous studies investigating the epidemiology of sepsis were conducted. However, significant limitations of these early sepsis consensus guidelines were soon recognized,[2,3] and the descriptions of the stages of sepsis syndrome were redefined during the 2001 Consensus Conference.[4] The introduction of these new criteria (predisposition, infection, response, and organ dysfunction [PIRO]) allowed for a better understanding of various stages of sepsis and aided in developing a better understanding of the various patient groups with sepsis and their outcomes.[5] Although the original understanding of sepsis syndromes placed the various syndromes (ie, SIRS, sepsis, severe sepsis, septic shock) along a linear path of progressive syndromes with increasing severity, this revised classification of sepsis placed these entities into a multidimensional staging system, similar to those systems used for cancer staging.[4]

Sepsis is now recognized worldwide as an important medical problem with significant morbidity and mortality.[6,7] In general, sepsis occurs in approximately 2% of hospitalized patients in developed countries, although rates for intensive care unit (ICU) patients are significantly higher (6%–30%).[8] Sepsis is among the most common causes of death in hospitalized patients and, together with septic shock, is the 11th leading cause of death in the United States.[9] Each year, in the United States alone, an estimated 1 million patients develop sepsis and/or severe sepsis with an associated mortality as high as 60%.[6,7,10,11] Similar data have been reported from other countries.[12,13] Despite significant improvements in diagnosis, treatment, care, and preventative measures,[14] the incidence of sepsis continues to increase by as much as 8.7%,[11] especially in patients admitted to a hospital ICU and in elderly patients, as the overall population continues to age.[6,15–18] Considering the implications on diagnosis and care for the individual patient with sepsis together with the overall large economic burden,[6,19] recently published guidelines emphasized the importance of rapid detection of the causative organisms together with prompt initiation of antimicrobial therapy and other supportive therapeutic measures.[20] This article provides an assessment of recent improvements in diagnostic methods, focusing on the usefulness of biomarkers and molecular methods for the diagnosis of sepsis.

THE CLINICAL CONTINUUM OF SEPSIS: CONSIDERATIONS FOR CURRENT DIAGNOSTIC METHODS

From a clinical perspective, sepsis is still defined and diagnosed based on the observation of physiologic changes in response to an infection (ie, changes in the patient's body temperature, heart rate, respiration rate, and changes in the white blood cell count [WBC]).[20] These criteria are known as the SIRS criteria. Although the clinical suspicion and preliminary diagnosis of sepsis are based on any combination of these criteria, the proof of the infection is provided by obtaining a blood culture (BC) that is positive for bacterial and/or fungal microorganisms.[21] However, bacteremia and/or fungemia alone, as defined by the identification of microorganisms in blood, do not designate sepsis and sepsis-related syndromes.[4] In this context, the collection of 2 to 3 sets of BCs at the time of initial suspicion of sepsis is considered the gold standard and cornerstone of many diagnostic algorithms.[22] BCs provide not only proof to establish the infectious cause of the patient's illness but also provide the organism for antimicrobial susceptibility testing (AST). The latter is essential to the continuum of clinical care in patients with sepsis because it provides the evidence to optimize antimicrobial therapy. On a larger scale, AST results are essential to support antimicrobial stewardship efforts in hospitals to decrease antimicrobial resistance rates. However, BCs and associated laboratory tests for diagnosis of bloodstream infection and sepsis are often limited by prolonged turnaround times (TAT) for results reporting. Despite being considered the gold standard for diagnosis, BCs have been described as having limited sensitivity, particularly when patients have already received antimicrobial therapy before BCs are collected, and they are subject to contamination by resident skin flora if BCs are not collected using an appropriate aseptic technique.[22–26] These diagnostic limitations and uncertainties are frequently compensated for by the liberal use of broad-spectrum antimicrobial therapy. Furthermore, physicians tend to have an equally liberal approach in ordering BCs for diagnostic purposes; as a result, only 4% to 7% of all BCs drawn in hospitals are positive.[27,28] In contrast, the positivity rate of BCs drawn from patients with a high index of suspicion for sepsis may be as high as 98% if BCs are drawn in duplicate or triplicate.[26]

The prevailing understanding of sepsis and related syndromes has been that sepsis, severe sepsis, and septic shock are stages of an uncontrolled inflammatory response to a bloodstream infection.[1,4] Although the clinical limitations of the SIRS concept were quickly recognized, additional studies investigating the pathophysiology of sepsis recognized that SIRS was accompanied by a compensatory antiinflammatory response syndrome (CARS), first described by Bone.[29,30] Studies leading to the current understanding of SIRS and CARS, or the combination thereof, known as the mixed inflammatory response syndrome have further recognized that patients with sepsis who present with an early hyperinflammatory state often evolve into a subsequent hypoinflammatory state, known as immunoparalysis.[31,32] As a result, there has been a renewed interest in, and better understanding of, the pathophysiology of sepsis during the past decade.[33–35] Further studies recognized that the immunosuppression caused by sepsis results not only in a decrease in the patient's ability to clear the primary bloodstream infection but also predisposes to developing secondary infections and overall significantly increased mortality; these findings are supported by patients who die from sepsis and multi organ failure having laboratory test–based evidence of being in a state of immunosuppression.[36]

Considering the previously mentioned diagnostic uncertainties of current laboratory tests for sepsis together with the evolving evidence of the immunologic concepts of sepsis, it is reasonable to search for and develop diagnostic approaches that target measurement of the immune response to sepsis. It is hoped that such newly developed tests will increase the sensitivity and positive predictive value (PPV) of established laboratory tests such as BCs, significantly reduce the TAT for test results compared with current gold standard methods, or provide means to better monitor the response to treatment and intervention. The usefulness of biomarkers and molecular laboratory tests currently available to improve sepsis diagnosis is discussed in the following sections.

BIOMARKERS

During the last decade, much effort has been directed toward identification of biomarkers that are useful in the differential diagnosis of sepsis and other infectious diseases. A biomarker is an analyte that can be used to assess a normal or pathologic process, or the response to a therapeutic intervention.[37] Aside from the recent advances in methodology for rapid organism detection, more sensitive methods have been developed for the measurement of various serum protein biomarkers for diagnosis and monitoring of sepsis. To be considered clinically useful, a biomarker must have high diagnostic accuracy, reflected by high sensitivity, specificity, and both PPVs and negative predictive values (NPVs).[38] Furthermore, the diagnostic accuracy of a test is assessed by calculating the positive and negative likelihood ratios. These statistical values are then typically expressed for various cutoff values by using a receiver operating characteristic curve. However, the accurate assessment of the clinical value for a biomarker is difficult, considering that various clinical and laboratory studies frequently use different cutoff values for the same marker and disease. In the 1970s to 1990s, 2 markers of inflammation were widely used for the diagnosis of sepsis: erythrocyte sedimentation rate (ESR) and C-reactive protein (CRP). However, in more recent years these markers proved less useful because of their lack of specificity for sepsis and even infection.[39] Although currently more than 100 potential biomarkers have been identified for the diagnosis of sepsis, their usefulness remains elusive.[40] In general, sepsis biomarkers can be classified based on their role as mediators of systemic inflammation; they can be acute-phase protein/biomarkers (eg, CRP, procalcitonin [PCT], lipopolysaccharide-binding protein), cytokine/chemokine biomarkers (eg, interleukin [IL]-6 and IL-8), or markers of other pathophysiologic processes that occur during sepsis. Markers of other pathophysiologic processes include coagulation biomarkers, soluble cell surface receptors, and adrenomedullin (ADM). Many of the older biomarkers such as ESR and CRP are nonspecific indicators of inflammation, and their discriminatory value for prediction and diagnosis of sepsis is doubtful. This article first discusses the advantages and disadvantages of several biomarkers currently applied for the diagnosis of sepsis, followed by a brief discussion of additional biomarkers that are currently considered for development and/or use in diagnostic algorithms. These concepts are summarized in **Table 1**.

CRP

CRP is a general acute-phase plasma protein in the pentraxin family of acute-phase reactants. It is primarily synthesized by hepatocytes and its plasma concentration increases significantly in response to inflammation and/or infection, mediated by cytokine stimulation.[38,41,42] Most healthy people have a plasma CRP concentration of less than or equal to 2 mg/L, although levels as high as 10 mg/L have been described. CRP has been used both as a diagnostic and prognostic marker for inflammation and infection in adult and pediatric patients. However, the sensitivity and specificity of CRP as a diagnostic marker of infection and sepsis varies greatly in the literature, largely dependent on the cutoff values chosen for these studies.[42] Although some investigators suggested that higher plasma CRP concentration may help in distinguishing bacterial from viral and other infections,[43,44] the clinical usefulness of such diagnostic approach remains unclear. Furthermore, a significant overlap in CRP values exists between patients with and without infection, which suggests that measurements of a single, absolute CRP level are not clinically useful. This limitation of the diagnostic usefulness of CRP is particularly apparent for ICU patients in whom other causes of inflammation may be present concomitant to sepsis.[45] Because of comorbidities associated with inflammation, many ICU patients, and particularly elderly patients, may already present with increased CRP levels on admission to the ICU; however, irrespective of this diagnostic limitation, a single increased CRP level may still support (together with other clinical indicators, such as fever and increased WBC) a strong clinical

Table 1
Biomarkers for diagnosis and prognosis of sepsis, identified by literature search, with select references

Biomarker	Commercially Available Assay	Biomarker Evaluated for Diagnostic Usefulness by Disease Category			Prognostic Usefulness	Patient Population		Health Care Setting		Study Design			Select References and Comments
		Sepsis	Severe Sepsis	Septic Shock		Adult	Pediatric	ED	Hospital (ICU)	Clinical, Observational	Clinical, Randomized-Controlled, Interventional	Experimental	
CRP	Yes	✓	✓	✓	(✓)	X	X	X	X	X	X	—	41–49
PCT	Yes	✓	✓	✓	(✓)	X	X	X	X	X	X	X	53,59–63,65–67,69 (meta-analyses)
IL-6, IL-8	Yes	✓	✓	✓	✓	✓	✓	X	X	X	X	X	95–99
ADM	Yes[a]	✓	(✓)	✓	✓	✓	—	—	X	X	—	X	84,86–93
LBP	Yes[a]	✓	✓	(✓)	—	—	—	—	X	X	—	—	77–81; higher in sepsis compared with no sepsis
PTX3	No	—	(✓)	(✓)	(✓)	✓	—	X	X	X	—	—	100,101; some predictive value for 28-d mortality
EAA	No	(✓)	(✓)	(✓)	(✓)	✓	—	—	X	X	—	X	102–104

✓, the test is useful; (✓), limited usefulness or insufficient data for evaluation; X, studies met specific patient care settings and study design characteristics as specified in the table; —, the studies had no usefulness or were not performed in this setting.

Abbreviations: ADM, adrenomedullin; CRP, C-reactive protein; EAA, endotoxin activity assay; IL, interleukin; LBP, lipopolysaccharide-binding protein; PCT, procalcitonin; PTX3, pentraxin 3.

[a] Not available in the United States.

suspicion of sepsis.[46,47] In one study, CRP levels greater than 200 mg/L were more likely to be associated with an acute infection.[48] More recently, Povoa and colleagues[49] suggested that, instead of single CRP levels, the use of daily monitoring of CRP levels may provide a better guidance tool for early detection of sepsis. In addition to the use as a diagnostic marker, CRP has been shown to have clinical usefulness for prognostic and therapeutic guidance. Similar to the limitations for diagnosis, a single CRP level has been shown to provide little information for prognostic purposes; instead, changes and trends of CRP levels over time have been reported to correlate with the level of severity of sepsis.[50] Two recent studies suggested that changes in CRP levels are good predictors for response to antimicrobial treatment and correlate with morbidity and mortality in patients with sepsis.[51,52] Failure of CRP levels to decline despite antimicrobial therapy were associated with increased morbidity and mortality and may indicate an inappropriate choice for antimicrobial therapy.[51] However, despite the continued and widespread use of CRP in various clinical situations, the lack of sensitivity and specificity is well recognized and continues to fuel the desire to identify newer and better biomarkers for sepsis.

PCT

For the past 20 years, PCT has been extensively, and with increasing frequency, subject to clinical investigations to define its clinical usefulness as a biomarker for the diagnosis of sepsis and other infectious diseases. A member of the *CAPA* protein family, PCT is a precursor peptide for the hormone calcitonin (CT), first mentioned in the medical literature in1975 and then again in 1981.[53] In 1993, Assicot and colleagues[54] recognized that serum levels of PCT and other CT-precursor molecules were significantly increased during microbial infections and other inflammatory conditions. In healthy individuals (ie, in noninfectious conditions), the transcription of the *CALC*-1 gene is restricted to neuroendocrine cells in the thyroid gland and the lung, and serum PCT levels are low, typically less than 0.1 ng/mL.[55] In contrast, during infections, and particularly during systemic infections such as sepsis, the gene expression of the *CALC*-I gene is upregulated and PCT is constitutively released from almost all tissues and cell types in the body.[56] PCT has a favorable kinetic profile for use as a diagnostic marker in clinical settings. On upregulation of the CT mRNA, serum PCT concentrations promptly increase within 6 to 12 hours.[57] On cessation of the expression of the CT mRNA (ie, when the infection and/or host immune responses are controlled), circulating PCT levels decrease by half within 24 hours. The rapid upregulation, sustainment, and decrease of serum PCT levels during infections and therapy makes it an ideal biomarker. Furthermore, it is important to recognize that the increase of PCT remains unaffected by the administration of immunosuppressive therapy (specifically corticosteroids) compared with other biomarkers such as CRP.[58] Data from a recently published prospective multicenter cohort study show that initial PCT levels in the emergency department accurately predicted BC positivity in patients with community-acquired pneumonia.[59] Two other studies, using a highly sensitive chemiluminescence sandwich immunoassay for PCT measurement, found that PCT is a valuable diagnostic biomarker for sepsis in febrile patients presenting to the emergency department.[60,61] DeKruif and colleagues[60] showed that the addition of PCT to clinical scoring criteria significantly increased the value of diagnostic algorithms for sepsis. Using a cutoff point of 0.1 ng/mL, Riedel and colleagues[61] showed that bacteremia and sepsis are unlikely in settings of low PCT levels; the NPV was 98.2% (sensitivity 75%, specificity 78%, and PPV 16.9%). Furthermore, PCT has proved to be a sensitive marker for diagnosing bacteremia and sepsis in the elderly as well as in the very young,[62,63] and has shown excellent correlation with bacterial load and could discriminate between BC contaminants and organisms representing bacteremia.[64] Despite the promising data on its usefulness as a diagnostic marker, several limitations to the use of PCT have also been described. First, there is no single cutoff value for PCT levels to define sepsis. Furthermore, many of the previously mentioned studies are single-center observational studies, with a great variation in analytical assays used for PCT measurement, as well as the clinical settings in which PCT was evaluated. Jones and colleagues[65] performed a meta-analysis evaluating the diagnostic performance of PCT for the diagnosis of sepsis in the emergency room setting. The investigators evaluated 150 published studies on this topic, including 17 for a final analysis. Most of these studies used 0.5 ng/mL as a cutoff value (range, 0.4–2 ng/mL); the prevalence of sepsis among these studies ranged from 4.2% to 53.7%. The investigators concluded from their analysis that PCT had a moderate diagnostic usefulness with a sensitivity of 76% and specificity of 70% for the detection of sepsis. They questioned the widespread use of PCT as a single diagnostic test for sepsis in an ambulatory care setting. A similar moderate performance of PCT as a diagnostic marker for sepsis was found in a meta-analysis by Tang and colleagues,[66] showing a sensitivity and specificity of 71%. In another meta-analysis of 33 studies with nearly 4000 patients, PCT was a superior biomarker for the diagnosis of sepsis compared with CRP.[67]

In addition to being a biomarker used for sepsis diagnosis, PCT has been evaluated as a prognostic test for the management of patients with sepsis. Although one study showed that PCT increases with increasing severity of sepsis and organ dysfunction,[68] another study showed that PCT, contrary to CRP and clinical indicators, failed to predict prognosis.[69] In contrast, PCT has been shown in clinical algorithms to safely reduce antimicrobial use for patients in the ICU and emergency room setting, suggesting that serial PCT measurements allow for a reduction of antimicrobial treatment duration without patient harm.[70–72] Several assays for measurement of PCT are commercially available; however, these assays vary in their performance characteristics and analytical sensitivities and are discussed in more detail elsewhere.[53] One of the first, and still widely used, assays is the immunoluminometric PCT assay (LUMItest, BRAHMS, Henningsdorf, Germany); this assay has a functional sensitivity of 0.5 ng/mL, with an analytical assay sensitivity of 0.08 ng/mL. Although this manual assay detects significantly increased serum levels of PCT, it may be too insensitive to detect mildly or moderately increased PCT levels during early stages of infections. The next generation of commercially available PCT assays is based on the principle of time-resolved amplified cryptate emission (TRACE) technology (KRYPTOR, BRAHMS, Henningsdorf, Germany); this assay has an analytical sensitivity of 0.019 ng/mL and a functional assay sensitivity of 0.06 ng/mL. Other commercially available PCT assays are the LIAISON BRAHMS PCT-immunoluminometric assay (DiaSorin, Saluggia, Italy) and the VIDAS enzyme-linked fluorescent immunoassay (bioMérieux, Durham, NC). The functional sensitivities for PCT for these two assays are 0.1 ng/mL and 0.09 ng/mL, respectively. At the time of this article's preparation, additional commercial assays by Siemens Healthcare Diagnostics (Tarrytown, NY), and Roche Diagnostics (Indianapolis, IN) are in development. Depending on the assay used in clinical studies, the cutoff value for PCT for the diagnosis of sepsis varies as stated earlier, ranging from 0.1 ng/mL to 0.5 ng/mL.[60,61,65]

Lipopolysaccharide-binding Protein

Like CRP and PCT, lipopolysaccharide-binding protein (LBP) is an acute-phase protein; on stimulation by IL-6 and IL-1, it is produced in hepatocytes, as well as by the epithelial cells of the lungs and the intestine.[73,74] LBP binds the lipopolysaccharide

(LPS) of gram-negative bacteria, forming a complex that in turn binds to CD14 and to Toll-like receptors, initiating a signal transduction and ultimately release of IL-1 and stimulation of macrophages and neutrophils.[73–76] In humans, LBP is constitutively present in serum at concentrations ranging between 5 and 10 ng/mL; however, during acute-phase reactions, peak levels of up to 200 µg/mL have been described.[73] A study in 1999 by Opal and colleagues[77] suggested that the quantitative level of endotoxin and LBP may have prognostic significance in patients with severe sepsis. Another study, comparing various biomarkers in patients with sepsis, found that CRP, IL-6, and LBP seemed to be superior to PCT as diagnostic markers of sepsis, whereas PCT seemed to be superior as a marker for disease severity.[78] However, the findings from these studies could not be confirmed by subsequent studies, which did not identify a significant predictive value of LBP for survival in sepsis.[79–81] Furthermore, LBP concentrations did not distinguish between sepsis caused by gram-positive and gram-negative bacteria. Considering this weak evidence for LBP as a biomarker, it is reasonable at this point to consider LBP as a less useful tool in diagnostic algorithms for sepsis. At present, there are no assays commercially available in the United States for measurement of LBP; however, assays for LBP, IL-6, and IL-2R are available on the Immulite 2000 XPi (Siemens Health care Diagnostics, GmbH, Eschborn, Germany). The investigators in studies referenced in this article used the Immulite 2000 XPi assay or home-made assays, not approved by the US Food and Drug Administration (FDA), for research use only.

Pro-ADM and Provasopressin

The early phases of severe sepsis and septic shock are dominated by severe alterations of the cardiovascular system.[82] The multitude of hemodynamic alterations, including ineffective tissue oxygenation, inappropriate peripheral vasodilatation, and myocardial dysfunction, ultimately lead to refractory hypotension to volume therapy. Two biomarkers related to regulation of the vasotonus have been described: vasopressin (AVP), and ADM. AVP is produced by the hypothalamus in response to hemodynamic and osmotic stimuli.[83] During the early phase of septic shock, serum levels of AVP are increased, but, during the later phases of septic shock, AVP levels are decreased.[83,84]

ADM is vasodilator that exhibits both natriuretic and diuretic properties.[85] This hormone was first identified in pheochromocytoma, but was subsequently shown to be increased in patients with sepsis.[86] Several subsequent studies confirmed that ADM is increased in early and late stages of severe sepsis and septic shock and has a pivotal role in the hyperdynamic responses during early sepsis.[87–89] A prospective, observational study of 101 consecutive, critically ill patients with SIRS, sepsis, severe sepsis, and shock evaluated the prognostic usefulness of pro-ADM compared with other biomarkers (PCT, CRP, IL-6).[90] Pro-ADM was an excellent prognostic biomarker for the severity and outcome of sepsis, similar to the predictive value of clinical scoring systems such as the Acute Physiology and Chronic Health Evaluation-II (APACHE II) scores, and superior to other biomarkers such as CRP and PCT. Furthermore, the prognostic value of pro-ADM was independent of the sepsis classification system used. In a recent study of 99 patients admitted to the ICU with septic shock, both pro-AVP and pro-ADM serum concentrations were significantly higher in nonsurvivors compared with survivors, and both biomarkers seemed to be good predictors of 28-day mortality after septic shock.[91] Furthermore, the predictive capacity was even higher when these biomarkers were assessed as a pair. Two additional recent studies showed similar promising results that pro-ADM and pro-AVP either alone or combined are good diagnostic and predictive markers for sepsis and septic shock.[92,93]

Other Biomarkers

Numerous other biomarkers belonging to various groups of biologic markers have been proposed for the diagnosis and prognosis of sepsis. To address all of these markers in a comprehensive manner is beyond the scope of this article, so only a few other biomarkers for which there is evidence of clinical usefulness are highlighted.

Cytokines are the major contributors in the pathophysiology of sepsis and have long been considered as diagnostic and prognostic markers of this disease. Cytokines are polypeptides produced by various cells and secreted in response to bacteria and other antigens that regulate inflammatory processes. Two cytokines have been of particular interest in recent years: IL-6 and IL-8.

IL-6 was proposed as a marker for the early diagnosis of sepsis in neonates and in patients presenting to the emergency department.[94,95] During a randomized, double-blinded, placebo-controlled interventional trial for evaluation of suppression of the cytokine response in patients with sepsis, IL-6 was a good predictor for 28-day mortality.[96] In a single-center prospective study of neonates with sepsis, IL-6 and IL-8 did not have a significant PPV for prediction of sepsis on day 1 or 2 of admission to the ICU. Both biomarkers had a better NPV for sepsis on day 1 (89%), despite the low sensitivity and PPV.[97] Andaluz-Ojeda and colleagues[98] investigated the usefulness of 17 various cytokines in a multiplex panel as predictors of outcome in adult patients with severe sepsis and septic shock. The proinflammatory cytokines IL-6 and IL-8, as well as the immunosuppressive cytokine IL-10, had higher serum levels during the early stages of severe sepsis in those patients with fatal outcome, as measured by 3-day and 28-day mortality. In addition, there have been other emerging cytokine biomarker candidates, including IL-27.[99] In a cohort study of 231 critically ill children (<10 years of age) compared with 61 healthy children, serum levels of IL-27 greater than or equal to 5 ng/mL during the first 24 hours of sepsis onset/SIRS strongly predicted bacteremia/sepsis.[99] However, the investigators did not find a correlation between IL-27 levels and severity of illness. In the same study, the combination of IL-27 with PCT further increased the PPV of these tests.

Pentraxin 3 (PTX3), an acute-phase protein, has also been studied as a biomarker for sepsis diagnosis. One study showed that serum levels of PTX3 were significantly higher in patients with septic shock compared with those with severe sepsis, and serum levels remained significantly higher within the first week of sepsis in nonsurvivors compared with survivors.[100] In another study, PTX3 correlated with severity of sepsis in febrile patients presenting to the emergency department with sepsis.[101]

Another interesting biomarker is endotoxin, which is an essential component of the cell membrane of gram-negative bacteria. The endotoxin activity assay (EAA) has been shown to be a useful in vitro diagnostic test, allowing rapid measurement of endotoxin activity (EA) at the patient's bedside, using whole blood.[102,103] EA is expressed in relative units based on the chemiluminescent measurement of LPS.[102] The assay was evaluated during the Multicenter Endotoxin Detection in Critical Illness (MEDIC) trial in 857 ICU patients suspected to have sepsis.[103] In this study, EAA results from patients with sepsis were also compared with 97 healthy volunteers, and 93% of those healthy subjects had an EA level of less than 0.4. In patients with sepsis, EA levels of greater than or equal to 0.6 were determined to be high, and EA levels greater than or equal to 0.4 but less than 0.6 were considered intermediate. High EA levels were associated with a significantly higher risk of developing severe sepsis. Another recent study investigated the diagnostic and prognostic usefulness of EAA together with other biomarkers, including PCT and CRP.[104] Again, high (≥0.6) levels of EA were strongly associated with gram-negative sepsis and a higher risk for developing severe sepsis. Increased PCT levels together with a left shift of the WBC allowed for further risk assessment in patients with intermediate EA levels.

Biomarker Summary

This article reviews the common and currently available biomarkers for the diagnosis of sepsis. Several other types of biomarkers are currently under investigation, including soluble cell surface receptors such as triggering receptor expressed on myeloid cells 1 (TREM-1), and leukocyte cell surface markers. In all studies conducted to date, no single biomarker has consistently been identified that could be used as a single marker with high diagnostic accuracy. Studies that used a combination of biomarkers showed promising data toward improving the sensitivity, specificity, and predictive values of diagnostic algorithms.[98,105,106] However, in another recent study, out of 4 commercially available biomarkers (PCT, IL-6, CRP, and LBP), PCT was the best single predictor of bacteremia/sepsis in febrile patients presenting to the emergency department.[107] Furthermore, the combination of PCT with any of the other three biomarkers did not significantly improve the diagnostic accuracy and predictive value of PCT.

The fundamental limitation of establishing clinically useful biomarker panels for the diagnosis of sepsis is based in the limited understanding of the underlying pathophysiologic processes of this complex disease syndrome referred to as sepsis. Future studies, including multicenter clinical trials, are necessary to better evaluate the clinical usefulness of old and new sepsis biomarkers.

MOLECULAR DIAGNOSTIC METHODS

Although BCs are still considered the gold standard in clinical practice for the detection of sepsis, several adjunctive test methods have been develop during the past 10 years that allow more rapid organism identification once a BC is positive for bacterial growth. Most of these tests are pathogen specific and can be divided into conventional methods and molecular methods. The latter can be further divided into nonamplified methodologies, nucleic acid amplification techniques, broad-based assays, and proteomic techniques such as matrix-assisted laser desorption-ionization time-of-flight mass spectroscopy (MALDI-TOF MS). Conventional and nonamplified methods for rapid organism identification from positive BCs, as well as MALDI-TOF MS, are discussed in more detail elsewhere in this issue. This article mainly discusses the nucleic acid amplified methods for organism identification from BCs.

Amplified Molecular Methods, Growth Required

There are a variety of pathogen-specific nucleic acid amplification tests or platforms available in the United States for differentiation of methicillin-susceptible *Staphylococcus aureus* (MSSA) from methicillin-resistant *S aureus* (MRSA), and in some cases coagulase-negative staphylococci (CoNS). The BD GeneOhm (San Diego, CA) StaphSR assay is a multiplex real-time polymerase chain reaction (PCR) test that is run on the SmartCycler instrument. The assay amplifies specific target sequences of *S. aureus* and a specific target near the *SCCmec* insertion site (*orfX* junction) in MRSA (**Table 2**). One clinical study[108] performed on 300 BCs reported excellent performance characteristics (sensitivity for MSSA and MRSA of 98.9% and 100%, respectively); however, others have noted some limitations. In a seeded study of 134 spiked BC bottles, Grobner and colleagues[109] compared the BD GeneOhm StaphSR with other molecular assays and standard laboratory procedures. The assay performed well for differentiating *S. aureus* from other gram-positive cocci (100%

Table 2
Molecular assays for identification of causes of bacteremia

Assay	Manufacturer	Principles of the Assay	Pathogens Detected	Turnaround Time (h)
Molecular Pathogen-specific Multiplex PCR Assays, Growth Required				
StaphSR	BD GeneOhm, Inc, San Diego, CA	A multiplex real-time PCR test assay that amplifies specific target sequences of S aureus and a specific target near the SCCmec insertion site (orfX junction) in MRSA	S. aureus: differentiates MSSA from MRSA	2.5–3
Xpert MRSA/SA	Cepheid Diagnostics, Inc, Sunnyvale CA	Real-time PCR assay that detects sequences in the staphylococcal protein A (spa) gene, the SCCmec inserted into the S aureus chromosomal attB insertion site, and the mecA gene	S. aureus: differentiates MSSA from MRSA	1
LightCycler Staphylococcus M^Grade	Roche Molecular, Indianapolis, IN	Multiplex real-time PCR using FRET probes and melt curve analysis	2 assays: one that detects and differentiates S. aureus from CoNS; another that detects mecA	3
StaphPlex	Qiagen, Inc, Valencia, CA	Target-enriched multiplex PCR combined with Luminex technology	S. aureus, 5 species CoNS, 18 specific genes in total, including resistance determinants and PVL	5
Broad-based Assays, Growth Amplification Required				
Verigene BC-GP	Nanosphere Inc, Northbrook, IL	Multiplex assay combined with signal-amplified gold nanoparticle array technology	13 gram-positive genera/species 3 resistance markers	2.5
Prove-it Sepsis	Mobidiag, Helsinki, Finland	Multiplex PCR combined with microarray	50 different pathogens	3
Hyplex BloodScreen	BAG Lich, Germany	PCR-ELISA	10 pathogens; mecA	6

(continued on next page)

		Principles of the	Pathogens	Turnaround
Assay	**Manufacturer**	**Assay**	**Detected**	**Time (h)**
Assays Performed Directly on Whole Blood				
SepsiTest	Molzym, Bremen, Germany	Broad-range PCR followed by sequencing	300 different pathogens	8–12
LightCycler SeptiFast	Roche Molecular Systems, Branchburg, NJ	A multiplex real-time PCR assay that uses dual-FRET probes targeting the species-specific internal transcribed spacer regions of bacteria and fungi	25 different pathogens	3–30
PLEX-ID BAC Spectrum	Ibis/Abbott Inc, Abbott Park, IL	Broad-range PCR combined with electrospray ionization mass spectrometry	Theoretically hundreds of pathogens and some resistance markers	8
VYOO	SIRS-Lab, Jena Germany	Multiplex PCR with gel electrophoresis	40 pathogens with some resistance genes	8

Table 2
(continued)

Abbreviations: ELISA, enzyme-linked immunosorbent assay; FRET, fluorescence resonance energy transfer.

sensitivity and specificity). However, for MRSA detection, the test was 95.6% sensitive and 95.3% specific.[109] The discrepant results were largely caused by methicillin-susceptible revertant strains.[106] Other studies have noted the failure to detect certain SCC*mec* types in addition to the misidentification of revertant strains.[110,111] Similar to other platforms that are pathogen specific (discussed later), other more practical considerations regarding this assay are the amount of time required to obtain results (2.5 hours) and the expense to the laboratory. The latter is particularly true when small sample sizes per test run are processed. It is likely that most laboratories batch test this particular assay. One group reported on a modification of this assay allowing less reagent waste by freezing master mix.[112] In 2013, the company will be modifying the assay to enable recognition and appropriate assignment of the *mecA* revertants and will be transitioning this assay to their new automated platform, the BD MAX.

Cepheid (Sunnyvale, CA) manufactures the real-time Xpert MRSA/MRSA BC assay that provides results within 1 hour. The primers and probes in the assay were designed to detect SCC*mec* cassette variants by detecting sequences in the staphylococcal protein A (*spa*) gene, the *S. aureus* chromosomal *attB* insertion site of the SCC*mec*-*orfX* junction, and the *mecA* gene.[113] A positive result for all three targets must be present for assignment of a sample as containing MRSA. In the study by Wolk and colleagues,[113] the sensitivity and specificity for *S aureus* detection was 100% and 98.6%, respectively, and for MRSA detection the values were 98.3% and 99.4%, respectively. Although false-positives caused by revertant strains in pure culture are not an issue with this assay, false-positives may occur when testing both a methicillin-resistant coagulase-negative *Staphylococcus* and an isolate with a SCC*mec* empty cassette variant together in the same sample.[113] The frequency with which this situation occurs varies by geographic location, but in general it is expected to be low.[22] Subsequent publications have confirmed the excellent PPV of the assay for *S. aureus* and sensitivity for MSSA.[114–116] At least one of the studies found false-negative results when testing a small number of clinical and spiked cultures with heterogeneous vancomycin intermediate *S. aureus* (hVISA)/vancomycin intermediate *S. aureus* (VISA) MRSA isolates.[115] In addition to the rapid turnaround time (60 minutes), the assay has the advantage of random access, but the price per test and initial capital expense are prohibitive to many laboratories. However, a small study by Parta and colleagues[117] showed a reduction in antistaphylococcal therapy for bacteremia in patients with gram-positive cocci in clusters that were not *S. aureus* and decreased use of MRSA therapy such as vancomycin in patients with MSSA. Larger prospective studies are needed to assess patient impact and potential institutional cost savings with the use of this and other single-pathogen assays. However, in January 2012, Cepheid recalled lots of this assay because of higher than expected ($\sim 5\%$) invalid rates and withdrew the product from the market. According to a November 2012 communication from the manufacturer, the assay will again be made available at the end of the second quarter of 2013.

Roche Molecular (Indianapolis, IN) has available, on a research-use-only basis in the United States, the LightCycler *Staphylococcus* kit M^GRADE. This assay detects and differentiates *S. aureus* and coagulase-negative *Staphylococcus* spp. It can be used in conjunction with the LightCycler MRSA research-use-only kit that detects *mecA*. This assay uses primers and probes that target the internal transcribed spacer (ITS) regions of the rRNA operon. There is an internal control that is amplified by the same primers as the target, but it is detected in a separate fluorescence channel.[118] Probe hybridization is detected using fluorescence resonance energy transfer[118] and *S aureus* is differentiated from CoNS using melting curve analysis.[118,119] Results are available in 3 hours. Several publications report sensitivities for detection of *S. aureus* of 100% and specificities ranging from 98.4% to 100%.[118–120] For CoNS, the reported sensitivities and specificities are 93.3% to 100% and 100%, respectively.[118,119]

The StaphPlex Research Use Only System (Qiagen Valencia, CA) is unique in that it simultaneously provides a species-level identification of *S. aureus* and 5 CoNS species, detects genes that encode Panton-Valentine leukocidin (PVL), and also detects resistance determinants to methicillin, aminoglycosides, macrolides, lincosamides, and tetracycline. In all, 18 *Staphylococcus*-specific genes are detected in 1 reaction.[121] Amplified products from this target-enriched multiplex PCR method are characterized by using the Luminex 100 suspension tray.[121] The procedure requires 5 hours to perform.[121] In the study by Tang and colleagues[121] using 360 positive BACTEC 9240 BCs, accurate detection for CoNS, MRSA, MSSA, and nonstaphylococci were 96.7%, 92.1%, 72.5%, and 66.7%, respectively. Resistance gene detection was less reliable than the comparative phenotypic methods with high major error rates reported.[121] PVL detection was not assessed in this study.[121] Further improvements are needed before this assay can be considered acceptable for clinical performance.

Broad-based Assays, Growth Required

Progress has been made in the availability of broad-based assays that target several different pathogens simultaneously. Several assays are available in Europe and there is at least 1 that is FDA-cleared in the United States and others that are in clinical trials. These assays can be classified into those assays that are applied to positive BC bottles and those assays that test directly from whole blood (see **Table 2**). A brief introduction to these technologies is presented later with more detailed discussion of those assays that are FDA-cleared.

The Verigene Gram-Positive Blood Culture Nucleic Acid Test (BC-GP) (Nanosphere, Inc. Northbrook, IL) is a nonamplified, qualitative, multiplex assay that detects and identifies the nucleic acids of 13 gram-positive bacterial genera/species and 3 resistance markers. The Verigene system consists of an extraction tray, utility tray, and a test cartridge, bench-top Processor SP where reagent trays are inserted and the testing occurs, and a Verigene Reader that has a touch-screen control panel and a barcode scanner. The Reader tracks the specimen and is used for automated imaging and analysis of the test cartridges after they are processed. The Reader interprets and displays the results; 1 Reader can control up to 32 Processor SP units. Testing can be performed on demand in real time with results available within 2.5 hours of BC positivity.[122]

After vortexing the patient's positive BC sample, 350 μL of blood are inoculated into the sample well of the extraction tray and, from that point on, the testing process is automated. Bacterial DNA is extracted, fragmented, and denatured in the extraction tray using a magnetic bead–based procedure, and then transferred to the self-contained test cartridge by pipette tips within the instrument. Within the test cartridge, if target nucleic acid is present, the single-stranded DNA hybridizes to complementary sequence-specific capture oligonucleotides arranged on the surface of a glass slide. A second mediator DNA oligonucleotide hybridizes to this complex. This mediator oligonucleotide also has a domain that attaches to a common nucleotide bound to a signal-generating gold nanoparticle.[119] At the end of the test cycle, the glass slide in its holder is removed and placed in an appropriate compartment within the Reader. Inside the Reader, the array is subjected to light and the presence of hybridized probes on the slide is determined by light scattering (optical array scanning).[122] Results are reported as detected or not detected for all 13 targets. For results to be valid, both the extraction control and the hybridization control must meet the detection criteria.

There are no publications summarizing the performance of the Verigene BC-GP assay. The package insert describes the method comparison study among 5 geographically diverse sites in the United States. Results of the Verigene BC-GP assay were compared with conventional methods at each site and bidirectional sequencing at a reference laboratory. A total of 1642 specimens were compliant. For the prospective clinical specimens, the overall positive agreement ranged from 93.1% for *Staphylococcus epidermidis* (N = 318) to 100% for the 3 *Listeria* sp, *Streptococcus pneumoniae* (N = 38), and *Streptococcus anginosus* (N = 12); the overall negative agreement ranged from 98.9% for *S. epidermidis* to 100% for *S. aureus, Staphylococcus lugdunensis, Listeria, Enterococcus faecium*, and the 2 beta-hemolytic streptococci.[122] For the prospective samples, the positive and negative agreements for *mecA* detection were 94.2% and 98.2%; for *vanA* they were 94.2% and 99.8%; and for *vanB* they were 100% and 100%.[122] There are a few caveats in terms of assay performance. The assay may not detect all organisms in a culture containing mixed gram-positive cocci and it does not link the *mecA* gene to a particular *Staphylococcus* spp in a mixed sample of CoNS and *S. aureus*.[122] Laboratories considering implementing this assay should also consult the package insert for information on organisms that were not verified in the FDA submission.[122]

Broad-range PCR assays that target universal genes (such as the 16SrRNA gene of bacteria) have the disadvantage that further identification procedures using sequencing, pathogen-specific PCR, or other methods must be performed after the initial amplification.[22] This complicates the performance of the tests, adds additional time to results and more costs, and may also lead to contamination depending on the configuration of the platform.[123] A few of these assays are discussed later.

The Prove-it sepsis assay (Mobidiag, Helsinki, Finland) uses multiplex PCR combined with a microarray after growth amplification in a BC system. Like the Verigene

BC-GP test, this assay requires growth amplification in a BC system; however, this assay is not FDA-cleared in the United States. According to the manufacturer, the assay is designed to detect the 50 most common gram-negative and gram-positive bacterial species encountered in positive BCs as well as the *mecA* gene. DNA is extracted from the positive BC bottles followed by broad-range PCR. The amplified products are detected in a proprietary tube that contains a microarray at the bottom, and an instrument with dedicated software interprets the results.[124] Two studies have evaluated the clinical performance of this assay.[124,125] Gaibani and colleagues[124] found 90% agreement with standard laboratory results for those organisms covered by the test. In the study performed in 2 large institutions in Europe using 2107 positive BCs, 86% of the bottles contained a pathogen covered by the assay.[125] Overall, this assay had a clinical sensitivity of 94.7% and a specificity of 98.8%. In both studies, results were also available12 to 21 hours sooner than with conventional methods.[124,125]

The Hyplex BloodScreen (BAG, Lich, Germany) is a PCR enzyme-linked immunosorbent assay for identification of gram-positive cocci (N = 6) and gram-negative bacilli (N = 4), as well as detection of the *mecA* gene from positive BCs. The assay requires up to 6 hours to perform and it is not currently available in the United States. In a study of 482 positive BACTEC 9240 (BD Diagnostics Inc, Sparks, MD), the Hyplex test showed an overall sensitivity of 100% for gram-negative rod identification and 96.6% to 100% sensitivity for the identification of gram-positive cocci.[126] Gene detection of *mecA* correlated with the results of oxacillin phenotypic susceptibility test results.[126]

Several other companies are working on amplified platforms that are both pathogen specific and broad based from positive BCs but at the time of this writing they have not entered clinical trials and are not discussed in this article.

Broad-based Whole-blood Assays

Several assays are now available outside the United States for detection and identification of pathogens directly from whole-blood samples without the culture-amplification step. The best described of these is the LightCycler SeptiFast test (Roche Molecular Systems, Branchburg, NJ), which is a multiplex real-time PCR assay that uses dual-fluorescence resonance energy transfer (FRET) probes targeting the species-specific ITS regions of bacteria and fungi. This assay has been available in Europe for several years and detects 25 commonly encountered pathogens including 10 bacteria to species level, several others at the genus level, 5 *Candida* spp, and *Aspergillus fumigatus*. This assay has been evaluated in children, adults, immunocompromised patients, and patients with endocarditis.[124,127–129] In the study by Wallet and colleagues,[127] the SeptiFast test was evaluated among 72 patients admitted for suspected sepsis to an ICU over a 6-month period. The clinical sensitivity was 78% and the specificity was 99%. Results were available 17 to 57 hours sooner than the conventional results. In 8 patients, initial antibiotic therapy was inadequate and antibiotic changes were made more quickly; in 4 others, therapy was changed based on Septi-Fast results alone because standard cultures were negative.[127] In the study by Bravo and colleagues,[128] the SeptiFast assay results were compared with the results of conventional BCs in both neutropenic patients and ICU patients. In the neutropenic cohort, the overall agreement between the SeptiFast assay and conventional BCs was 69% and the sensitivity was 62% after contaminants and microorganisms not detected by the assay were excluded.[128] Similar results were seen among the ICU patients suspected of having sepsis (75% agreement, sensitivity of 70%).[128] In a large study of 1673 samples from 803 children, the SeptiFast assay had a sensitivity of

85.0% and a specificity of 93.5% compared with clinical information and standard conventional BC results.[129] More clinically relevant positive results were detected with the SeptiFast assay, especially among patients receiving antibiotic therapy.[129] All of these studies highlight that the assay in its current format may be a useful ancillary test, especially in patients with culture-negative endocarditis and who have negative BCs because of treatment. Pitfalls include failure to amplify organisms that are in the database, inability to detect those pathogens not in the database, amplification of dead organisms, and, like other methods, the potential for contamination.[127–129]

The SepsiTest (Molzym, Bremen, Germany) uses broad-range PCR targeting 16SrDNA of bacteria and 18SrDNA of fungi. After PCR, the samples are run on an agarose gel and sequencing is performed, making the test vulnerable to contamination.[130] The TAT is longer with this assay than with the LightCycler test; however, this assay allows for a broader approach to pathogen detection. A recent study examined the usefulness of this test for the diagnosis of infectious endocarditis (IE) in 20 patients who met the modified Duke criteria for definitive disease.[131] The PCR assay detected almost double the number of true cases of IE compared with culture.[131] Combining PCR on whole blood and heart valve tissue improved the overall diagnostic usefulness of PCR in this study.[131] However, in practice, heart valve tissue may not always be available.

The VYOO (SIRS-Lab, Jena, Germany) is a multiplex PCR-based assay targeting 34 bacterial species, 6 fungal species, and 5 resistance markers including mecA, vanA, vanB, β-lactamase blaSHV, and β-lactamase blaCTX-M.[132,133] Fitting and colleagues[133] found a 46.2% correlation between this test and the results of positive microbiology from all sources. False-positive results were seen in patients who had noninfectious causes of SIRS.[133] The investigators concluded that improvements are still needed with this assay.[133]

Of the available broad-range commercial assays that can be used directly on whole blood, the PLEX-ID BAC Spectrum assay (Abbott/Ibis, Abbott Park, IL) offers the most comprehensive test menu and the most expensive platform. The assay uses broad-based PCR using 9 primer pairs targeting 16SrDNA, 23SrDNA, and 4 housekeeping genes followed by analysis of the base composition of the amplified targets using high-performance electrospray ionization mass spectrometry.[134] In theory, hundreds of pathogens and 4 resistance markers (mecA, vanA, vanB, and blaKPC) can be detected by this assay, which takes 8 hours to perform and is highly complex.[22,134,135]

To date, the published performance of this assay has been assessed on positive BC bottles in 1 study[135] and for the direct detection of Ehrlichia species in blood in a second study. In the study by Kaleta and colleagues,[135] the BAC assay showed 98.7% concordance at the genus level and 96.6% concordance at the species level with standard methods using 234 positive BacT-Alert (bioMerieux, Durham, NC) BC bottles. In a separate study, rapid detection and identification of Ehrlichia species directly from whole-blood samples showed 95% sensitivity and 98.8% specificity compared with a laboratory-developed PCR-enzyme immunoassay (PCR-EIA) method.[136] In addition to its broad range, other advantages of this assay include its high throughput, accurate detection of mixed cultures, and that it can be quantitative.[134] Limitations include the size of the platform, the requirement for batch mode given the TAT of 8 hours, and the cost of the instrumentation. The analytical sensitivities of the assays discussed earlier range from 3 CFU/mL to 40 CFU/mL.[123,132] They are all limited by high cost and, as mentioned for some, by the long TAT and potential for contamination.

In summary, molecular technologies have provided a significant improvement for more rapid organism identification from positive blood and BCs in patients with bacteremia/sepsis. Future refinements of these technologies will likely allow a broader range of organism detection. Other diagnostic improvements will rely on the development of assays for detection of resistance markers and virulence factors, leading to further improvement of the diagnostic and therapeutic approaches to management of patients with bacteremia/sepsis.

SUMMARY

This article presents and discusses various novel approaches for the improvement of sepsis diagnosis. Considering the diagnostic uncertainties of using gold standard laboratory methods such as BCs alone, the development of robust diagnostic algorithms, incorporating biomarker panels and other surrogate methods for organism identification, has the potential not only to improve the diagnosis of sepsis itself but also to improve the TAT for test results. Reduction of TAT of test results is particularly desirable because it will lead to improvements of therapeutic interventions, antimicrobial therapy, and outcomes. In the past 2 decades, numerous observational studies have been published on the usefulness of biomarkers and adjunctive test methods for more rapid diagnosis of sepsis. In conventional diagnostic accuracy studies, the usefulness of a novel test method is determined by comparison of test results with the definitive diagnosis as it is established by use of a gold standard method. As mentioned earlier, sepsis is a heterogeneous group of disease states and syndromes rather than a single final diagnosis, and therefore it lacks a gold standard definition. In this case, 2 fundamentally different approaches can be used to investigate novel tests.[137] One approach ignores the existence of the gold standard dilemma and the assumption is made that a well-defined clinical disease exists, based on a clinical diagnosis or the results of the alleged gold standard. Because many of the clinical studies and subsequent meta-analyses referenced in this article have used such an approach, there are conflicting results and opinions on the usefulness of biomarkers and other tests. The other approach to solving the diagnostic dilemma is based on discarding the use of a gold standard all together. Such studies typically focus on clinical outcomes instead of using a reference test result/definition provided by a gold standard test method.

Despite the improvements in understanding the pathophysiology of sepsis and in the development of advanced diagnostic methodologies, the initial and early diagnosis of sepsis remains a challenge for both physicians and laboratories.[138] While critical clinical awareness together with biomarker assays can improve the initial pathway to establishing the (clinical) diagnosis of sepsis, the gold standard and confirmatory (laboratory) diagnosis of sepsis remains the proof of bacteremia established by collection and preparation of BCs. Additional laboratory and molecular test methods provide improvements of TAT of results to demonstrate and identify the microorganisms present in the patient's blood. Further research and improvements of test methods may lead to the ability to predict and detect sepsis at the bedside. Until that is possible, the final diagnosis of sepsis will most likely continue to be based on a combination of clinical findings, biomarkers, and microbiological tests, because the diagnosis "sepsis", too, remains a blend of various clinical syndromes.

REFERENCES

1. Bone RC, Balk RA, Cerra FB, et al. Definitions for sepsis and organ failure and guidelines for the use of innovative therapies in sepsis. The ACCP/SCCM Consensus Conference Committee. American College of Chest Physicians/Society of Critical Care Medicine. Chest 1992;101:1656–62.

2. Vincent JL. Dear SIRS, I'm sorry to say that I don't like you.... Crit Care Med 1997;25:372–4.
3. Trzeciak S, Zanotti-Cavazzoni S, Parrillo JE, et al. Inclusion criteria for clinical trials in sepsis: did the American College of Chest Physicians/Society of Critical care Medicine consensus conference definitions of sepsis have an impact? Chest 2005;127:242–5.
4. Levy MM, Fink MP, Marshall JC, et al. 2001 SCCM/ESICM/ACCP/ATS/SIS International Sepsis Definition Conference. Crit Care Med 2003;31:1250–6.
5. Howell MD, Talmor D, Schuetz P, et al. Proof of principle: the predisposition, infection, response, organ failure sepsis staging system. Crit Care Med 2011;39:322–7.
6. Angus DC, Linde-Zwirble WT, Lidicker J, et al. Epidemiology of severe sepsis in the United States: analysis of incidence, outcome, and associated costs of care. Crit Care Med 2001;29:1303–10.
7. Engel C, Brunkhorst FM, Bone HC, et al. Epidemiology of sepsis in Germany: results from a national prospective multicenter study. Intensive Care Med 2007;33:606–18.
8. Vincent JL, Sakr Y, Sprung CL, et al. Sepsis in European intensive care units: results of the SOAP study. Crit Care Med 2006;34:344–53.
9. Hoyert DL, Xu J. Deaths: preliminary data for 2011. Natl Vital Stat Rep 2012;61:1–65.
10. Diekema DJ, Beekmann SE, Chapin KC, et al. Epidemiology and outcome of nosocomial and community-acquired bloodstream infection. J Clin Microbiol 2003;41:3655–60.
11. Martin GS, Mannino DM, Eaton S, et al. The epidemiology of sepsis in the United States from 1979 through 2000. N Engl J Med 2003;348:1546–54.
12. Finfer S, Bellomo R, Lipman J, et al. Adult-population incidence of severe sepsis in Australian and New Zealand intensive care units. Intensive Care Med 2004;30:589–96.
13. Harrison DA, Welch CA, Eddleston JM. The epidemiology of severe sepsis in England, Wales and Northern Ireland, 1996-2004: secondary analysis of a high quality clinical database, the ICNARC case mix programme database. Crit Care 2006;10:R42.
14. Levy MM, Dellinger RP, Townsend SR, et al. The surviving sepsis campaign: results of an international guideline-based performance improvement program targeting severe sepsis. Crit Care Med 2010;38:367–74.
15. Hall MJ, Williams SN, DeFrances CJ, et al. Inpatient care for septicemia or sepsis: a challenge for patients and hospitals. NCHS Data Brief 2011;(62):1–8 National Center for Health Statistics, Hyattsville (MD).
16. Moore LJ, Moore FA. Epidemiology of sepsis in surgical patients. Surg Clin North Am 2012;92:1425–43.
17. McBean M, Rajamani S. Increasing rates of hospitalization due to septicemia in the US elderly population, 1986-1997. J Infect Dis 2001;183:596–603.
18. Baine WB, Yu W, Summe JP. The epidemiology of hospitalization of elderly Americans for septicemia or bacteremia in 1991-1998: application of Medicare claims data. Ann Epidemiol 2001;11:118–26.
19. Burchardi H, Schneider H. Economic aspects of severe sepsis. Pharmacoeconomics 2004;22:793–813.
20. Dellinger RP, Levy MM, Carlet JM, et al. Surviving sepsis campaign: international guidelines for management of severe sepsis and septic shock. Crit Care Med 2008;36:296–327.

21. Magadia RR, Weinstein MP. Laboratory diagnosis of bacteremia and fungemia. Infect Dis Clin North Am 2001;15:1009–24.
22. Riedel S, Carroll KC. Blood cultures: key elements for best practices and future directions. J Infect Chemother 2010;16:301–16.
23. Schifman AB, Strand CL, Meier FA, et al. Blood culture contamination: a College of American Pathologists Q-Probes study involving 640 institutions and 497134 specimens from adult patients. Arch Pathol Lab Med 1998;122:216–21.
24. Lee CC, Lin WJ, Shih HI, et al. Clinical significance of potential contaminants in blood cultures among patients in a medical center. J Microbiol Immunol Infect 2007;40:438–44.
25. Tokars JI. Predictive value of blood cultures positive for coagulase-negative staphylococci: implications for patient care and health care quality assurance. Clin Infect Dis 2004;39:333–41.
26. Lee A, Mirrett S, Reller LB, et al. Detection of bloodstream infection in adults: how many blood cultures are needed? J Clin Microbiol 2007;45:3546–8.
27. Bates DW, Cook EF, Goldman L, et al. Predicting bacteremia in hospitalized patients: a prospective validated model. Ann Intern Med 1990;113:495–500.
28. Roth A, Wiklund AE, Palsson AS, et al. Reducing blood culture contamination by a simple informational intervention. J Clin Microbiol 2010;48:4552–8.
29. Bone RC. Sir Isaac Newton, sepsis, SIRS, and CARS. Crit Care Med 1996;24:1125–8.
30. Ward NS, Casserly B, Ayala A. The compensatory anti-inflammatory response syndrome (CARS) in critically ill patients. Clin Chest Med 2008;29:617–25.
31. Volk HD, Reinke P, Docke WD. Clinical aspects: from systemic inflammation to "immuneparalysis". Chem Immunol 2000;74:162–77.
32. Wolk K, Docke WD, von Baehr V, et al. Impaired antigen presentation by human monocytes during endotoxin tolerance. Blood 2000;96:218–23.
33. Hotchkiss RS, Karl IE. The pathophysiology and treatment of sepsis. N Engl J Med 2003;348:138–50.
34. Remick DG. Biological perspectives: pathophysiology of sepsis. Am J Pathol 2007;170:1435–44.
35. Rittirsch D, Flierl M, Ward PA. Harmful molecular mechanisms in sepsis. Nat Rev Immunol 2008;8:776–87.
36. Boomer JS, To K, Chang KC, et al. Immunosuppression in patients who die of sepsis and multiple organ failure. JAMA 2011;306:2594–605.
37. Biomarkers Definitions Working Group, Bethesda, MD. Biomarkers and surrogate endpoints: preferred definitions and conceptual framework. Clin Pharmacol Ther 2001;69:89–95.
38. Marshall JC, Reinhart K, International Sepsis Forum. Biomarkers of sepsis. Crit Care Med 2009;37(7):2290–8.
39. Limper M, de Kruif MD, Duits AJ, et al. The diagnostic role of procalcitonin and other biomarkers in discriminating infectious from non-infectious fever. J Infect 2010;60:409–16.
40. Marshall JC, Vincent JL, Mitchell PF, et al. Measures, markers, and mediators: toward a staging system for clinical sepsis: a report of the Fifth Toronto Sepsis Roundtable, Ontario, Canada, October 25–26, 2000. Crit Care Med 2003;31:1560–7.
41. Simon L, Gauvin F, Amre DK, et al. Serum procalcitonin and C-reactive protein levels as markers of bacterial infection: a systematic review and meta-analysis. Clin Infect Dis 2004;39:206–17.

42. Vincent JL, Donadello K, Schmidt X. Biomarkers in the critically ill patient: C-reactive protein. Crit Care Clin 2011;27:241–51.

43. Timonen TT, Koistinen P. C-reactive protein for detection and follow-up of bacterial and fungal infections in severely neutropenic patients with acute leukemia. Eur J Cancer Clin Oncol 1985;21:557–62.

44. Flood RG, Badik J, Aronoff SC. The utility of serum C-reactive protein in differentiating bacterial from nonbacterial pneumonia in children: a meta-analysis of 1230 children. Pediatr Infect Dis J 2008;27:95–9.

45. Lannergard A, Friman G, Ewald U, et al. Serum amyloid A (SAA) protein and high-sensitivity C-reactive protein (hsCRP) in healthy newborn infants and healthy young through elderly adults. Acta Paediatr 2005;94:1198–202.

46. Povoa P, Coelho L, Almeida E, et al. C-reactive protein as a marker of infection in critically ill patients. Clin Microbiol Infect 2005;11:101–8.

47. Ho KM, Lipman J. An update on C-reactive protein for intensivists. Anaesth Intensive Care 2009;37:234–41.

48. Martini A, Gottin L, Melot C, et al. A prospective evaluation of the Infection Probability Score (IPS) in the intensive care unit. J Infect 2008;56:313–8.

49. Povoa P, Coelho L, Almeida E, et al. Early identification of intensive care unit-acquired infections with daily monitoring of C-reactive protein: a prospective observational study. Crit Care 2006;10:R63.

50. Silvestre J, Povoa P, Coelho L, et al. Is C-reactive protein a good prognostic marker in septic patients? Intensive Care Med 2009;35:909–13.

51. Reny JL, Vuagnat A, Ract C, et al. Diagnosis and follow-up of infections in intensive care patients: value of C-reactive protein compared with other clinical and biological variables. Crit Care Med 2002;30:529–35.

52. Schmidt X, Vincent JL. The time course of blood C-reactive protein concentrations in relation to the response to initial antimicrobial therapy in patients with sepsis. Infection 2008;36:213–9.

53. Riedel S. Procalcitonin and the role of biomarkers in the diagnosis and management of sepsis. Diagn Microbiol Infect Dis 2012;73:221–7.

54. Assicot M, Gendrel D, Carsin H, et al. High serum procalcitonin concentrations in patients with sepsis and infection. Lancet 1993;341:515–8.

55. Linscheid P, Seboek D, Nylen ES, et al. In vitro and in vivo calcitonin I gene expression in parenchymal cells: a novel product of human adipose tissue. Endocrinology 2003;144:5578–84.

56. Mueller B, White JC, Nylen ES, et al. Ubiquitous expression of the calcitonin I gene in multiple tissues in response to sepsis. J Clin Endocrinol Metab 2001; 86:396–404.

57. Becker KL, Nylen ES, White JC, et al. Procalcitonin and the calcitonin gene family of peptides in inflammation, infection, and sepsis: a journey from calcitonin back to its precursors. J Clin Endocrinol Metab 2004;89: 1512–25.

58. Mueller B, Peri G, Doni A, et al. High circulating levels of the IL-1 type II decoy receptor in critically ill patients with sepsis: association of high decoy receptor levels with glucocorticoid administration. J Leukoc Biol 2002;72:643–9.

59. Mueller F, Christ-Crain M, Bregenzer T, et al. Procalcitonin levels predict bacteremia in patients with community-acquired pneumonia: a prospective cohort trial. Chest 2010;138:121–9.

60. De Kruif M, Limper M, Gerritsen H, et al. Additional value of procalcitonin for diagnosis of infection in patients with fever at the emergency department. Crit Care Med 2010;38:457–63.

61. Riedel S, Melendez JH, An AT, et al. Procalcitonin as a marker for the detection of bacteremia and sepsis in the emergency department. Am J Clin Pathol 2011; 135:182–9.
62. Lai CC, Chen SY, Wang CY, et al. Diagnostic value of procalcitonin for bacterial infection in elderly patients in the emergency department. J Am Geriatr Soc 2010;58:518–22.
63. Fioretto JR, Martin JG, Kurokawa CS, et al. Comparison between procalcitonin and C-reactive protein for early diagnosis of children with sepsis and septic shock. Inflamm Res 2010;59:581–6.
64. Schuetz P, Mueller B, Trampuz A. Serum procalcitonin for discrimination of blood contamination from bloodstream infection due to coagulase-negative staphylo-cocci. Infection 2007;35:352–5.
65. Jones AE, Fiechtl JF, Brown MD, et al. Procalcitonin test in the diagnosis of bacteremia: a meta-analysis. Ann Emerg Med 2007;50:34–41.
66. Tang BM, Eslick GD, Craig JC, et al. Accuracy of procalcitonin for sepsis diagnosis in critically ill patients: systematic review and meta-analysis. Lancet Infect Dis 2007;7:210–7.
67. Uzzan B, Cohen R, Nicolas P, et al. Procalcitonin as a diagnostic test for sepsis in critically ill adults and after surgery or trauma: a systematic review and meta-analysis. Crit Care Med 2006;34:1996–2003.
68. Kibe S, Adams K, Barlow G. Diagnostic and prognostic biomarkers of sepsis in critical care. J Antimicrob Chemother 2011;66(Suppl 2):33–40.
69. Ruiz-Alvarez MJ, Garcia-Valdecasas S, De Pablo R, et al. Diagnostic efficacy and prognostic value of serum procalcitonin concentration in patients with suspected sepsis. J Intensive Care Med 2009;24:63–71.
70. Nobre V, Harbath S, Graf JD, et al. Use of procalcitonin to shorten antibiotic treatment duration in septic patients. Am J Respir Crit Care Med 2008;177: 498–505.
71. Agarwal R, Schwartz DN. Procalcitonin to guide duration of antimicrobial therapy in intensive care units: a systematic review. Clin Infect Dis 2011;53:379–87.
72. Schuetz P, Chiappa V, Briel M, et al. Procalcitonin algorithms for antibiotic therapy decisions: a systematic review of randomized controlled trials and recommendations for clinical algorithms. Arch Intern Med 2011;171:1322–31.
73. Tobias PS, Mathison J, Mintz D, et al. Participation of lipopolysaccharide-binding protein in lipopolysaccharide-dependent macrophage activation. Am J Respir Cell Mol Biol 1992;7:239–45.
74. Wurfel MM, Kunitake ST, Lichenstein H, et al. Lipopolysaccharide (LPS)-binding protein is carried on lipoproteins and acts as a cofactor in the neutralization of LPS. J Exp Med 1994;180:1025 35.
75. Worthen GS, Avdi N, Vukajlovich S, et al. Neutrophil adherence induced by lipopolysaccharide in vitro. Role of plasma component interaction with lipopolysaccharide. J Clin Invest 1992;90:2526–35.
76. Mathison J, Tobias PS, Wolfson E, et al. Plasma lipopolysaccharide (LPS)-binding protein. A key component in macrophage recognition of gram-negative LPS. J Immunol 1992;149:200–6.
77. Opal SM, Scannon PJ, Vincent JL, et al. Relationship between plasma levels of lipopolysaccharide (LPS) and LPS-binding protein in patients with severe sepsis and septic shock. J Infect Dis 1999;180:1584–9.
78. Gaini S, Koldkjaer OG, Pedersen C, et al. Procalcitonin, lipopolysaccharide-binding protein, interleukin-6 and C-reactive protein in community-acquired infections and sepsis: a prospective study. Crit Care 2006;10:R53.

79. Tschaikowsky K, Hedwig-Geissing M, Schmidt J, et al. Lipopolysaccharide-binding protein for monitoring of post-operative sepsis: complemental to C-reactive protein or redundant? PLoS One 2011;6:e23615.

80. Villar J, Perez-Mendez L, Espinosa E, et al. Serum lipopolysaccharide-binding protein levels predict severity of lung injury and mortality in patients with severe sepsis. PLoS One 2009;4:e6818.

81. Sakr Y, Burgett U, Nacul FE, et al. Lipopolysaccharide binding protein in a surgical intensive care unit: a marker of sepsis? Crit Care Med 2008;36:2014–22.

82. Hollenberg SM, Ahrens TS, Annane D, et al. Practice parameters for hemodynamic support of sepsis in adult patients: 2004 update. Crit Care Med 2004; 32:1928–48.

83. Treschan TA, Peters J. The vasopressin system: physiology and clinical strategies. Anesthesiology 2006;105:599–612.

84. Sharshar T, Blanchard A, Paillard M, et al. Circulating vasopressin levels in septic shock. Crit Care Med 2003;31:1752–8.

85. Hinson JP, Kapas S, Smith DM. Adrenomedullin, a multifunctional regulatory peptide. Endocr Rev 2000;21:138–67.

86. Hirata Y, Mitaka C, Sato K, et al. Increased circulating adrenomedullin, a novel vasodilatory peptide, in sepsis. J Clin Endocrinol Metab 1996;81: 1449–53.

87. Wang P, Ba ZF, Cioffi WG, et al. The pivotal role of adrenomedullin in producing hyperdynamic circulation during the early stage of sepsis. Arch Surg 1998;133: 1298–304.

88. Ornan DA, Chaudry IA, Wang P. Pulmonary clearance of adrenomedullin is reduced during the late stage of sepsis. Biochim Biophys Acta 1999;1427: 315–21.

89. Ueda S, Nishio K, Minamino N, et al. Increased plasma levels of adrenomedullin in patients with systemic inflammatory response syndrome. Am J Respir Crit Care Med 1999;160:132–6.

90. Christ-Crain M, Morgenthaler NG, Struck J, et al. Mid-regional pro-adrenomedullin as a prognostic marker in sepsis: an observational study. Crit Care 2005;9:R816–24.

91. Guignant C, Voirin N, Venet F, et al. Assessment of pro-vasopressin and pro-adrenomedullin as predictors of 28-day mortality in septic shock patients. Intensive Care Med 2009;35:1859–67.

92. Travaglino F, De Berardinis B, Magrini L, et al. Utility of procalcitonin (PCT) and mid regional pro-adrenomedullin (MR-proADM) in risk stratification of critically ill febrile patients in emergency department (ED). A comparison with APACHE II score. BMC Infect Dis 2012;12:184.

93. Angeletti S, Battistoni F, Fioravanti M, et al. Procalcitonin and mid-regional pro-adrenomedullin test combination in sepsis diagnosis. Clin Chem Lab Med 2012. [Epub ahead of print]. http://dx.doi.org/10.1515/cclm-2012-0595.

94. Kuster H, Weiss M, Willeitner AE, et al. Interleukin-1 receptor antagonist and interleukin-6 for early diagnosis of neonatal sepsis 2 days before clinical manifestation. Lancet 1998;352:1271–7.

95. Uusitalo-Seppala R, Koskinen P, Leino A, et al. Early detection of severe sepsis in the emergency room: diagnostic value of C-reactive protein, procalcitonin, and interleukin-6. Scand J Infect Dis 2011;43:883–90.

96. Rice TW, Wheeler AP, Bernard GW, et al. A randomized, double-blind, placebo-controlled trial of TAK-242 for the treatment of severe sepsis. Crit Care Med 2010;38:1685–94.

97. Urbonas V, Eidukaite A, Tamuliene I. The diagnostic value of interleukin-6 and interleukin-8 for early prediction of bacteremia and sepsis in children with febrile neutropenia and cancer. J Pediatr Hematol Oncol 2012;34:122–7.
98. Andaluz-Ojeda D, Bobillo F, Iglesias V, et al. A combined score of pro- and anti-inflammatory interleukins improves mortality prediction in severe sepsis. Cytokine 2012;57:332–6.
99. Wong HR, Cvijanovich NZ, Hall M, et al. Interleukin-27 is a novel candidate diagnostic biomarker for bacterial infection in critically ill children. Crit Care 2012;16: R213.
100. Mauri T, Bellani G, Patroniti N, et al. Persisting high levels of plasma pentraxin 3 over the first days after severe sepsis and septic shock onset are associated with mortality. Intensive Care Med 2010;36:621–9.
101. deKriuf MD, Limper M, Sierhuis K, et al. PTX3 predicts severe disease in febrile patients in the emergency department. J Infect 2010;60:122–7.
102. Romaschin AD, Harris DM, Ribeiro MB, et al. A rapid assay of endotoxin in whole blood using autologous neutrophil dependent chemiluminescence. J Immunol Methods 1998;212:169–85.
103. Marshall JC, Foster D, Vincent JL, et al. Diagnostic and prognostic implications of endotoxemia in critical illness: results of the MEDIC study. J Infect Dis 2004; 190:527–34.
104. Yaguchi A, Yuzawa J, Klein DJ, et al. Combining intermediate levels of the endotoxin activity assay (EAA) with other biomarkers in the assessment of patients with sepsis: results of an observational study. Crit Care 2012;16:R88.
105. Ventetuolo CE, Levy MM. Biomarkers: diagnosis and risk assessment in sepsis. Clin Chest Med 2008;29:591–603.
106. Casserly B, Read R, Levy MM. Multimarker panels in sepsis. Crit Care Clin 2011; 27:391–405.
107. Tromp M, Lansdorp B, Bleeker-Rovers CP, et al. Serial and panel analyses of biomarkers do not improve the prediction of bacteremia compared to one procalcitonin measurement. J Infect 2012;65:292–301.
108. Stamper PS, Cai M, Howard T, et al. Clinical validation of the molecular-based BD GeneOhmTM StaphSR for the direct detection of *Staphylococcus aureus* and methicillin resistant *Staphylococcus aureus* in positive blood cultures. J Clin Microbiol 2007;45:2191–6.
109. Grobner S, Dion M, Plante M, et al. Evaluation of the BD GeneOhm StaphSR assay for detection of methicillin resistant and methicillin-susceptible *Staphylococcus aureus* isolates from spiked positive blood culture bottles. J Clin Microbiol 2009;47:1689–94.
110. Snyder JW, Munier GK, Heckman SA, et al. Failure of the BD GeneOhm StaphSR assay for direct detection of methicillin-resistant and methicillin-susceptible *Staphylococcus aureus* isolates in positive blood cultures collected in the United States. J Clin Microbiol 2009;47:3747–8.
111. Stamper PD, Louie L, Wong H, et al. Genotypic and phenotypic characterization of methicillin-susceptible *Staphylococcus aureus* isolates misidentified as methicillin-resistant *Staphylococcus aureus* by the BD GeneOhm MRSA assay. J Clin Microbiol 2011;49:1240–4.
112. Munson E, Kramme T, Culver A, et al. Cost effective modification of a commercial PCR-assay for detection of methicillin-resistant/susceptible *Staphylococcus aureus* from positive blood cultures. J Clin Microbiol 2010;48:1408–12.
113. Wolk DM, Struelens MJ, Pancholi P, et al. Rapid detection of *Staphylococcus aureus* and methicillin-resistant *S. aureus* (MRSA) in wound specimens and

blood cultures: multicenter preclinical evaluation of the Cepheid Xpert MRSA/SA skin and soft tissue and blood cultures assays. J Clin Microbiol 2009;47:823–6.

114. Spencer DH, Sellenriek P, Burnham CA. Validation and implementation of the GeneXpert MRSA/SA blood culture assay in a pediatric setting. Am J Clin Pathol 2011;136:690–4.

115. Kelley PG, Grabsch EA, Farrell J, et al. Evaluation of the Xpert MRSA/SA blood culture assay for the detection of *Staphylococcus aureus* including strains with reduced vancomycin susceptibility from blood culture specimens. Diagn Microbiol Infect Dis 2012;70:404–7.

116. Biendo M, Mammeri H, Pluquet E, et al. Value of Xpert MRSA/SA blood culture assay on the GeneXpert Dx system for rapid detection of *Staphylococcus aureus* and coagulase-negative staphylococci in patients with staphylococcal bacteremia. Diagn Microbiol Infect Dis 2013;75:139–43.

117. Parta M, Goebel M, Thomas J, et al. Impact of an assay that enables rapid determination of *Staphylococcus* species and their drug susceptibility on the treatment of patients with positive blood culture results. Infect Control Hosp Epidemiol 2010;31:1043–8.

118. Liberto MC, Puccio R, Matera G, et al. Applications of LightCycler *Staphylococcus* M-GRADE assay to detect *Staphylococcus aureus* and coagulase-negative staphylococci in clinical samples and in blood culture bottles. Infez Med 2006;14:71–6.

119. Shrestha NK, Tuohy MJ, Padmanabhan RA, et al. Evaluation of the LightCycler *Staphylococcus* M GRADE kits on positive blood cultures that contained gram-positive cocci in clusters. J Clin Microbiol 2005;43:6144–6.

120. Ozen NS, Ogunc D, Mutlu D, et al. Comparison of four methods for rapid identification of *Staphylococcus aureus* from BACTEC 9240 blood culture system. Indian J Med Microbiol 2011;29:42–6.

121. Tang YW, Kilic A, Yang Q, et al. StaphPlex System for rapid and simultaneous identification of antibiotic resistance determinants and Panton-Valentine leukocidin detection of staphylococci from positive blood cultures. J Clin Microbiol 2007;45:1867–73.

122. Nanosphere product [package insert]. 2012. Verigene Gram-Positive Blood Culture Nucleic Acid Test (BC-GP) Nanosphere, Inc. Northbrook, IL.

123. Mancini N, Clerici N, Diotti R, et al. Molecular diagnosis of sepsis in neutropenic patients with haematological malignancies. J Med Microbiol 2008;57:601–4.

124. Gaibani P, Rossini G, Ambretti S, et al. Blood culture systems: rapid detection–how and why? Int J Antimicrob Agents 2009;34:S13–5.

125. Tissari P, Zumla A, Tarkka E, et al. Accurate and rapid identification of bacterial species from positive blood cultures with a DNA-based microarray platform: an observational study. Lancet 2010;375:224–30.

126. Wellinghausen N, Wirths B, Essig A, et al. Evaluation of the Hyplex BloodScreen multiplex PCR-enzyme-linked immunosorbent assay system for direct identification of gram-positive cocci and gram-negative bacilli from positive blood cultures. J Clin Microbiol 2004;42:3147–52.

127. Wallet F, Nseir S, Baumann L, et al. Preliminary clinical study using a multiplex real-time PCR test for the detection of bacterial and fungal DNA directly in blood. Clin Microbiol Infect 2010;16:774–9.

128. Bravo D, Blanquer J, Tormo M, et al. Diagnostic accuracy and potential clinical value of the LightCycler SeptiFast assay in the management of bloodstream infections occurring in neutropenic and critically ill patients. Int J Infect Dis 2011; 15:e326–31.

129. Lucignano B, Ranno S, Liessenfeld O, et al. Multiplex PCR allows rapid and accurate diagnosis of bloodstream infections in newborns and children with suspected sepsis. J Clin Microbiol 2011;49:2252–8.
130. Wellinghausen N, Kochem AJ, Disqué C, et al. Diagnosis of bacteremia in whole-blood samples by use of a commercial universal 16S rRNA gene-based PCR and sequence analysis. J Clin Microbiol 2009;47:2759–65.
131. Kuhn C, Disque C, Muhl H, et al. Evaluation of commercial universal rRNA gene PCR plus sequencing tests for identification of bacteria and fungi associated with infectious endocarditis. J Clin Microbiol 2011;49:2919–23.
132. Mancini N, Carletti S, Ghidoli N, et al. The era of molecular and other non-culture based methods in diagnosis of sepsis. Clin Microbiol Rev 2010;23:235–51.
133. Fitting C, Parlato M, Adib-Conquy M, et al. DNAemia detection by multiplex PCR and biomarkers for infection in systemic inflammatory response syndrome patients. PLoS One 2012;7:338916.
134. Ecker DJ, Sampath R, Li H, et al. New technology for rapid molecular diagnosis of bloodstream infections. Expert Rev Mol Diagn 2010;10:399–415.
135. Kaleta EJ, Clark AE, Johnson DR, et al. Use of PCR coupled with electrospray ionization mass spectrometry for rapid identification of bacterial and yeast bloodstream pathogens from blood culture bottles. J Clin Microbiol 2011;49:345–53.
136. Eshoo MW, Crowder CD, Li H, et al. Detection and identification of *Ehrlichia* species in blood by use of PCR and electrospray ionization mass spectrometry. J Clin Microbiol 2010;48:472–8.
137. Bachmann LM, Juni P, Reichenbach S, et al. Consequences of different diagnostic "gold standards" in test accuracy research: carpal tunnel syndrome as an example. Int J Epidemiol 2005;34:953–5.
138. Marshall JC. Sepsis: rethinking the approach to clinical research. J Leukoc Biol 2008;83:471–82.

Molecular Detection of Respiratory Viruses

Richard S. Buller, PhD, D(ABMM)

KEYWORDS

- Respiratory viruses • Laboratory diagnosis • Molecular methods
- Polymerase chain reaction

KEY POINTS

- Molecular tests for the detection of respiratory viruses are more sensitive and can detect more viruses than the traditional methods of culture and antigen detection.
- There are now several molecular assays available, cleared by the Food and Drug Administration, which differ with respect to the viruses detected, instrumentation, throughput, hands-on time, the need for separate nucleic acid extraction, and sensitivity for certain groups of viruses.
- Issues associated with molecular tests for respiratory viruses include: possible false-negative results due to sequence variants; the inability of many assays to discriminate rhinoviruses from enteroviruses; the ability to detect viral nucleic acids in asymptomatic individuals; and the increased prevalence of coinfections.

INTRODUCTION

The purpose of this review is to provide an update on recent advances in molecular testing for respiratory viruses, focusing primarily on commercially available assays that have been cleared by the Food and Drug Administration (FDA) for use in the United States. Rather than a detailed look at technical aspects of the assays, attention is paid herein to practical aspects of the tests such as viruses detected, nucleic acid extraction requirements, throughput, and so forth. References are provided for more detailed descriptions of sensitivity and specificity, as well as technical aspects. Issues pertinent to both clinicians and laboratorians regarding molecular assays in general for respiratory virus detection are also discussed.

For the purposes of this article, the following viruses are considered agents of viral respiratory tract infections: influenza A and B; respiratory syncytial virus (RSV); parainfluenza virus types 1 to 4; rhinoviruses; human coronaviruses (NL63, HKU1, 229E, OC43); human metapneumovirus; and adenoviruses. Although other viruses such as

Department of Pediatrics, Washington University School of Medicine, 660 South Euclid Avenue, St Louis, MO 63110, USA
E-mail address: buller@kids.wustl.edu

Clin Lab Med 33 (2013) 439–460
http://dx.doi.org/10.1016/j.cll.2013.03.007
0272-2712/13/$ – see front matter © 2013 Elsevier Inc. All rights reserved.

human bocavirus and the WU and KI polyomaviruses may be detected in human respiratory tract specimens, their role in causing respiratory tract disease has not been firmly established, and therefore is not covered.

Respiratory tract disease caused by infection with these viruses imposes a significant burden on human society. Community-based studies have revealed the high prevalence of viral respiratory infections, with young children experiencing the greatest number of infections annually and the number of infections decreasing with age. Such studies have also noted that rhinoviruses, influenza viruses and coronaviruses tend to cause the highest number of infections.[1,2] Viral respiratory tract infections are also an important cause of morbidity and mortality in adults, with the elderly being particularly at risk.[3,4] In addition to the very young and elderly, other groups with underlying conditions such as solid-organ and hematopoietic stem-cell transplant recipients,[5,6] patients with chronic obstructive pulmonary disease,[7] and those with asthma[8,9] are also known to be at higher risk for severe complications from viral respiratory tract infections. As an example of the importance of viral respiratory infections, in the relatively small country of the Netherlands, a country-wide study led to the estimate that 900,000 individuals visit their physicians annually with an acute respiratory tract infection.[2]

Because they are obligate intracellular pathogens, the ability to provide a useful laboratory diagnosis for viruses has historically lagged behind that for bacterial infections. Before the introduction of molecular methods into the diagnostic virology laboratory, the traditional methods of cell culture and antigen detection were the predominant methods for the detection of respiratory viruses in clinical specimens. Conventional cell-culture detection of respiratory viruses involves the selection of a range of cell types known to support the growth of respiratory viruses, then observation of the cells by microscopy to look for morphologic changes, referred to as cytopathic effects, which are characteristic for different viruses. A major drawback to conventional viral culture is that it can take as long as 2 weeks for results, seriously compromising the clinical usefulness of this method.[10] Although variations of conventional cell culture have been developed that shorten the time to detection,[11] there are still several respiratory viruses that grow poorly or not at all in culture, also limiting the usefulness of these methods.

The development of antigen-detection methods was considered to be a major advance in the laboratory diagnosis of viral respiratory infections. By detecting viral antigens directly in patient specimens, either by fluorescent antibody methods or enzyme immunoassay–based techniques, it was possible to obtain a result within a clinically useful time period. Antigen-detection tests remain an important tool in viral diagnostics; however, this method also has shortcomings, with some methods having poor sensitivity for some viral targets, particularly in adult populations. In addition, owing to the lack of conserved antigens there are several respiratory viruses, such as rhinoviruses and coronaviruses, for which antigen-detection assays do not exist.

Molecular detection of viral nucleic acids has revolutionized the laboratory diagnosis of viral infections. Before the development of nucleic acid amplification technologies there were attempts to detect viral nucleic acids in clinical specimens by methods such as dot-blot hybridization, but these were largely unsuccessful because of a lack of sensitivity. The publication of the first description of a nucleic acid amplification method, the polymerase chain reaction (PCR), in 1986,[12] describing how nucleic acids could be specifically and exponentially amplified to a readily detected level, was soon followed by numerous publications describing the successful application of this method to the detection of viral nucleic acids in clinical specimens. Today, PCR and other nucleic acid amplification tests (NAATs) are beginning to supplant the traditional laboratory methods to the point that in the future, these methods will likely be the primary laboratory methods in viral diagnostics.

There are advantages and disadvantages associated with the use of NAATs for the diagnosis of viral respiratory infections (**Box 1**). Advantages include the extreme sensitivity of these techniques and the fact that viral viability does not have to be maintained prior to testing, allowing for the potential to ship specimens long distances to testing laboratories; this is in contrast to the problems associated with shipping of specimens for culture, especially for viruses such as RSV, which is known to rapidly lose viability. Another advantage is the ability to detect viruses, such as the human coronaviruses, for which no practical culture or antigen-detection methods exist. The rapid, sensitive, and specific results afforded by molecular testing also allow for the timely institution of antiviral therapy and the proper cohorting of patients admitted to the hospital. There are, however, disadvantages associated with NAAT testing as well. For example, there is the potential for the appearance of sequence variants, which can produce false-negative results. It has also become well established that molecular tests can detect viral nucleic acids in respiratory specimens obtained from asymptomatic individuals, complicating the interpretation of results. NAAT assays can also be more expensive than nonmolecular methods, although with the introduction of ever more assays to the market it is expected that prices will drop. These and other molecular testing issues are discussed in greater depth later.

NAATS FOR THE DETECTION OF RESPIRATORY VIRUSES

NAATs for the detection of respiratory viruses have evolved from user-developed and laboratory-developed tests using conventional PCR technology with electrophoresis-gel detection of products, to user-developed real-time PCR-based tests whereby amplified products are detected by technologies primarily involving the production of luminescent signals that are proportional to the amount of target amplified. A problem with these technologies is that they are limited with respect to the number of targets that can practically be amplified and detected, or "multiplexed," in a single reaction. For many of the traditional real-time platforms 3 or 4 targets are the maximum, a real drawback when one wants to comprehensively detect up to 20 or more different targets.

Box 1
Advantages and disadvantages of NAATs for the detection of respiratory viruses

Advantages of NAATs for the detection of respiratory viruses

- The ability to identify viruses that are not detected by conventional culture and antigen detection methods

- Extreme sensitivity

- Rapidity and accuracy of results allow for timely institution of antiviral therapy and appropriate infection control

- Because viral viability does not need to be maintained, specimen transport conditions can be relaxed, allowing specimens to be sent to distant testing sites

Disadvantages of NAATs for the detection of respiratory viruses

- False-negative results due to the existence of sequence variants

- NAATs more often result in detection of viruses in asymptomatic individuals than other methods

- Higher cost

Other technologies have now appeared in commercial formats, which are able to surmount the limitations of the other platforms. For a detailed description of these technologies, the reader is referred to an excellent review dealing with this topic.[13]

There is an extensive literature describing noncommercial user-developed NAATs for the detection of respiratory viruses. Because this review deals with commercially available assays for the detection of respiratory viruses, the reader is referred to reviews dealing with this topic.[14,15] However, some brief observations can be made concerning such assays. There are many examples in the literature of comparisons of molecular assays for a particular virus with conventional methods such as culture and/or antigen detection. For some viruses, such as RSV and influenza viruses, there appears to be a modest but real increase in sensitivity, whereas for others such as human metapneumovirus (hMPV) and human rhinoviruses, there is a more significant increase in detection by molecular methods. In addition, user-developed assays tend to be developed to detect one virus, or one group of related viruses, and are constrained by the previously mentioned limitations of conventional real-time assays to a maximum of 3 or 4 targets. Because the signs and symptoms of respiratory virus infections can overlap between the different viruses, to confidently rule out all potential viruses it would be necessary to run a battery of assays. One instance in which single directed assays may be useful is in geographic areas where there are annual epidemics of influenza and RSV. During such epidemics it may make sense to test just for these viruses before testing for other agents.

COMMERCIALLY AVAILABLE NAATS FOR RESPIRATORY VIRUSES
Hologic Assays

The company starting out as Prodesse, later acquired by Gen-Probe and now Hologic (Hologic Gen-Probe Inc, San Diego, CA), offers 5 assays for molecular detection of respiratory viruses (**Box 2**). The assays are all based on TaqMan real-time PCR technology; require that nucleic acids be extracted by either the Roche MagNA Pure (Roche Diagnostics, Indianapolis, IN) or bioMerieux easyMAG (bioMerieux Inc, Durham, NC) automated extractors; and require that the reactions be run on a Cepheid SmartCycler

---

Box 2
Respiratory virus NAAT kits offered by Hologic (Gen-Probe/Prodesse)

- Prodesse Pro hMPV+ Assay
  - Detects human metapneumovirus
- Prodesse ProAdeno+ Assay
  - Detects human adenoviruses associated with respiratory infections
- Prodesse ProFAST+
  - Discriminates subtypes of Influenza A including:
    - Seasonal influenza A/H1
    - Seasonal influenza A/H3
    - 2009 H1N1 influenza A
- Prodesse ProFlu+ Assay
  - Detects influenza A, influenza B, and RSV
- Prodesse ProParaflu+ Assay
  - Detects and differentiates human parainfluenza virus 1, 2, and 3

(Cepheid, Sunnyvale, CA). The kits contain all of the reagents necessary to run the reaction, including an internal control, and have the benefit of being cleared for in vitro diagnostic use by the FDA. Publications have described the use of the assays as comparators for other tests, with favorable results.[16,17] In a comparison of 3 influenza PCR assays the ProFlu+ failed to detect 2 of 29 seasonal influenza A H1 viruses but was 100% sensitive for similar numbers of influenza H3, 2009 H1N1, and influenza B specimens.[18] In addition, the company Web site provides performance data and links to data presented in poster presentations. These assays might be particularly useful for those wishing to screen during yearly epidemics of influenza and RSV, or to determine the cause of RSV-like illness in young children testing negative for RSV for which hMPV or parainfluenza virus might be a consideration. The ProFAST+ assay that subtypes influenza A could be useful for guiding antiviral therapy. Drawbacks to these assays include the necessity to run 4 separate assays to rule out all of the targets, and the fact that they do not detect parainfluenza type 4 or any of the coronaviruses. In addition, the requirement to use the Cepheid SmartCycler would limit throughput to 16 samples per SmartCycler module.

Quidel Assays

Quidel Corp (San Diego, CA) markets 2 FDA-cleared assays for the detection of respiratory viruses. The Influenza A+B assay detects both influenza A and B viruses, and the hMPV Assay detects human metapneumovirus. Both assays are sold in a kit format containing primers and fluorescently labeled probes, master mix, and an internal processing control. Quidel recommends the inclusion of a positive control for each assay, either in the form of a commercial product, which they sell separately, or through the use of known previously positive specimens. Both assays are approved for nasal or nasopharyngeal swab specimens extracted on the bioMerieux NucliSENS easyMAG automated extractor, and require amplification on either a Cepheid Smart-Cycler or ABI 7500 Fast Dx for the Influenza A+B assay or the ABI 7500 Fast Dx for the hMPV test.

To date there are no peer-reviewed evaluations of the Quidel assays available, but performance data are available for download from the company Web site.[19] Advantages of the assays include: molecular detection of 3 important and common respiratory viruses; 2° to 8°C kit storage temperature (no need to store frozen); room temperature setup; and 2-year shelf-life of reagents. Disadvantages include inability to detect other respiratory viruses and the lack of peer-reviewed evaluations of the assays.

Cepheid Assay

The Cepheid GeneXpert Flu Assay (Cepheid, Sunnyvale, CA) consists of a single-use disposable cartridge and associated instrument, including a computer with analysis software (**Fig. 1**). Following addition of specimen and placement in the instrument, extraction of nucleic acids and PCR take place within the cartridge. An independent evaluation of the Xpert Flu test reported that the assay has 2 minutes of hands-on time, with the run being completed in 76 minutes.[20] The assay detects and differentiates influenza A and B, identifies influenza A 2009 H1N1 if present, and includes an internal control. The assay is FDA-cleared for use with nasal aspirates and washes, as well as nasopharyngeal swabs. The instrument itself comes in different iterations capable of accommodating 1, 2, 4, or 16 cartridges at a time. In addition to the influenza assay, Cepheid offers several cartridges for the detection of other targets.

The Cepheid GeneXpert system was the first technology to allow for democratization of molecular testing. When molecular testing was first introduced into the diagnostic virology laboratory it was viewed as a technically demanding method that required

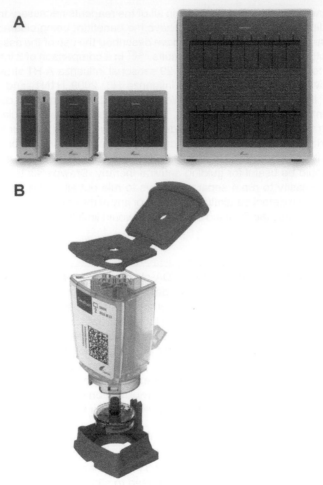

Fig. 1. Cepheid GenXpert system. (*A*) Instruments with 1- to 16-cartridge capacity. (*B*) Exploded view of GenXpert cartridge. (*Courtesy of* Cepheid, Sunnyvale, CA; with permission.)

highly trained technologists. The "specimen in, answer out" format of the GeneXpert system allows for molecular testing by laboratories with little or no previous experience in the area, with Clinical Laboratory Improvement Amendments classifying the Xpert Flu assay as "moderately complex."

To facilitate testing during the outbreak of 2009 H1N1 influenza A, an initial version of the Xpert Flu assay detecting only influenza A with differentiation of 2009 H1N1 influenza A was granted Emergency Use Authorization in December 2009. Published comparisons of this version of the Xpert Flu assay with conventional methods, laboratory-developed techniques, and commercial PCR assays for the detection of influenza A viruses revealed acceptable sensitivity and specificity, with somewhat reduced sensitivity for the detection of 2009 H1N1 viruses.[21–23] An evaluation using a collection of retrospectively tested respiratory specimens and a subsequent FDA-cleared version of the Xpert Flu assay with the added ability to detect influenza B reported 100% sensitivities for the detection of seasonal H1N1 and H3N2 influenza A viruses and influenza B viruses, but only 77% sensitivity for 2009 H1N1, compared with a laboratory-developed

PCR test with up-front automated nucleic acid extraction.[20] Despite the reduced sensitivity for 2009 H1N1 viruses, the investigators indicated that the rapid turnaround time of the Xpert Flu assay make it a reasonable option for laboratory testing. Two other peer-reviewed studies comparing the FDA-cleared version of the Xpert Flu assay with culture, direct fluorescent antibody staining, antigen immunoassays, and reference molecular tests report generally enhanced sensitivity relative to conventional methods and acceptable performance relative to reference molecular methods, with both studies supporting the use of the Xpert Flu assay for the rapid diagnosis of influenza.[24,25]

The Cepheid Xpert Flu assay offers laboratories the advantage of a rapid, sensitive molecular test for influenza that is simple to perform. The disposable, self-contained cartridge system, in addition to abrogating the need for up-front nucleic acid extraction, also greatly reduces the opportunity for false positives attributable to amplicon contamination that can affect other NAATs. Disadvantages of the assay include, depending on the instrument configuration, limited throughput and the fact that the assay only detects influenza viruses.

IQuum Assay

IQuum (Marlborough, MA) offers a molecular assay called the Liat Influenza A/B assay. The assay is FDA-cleared for nasopharyngeal swabs, and detects and differentiates influenza A and B. The assay is in a sample-in-answer-out format, and has a turnaround time of only 20 minutes with about 1 minute of hands-on time, according to information provided by the company.[26] The assay consists of a single-use disposable Liat Influenza A/B Assay Tube containing all the test reagents and the associated instrument, called the Liat Analyzer. The assay uses TaqMan probe real-time PCR chemistry and includes all appropriate controls. Because of the simplicity of operation and rapidity of results, the assay is being considered for possible use as a point-of-care test. Performance data provided by the manufacturer indicate a sensitivity and specificity relative to culture of 100% and 96.8% for influenza A and 100% and 94.1% for influenza B. At the time of writing there were no peer-reviewed evaluations of the assay available.

Focus Diagnostics Assays

Focus Diagnostics Inc (Cypress, CA) markets 3 FDA-cleared molecular diagnostic assays for the detection of influenza viruses and RSV. The Simplexa Influenza A H1N1 (2009) assay detects influenza A viruses and differentiates 2009 influenza A H1N1. The Simplexa Flu A/B & RSV assay detects and differentiates influenza A and B viruses and RSV. Both assays require the use of the 3M Integrated Cycler and its associated computer and analysis software (**Fig. 2**). The assays are real-time PCR assays that use a bifunctional fluorescent probe-primer combined with a reverse primer, to specifically amplify and detect viral sequences and include an internal control. Both assays have requirements regarding acceptable specimen types and nucleic acid extraction methods (**Box 3**). The 3M Integrated Cycler uses a novel single-use Universal Disk that contains 96 reaction positions. Of note, Focus markets other molecular assays, all of which use the same reaction conditions so that different assays can be simultaneously run on the same disk. The single independent evaluation of the Simplexa Flu A/B & RSV available at this time reported that the test requires 45 minutes of hands-on time, with results being available in approximately 2.5 hours.[27] The same investigators reported that in a comparison with another FDA-cleared NAAT (Nanosphere Verigene RV+) using both retrospective and prospective specimens, the Simplexa assay had lower a sensitivity for all 3 targets, which was statistically significant for influenza A and B.[27] This result was noted to be at odds with the manufacturer's sensitivity

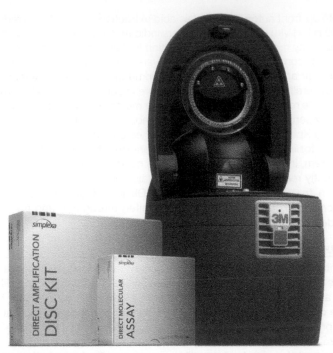

Fig. 2. 3M Integrated Cycler and Focus Simplexa kit. (*Courtesy of* Focus Diagnostics, Cypress, CA; with permission.)

data, with the investigators indicating that strain differences could be the explanation for their observation. The manufacturer's performance data are available for download from the company Web site.[28]

Focus Diagnostics also offers the Simplexa Flu A/B & RSV Direct assay, which uses their Direct Amplification Disk, a disk with 8 sample positions that both extracts nucleic acids and amplifies viral sequences for influenza A and B and RSV. Through the use of adhesive foil covers for the reaction positions, it is not necessary to choose between having to run 8 specimens or waste unused positions; rather, the disk can be reused until 8 specimens have been run. The assay uses the same method as the other Simplexa assays, and requires the 3M Integrated Cycler. At the time of writing there were no independent evaluations of the assay, but manufacturer's data are available for download from the Web site.[28]

The Simplexa assays offer the advantage of a multiplex assay for 2 of the most prevalent respiratory viruses, a high throughput using the 96-well disk, and a cycling program that allows for the simultaneous running of other Focus Diagnostic assays. The Simplexa Direct assay represents another choice for laboratories considering a sample-in-answer-out platform. Disadvantages include that the assays only test for influenza and RSV, and that there are only minimal peer-reviewed data available.

Nanosphere Assay

In addition to other infectious disease and genetics targets, Nanosphere Inc (Northbrook, IL) offers a commercial FDA-cleared assay, called the Verigene RV+, which detects influenza and RSV in nasopharyngeal swab specimens. The assay detects and differentiates influenza A and B and RSV, and also provides influenza A subtyping information (seasonal H1 and H3 and 2009 H1N1). In addition, the assay subtypes

---

Box 3
Respiratory NAAT kits offered by Focus Diagnostics

- Simplexa Influenza A H1N1 (2009)
  - Detects influenza A with differentiation of 2009 H1N1
  - FDA-cleared for nasopharyngeal swabs and aspirates
  - Requires nucleic acid extraction with either:
    - Automated Roche MagNA Pure LC System
    - Manual Qiagen QIAamp Viral RNA Mini Kit (Qiagen Inc, Valencia, CA)
  - Uses 96-well Universal Disk and 3M Integrated Cycler
- Simplexa Flu A/B & RSV
  - Detects and differentiates influenza A and B and RSV
  - FDA-cleared for nasopharyngeal swabs
  - Requires nucleic acid extraction with either:
    - Automated Roche MagNA Pure LC System
    - Automated bioMerieux NucliSENS easyMag
  - Uses 96-well Universal Disk and 3M Integrated Cycler
- Simplexa Flu A/B & RSV Direct
  - Detects and differentiates influenza A and B and RSV
  - FDA-cleared for nasopharyngeal swabs
  - Does not require up-front nucleic acid extraction
  - Uses 8-well Direct Amplification Disk and 3M Integrated Cycler

---

RSV, and a version of the product available outside the United States includes detection of the H275Y mutation conferring oseltamivir resistance in influenza A viruses. The assay is in a sample-in-answer-out format, therefore it does not require nucleic acid extraction and includes all the necessary reagents, including processing and inhibition controls.

The assay, using a novel detection technology, takes place in a single-use cartridge that is placed in a Verigene Processor SP instrument where nucleic acids are extracted, purified, and target-amplified if present (**Fig. 3**). A hybridization step involving gold nanoparticles to which are bound probes specific for the amplified product is used as part of the detection process. The cartridge is then placed in the Verigene Reader, which reads the result by the detection of light scatter rather than other methods such as fluorescence. For those interested, Thaxton and colleagues[29] have published a detailed description of the technology. An independent evaluation reported that the assay requires 5 minutes of hands-on time, and the results are ready in 2.5 hours.[27]

In the single peer-reviewed evaluation of the Verigene RV+, the assay had 97% sensitivity for influenza A, 100% sensitivity for influenza B, and 100% sensitivity for RSV, with good specificities for all targets as determined using a set of several hundred retrospective and prospective specimens that were tested with other commercial assays, with discrepant results resolved using a laboratory-developed NAAT.[27]

Advantages of the Verigene RV+ include offering another choice in the sample-in-answer-out format, with limited labor time as well as the reduced risk of contamination previously mentioned for other self-contained disposable systems. The ability to

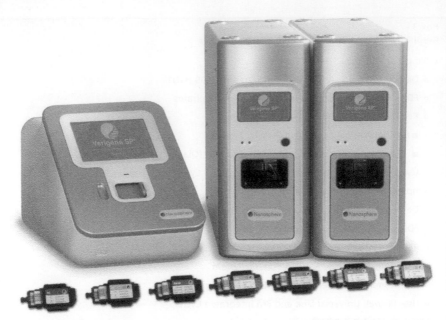

Fig. 3. Nanosphere Verigene system. Verigene processor on the right, reader and cartridges on the left. Instrument footprints in inches: Processor, 7.6 width × 18.7 height × 22.9 depth; reader, 11.7 width × 12.4 height × 20.5 depth. Processors are stackable. No computer is required for operation. (*Courtesy of* Nanosphere, Northbrook, IL; with permission.)

detect the most common epidemic respiratory viruses and the ability to subtype influenza A viruses are other assets. Disadvantages include the low throughput, although this can be increased by having more processor modules, and the fact that only influenza and RSV are detected by the assay.

GenMark Assay

The GenMark eSensor Respiratory Viral Panel (GenMark Diagnostics, Carlsbad, CA) is a multiplex PCR assay, cleared by the FDA for nasopharyngeal swabs for the detection of 14 respiratory viruses (influenza A [seasonal H1, H3, 2009 H1], influenza B, RSV A and B, parainfluenza 1, 2, and 3, human metapneumovirus, rhinovirus, and adenovirus B/E and C). The kit provides all the reagents for performing the assay, and requires nucleic acid to be extracted on a bioMerieux NucliSENS easyMAG followed by amplification with a thermocycler using 0.2-mL tubes. Following amplification, potential amplicons are loaded into an eSensor cartridge, which is then placed in the XT-8 instrument where detection takes place by a novel technology involving production of electric current through specific binding of amplicons to a gold-plated electrode (**Fig. 4**). The instrument is of random access with spaces for up to 24 cartridges, and has an integrated computer with analysis software. An independent evaluation found that the assay required about 6.5 hours to test 6 specimens, with hands-on time of about 1 hour.[30]

A single peer-reviewed study evaluated the eSensor by testing 250 frozen specimens from pediatric patients and comparing the results with a panel of laboratory-developed PCR assays, with overall agreement between the methods being reported as 99.2%.[30] Of note, the investigators reported that the GenMark assay was more sensitive and specific than their laboratory assay for the detection of rhinoviruses and, although they found that the assay may have higher sensitivity for some adenovirus types, the assay showed some cross-reactivity for adenoviruses other than those found in species B, C, and E.

Advantages of the eSensor Respiratory Viral Panel include: the ability to detect a wide range of respiratory viruses in a single assay; the ability to subtype influenza A and RSV viruses; potentially higher sensitivity for some adenovirus types; and higher specificity for rhinoviruses. Potential disadvantages to the assay include: the inability to detect coronaviruses and parainfluenza type 4; the requirement for up-front nucleic acid extraction; and potential contamination issues raised by the need to manipulate PCR products following amplification.

Luminex Assays

Luminex (Austin, TX) offers 2 multiplex molecular assays for the detection of respiratory viruses, the xTAG Respiratory Virus Panel (RVP) and the xTAG RVP *FAST* assays.

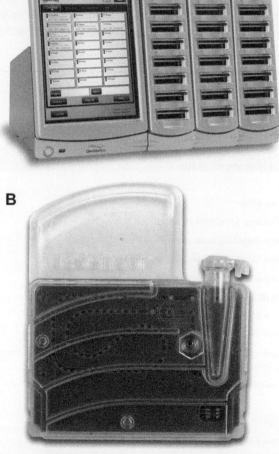

Fig. 4. GenMark eSensor system. (*A*) XT-8 instrument. (*B*) eSensor cartridge. Instrument footprint in inches: 15.75 width × 18.11 height × 16.14 depth. A computer is not required for operation. (*Courtesy of* GenMark Diagnostics, Carlsbad, CA; with permission.)

The assays detect different numbers of respiratory viruses and are cleared for specific nucleic acid extraction methods (**Box 4**). Other versions of these assays that detect different targets are available in other global markets outside the United States.

Both assays use a multiplex real-time PCR performed in a thermocycler using 0.2-mL reaction tubes, and include extraction and assay controls. To overcome the technical issues associated with detecting products of large multiplex PCR assays, both assays use the proprietary Universal Tag sorting system whereby virus-specific oligonucleotide tags are added to viral amplicons, after which the tagged amplicons are hybridized to a liquid suspension of microsphere bead sets in a 96-well plate. Each bead set has a virus-specific antitag bound to its surface, with each bead set uniquely identified by the ratio of dyes impregnated into the beads. Each colored bead set thus represents a specific virus through the bead-antitag-tag-amplicon interaction. Following hybridization, the beads are then read by the Luminex 100/200 instrument (**Fig. 5**), a flow cell using dual lasers, one identifying the bead set and the other determining whether or not an amplicon is bound to the bead through the emission of a phycoerythrin reporter. The run time for the RVP assay is about 8.5 hours, including extraction. The RVP *FAST* assay decreases run time through the elimination of some of the assay steps; an independent assessment reports hands-on time for the *FAST* assay of 60 to 80 min, with the time to results, including extraction, requiring 5 hours.[31] For those wishing more information, a detailed description of RVP technology has been published by the company.[32]

Box 4
Luminex assays

- Luminex xTAG RVP Assay
    - 12 targets including: RSV A and B; influenza A (H1, H3); influenza B; parainfluenza 1, 2, and 3; human metapneumovirus; adenoviruses; rhinovirus/enterovirus
    - Cleared for nasopharyngeal swabs
    - Requires:
        - Extraction on either:
            - Qiagen QIAamp MiniElute (manual)
            - bioMerieux EasyMAG (automated)
            - bioMerieux MiniMAG (manual)
        - Thermocycler accommodating 0.2-mL tubes and 96-well plates
        - Specific lots of *TAQ* enzyme
    - Time to result ~8.5 hours (including extraction)
- Luminex xTAG RVP FAST Assay
    - 8 targets including: RSV; influenza A (H1, H3); influenza B; human metapneumovirus; adenoviruses; rhinovirus/enterovirus
    - Cleared for nasopharyngeal swabs
    - Requires:
        - Extraction on:
            - bioMerieux EasyMAG
        - Thermocycler accommodating 0.2-mL tubes and 96-well plates
    - Time to result ~5 hours (including extraction)

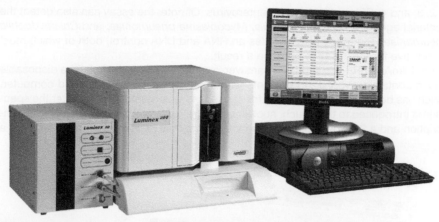

Fig. 5. Luminex 200 instrument. Luminex 200 (*right*) and SD sheath fluid module (*left*). Instrument footprints in inches: Luminex 200, 17.00 width × 9.50 height × 20.00 depth; SD Module, 8.00 width × 9.75 height × 11.75 depth. A computer is required for operation. (*Courtesy of* Luminex Corporation, Austin, Texas; with permission.)

The xTAG RVP assay was the first large multiplex respiratory virus assay to enter the market as an FDA-cleared assay, and as such there are several reports demonstrating increased or comparable sensitivity for the detection of respiratory viruses relative to antigen detection/culture methods and other molecular methods.[33-36] Other studies have demonstrated cost savings realized by implementing the RVP assay in place of conventional methods.[37,38]

Although the RVP assay has increased sensitivity relative to conventional methods, when compared with other multiplex molecular assays the RVP assay has demonstrated reduced sensitivity for some targets such as parainfluenza viruses[39] and RSV.[40] Likewise, the RVP *FAST* assay, although demonstrating increased sensitivity relative to antigen detection/culture methods, has been reported to have reduced sensitivity for some targets relative to other molecular assays. Gharabaghi and colleagues[39] reported reduced sensitivity for influenza B and adenoviruses, with another study also reporting lower sensitivity for adenoviruses.[41] A recent study noted lower sensitivity for influenza B and RSV in comparison with the BioFire FilmArray.[31]

Advantages of the xTAG RVP assay include: the ability to detect a wide array of viruses in a single assay; high throughput; increased sensitivity relative to traditional methods; and the potential for cost savings. Disadvantages include: inability to detect some viruses such as the coronaviruses; a relatively large amount of hands-on time; reported reduced sensitivity for some targets relative to other assays; and the need for multiple user interventions, including opening tubes containing amplicons, which increase the potential for contamination to occur. The xTAG RVP *FAST* has the obvious advantage of requiring less hands-on time, but has the disadvantage that the current FDA-cleared version has fewer viral targets.

BioFire Assay

The BioFire (formerly Idaho Technology) FilmArray Respiratory Panel (RP) (BioFire Diagnostics, Salt Lake City, UT) is a multiplex real-time PCR assay capable of detecting 17 viral respiratory agents including: adenovirus; coronaviruses 229E, OC43, NL63 and HKU1; metapneumovirus; influenza A, H3, H1, and 2009 H1; parainfluenza viruses

1, 2, 3, and 4; RSV; and rhinovirus/enterovirus. Of note, the assay can also detect the bacterial agents *Bordetella pertussis, Mycoplasma pneumoniae,* and *Chlamydophila pneumoniae.* The assay also includes an RNA and DNA control, both of which must be positive for the assay to produce a result.

The FilmArray RP is a sample-in-answer-out test that uses a single-use disposable pouch containing lyophilized reagents with an associated instrument and computer, which has been cleared by the FDA for nasopharyngeal swabs (**Fig. 6**). After the specimen is introduced to the pouch, nucleic acids are extracted followed by reverse transcription and a 2-stage nested PCR reaction. The final PCR reaction takes place in a

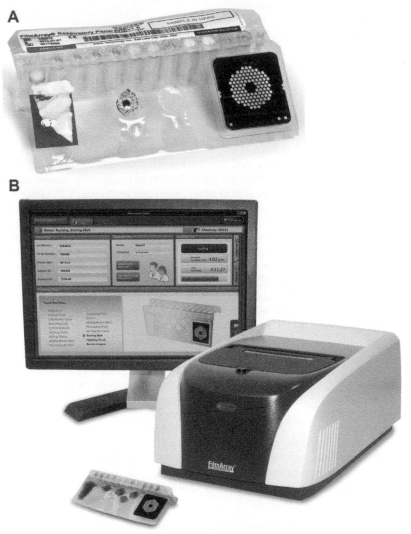

Fig. 6. BioFire FilmArray respiratory panel assay. (*A*) FilmArray RP Pouch. (*B*) FilmArray instrument and pouch. Instrument footprint in inches: 10.00 width × 6.5 height × 15.5 depth. A computer is required for operation. (*Courtesy of* BioFire Diagnostics Inc, Salt Lake City, UT; with permission.)

multiwell array, with products detected by melt-curve analysis. The associated instrument has room for a single pouch at a time. For those interested, a detailed description of the FilmArray technology has been published.[42] The manufacturer notes that the RP assay cannot reliably discriminate rhinoviruses from enteroviruses, that the coronavirus OC43 component may cross-react with some strains of coronavirus HKU1, and that the assay has reduced sensitivity for adenovirus species C serotypes 2 and 6. An updated version of the assay with increased sensitivity for the detection of the adenovirus C serotypes is due out in 2013 (BioFire, personal communication, 2012).

Several studies have demonstrated that the FilmArray RP has greater sensitivity than antigen detection/culture methods and/or sensitivity generally comparable to that of other molecular methods.[16,31,40,43–45] Confirming the manufacturer's information, some studies have noted decreased sensitivity of the FilmArray FP for adenoviruses.[16,44] Pierce and colleagues[44] also reported that, using a collection of previously characterized adenovirus types, in addition to types 2 and 6 the FilmArray RP also had reduced sensitivity for detection of adenovirus types 20, 35, 37, and 41, although the investigators noted that these types have not been considered important causes of respiratory illnesses. Some of these same studies also noted increased sensitivity of the RP assay relative to other molecular tests for targets such as RSV, parainfluenza viruses, and influenza B.[16,31,40]

Advantages of the FilmArray RP include: sample-in-answer-out format for the largest number of viral respiratory agents currently on the market; rapid result with minimal hands-on time; performance generally comparable to that of other molecular methods. Disadvantages include: limited throughput; decreased sensitivity for some adenovirus types.

ISSUES ASSOCIATED WITH MOLECULAR TESTING FOR RESPIRATORY VIRUSES
False-Negative Results due to Sequence Variants

With the exception of the adenoviruses, the majority of the known viruses causing respiratory tract disease are RNA viruses, a group of viruses whose genomes are generally considered to exhibit higher rates of mutations. Mutation rates for some RNA viruses such as HIV1 and influenza A have been extensively studied, and there exist large sequence databases for these viruses. However, for some important respiratory viruses such as RSV and parainfluenza 1 the number of available sequences, and hence knowledge of sequence variation, is very limited, with some groups now undertaking projects sequencing more genomes of these important agents.[46,47] Because most molecular assays rely on hybridization between a primer and target sequence to detect the virus, lack of knowledge of the full extent of sequence variation could result in the inability to detect a particular viral strain or newly arising mutant. Such an event has already occurred in Sweden, where a strain of *Chlamydia trachomatis* with a deletion mutation rendering it nondetectable by 2 widely used commercial molecular assays spread around the country, likely aided by the production of false-negative results by what were presumed to be gold-standard diagnostic tests.[48] With more laboratories switching to molecular assays for the detection of respiratory agents, it will be necessary for both laboratorians and clinicians to remain vigilant for cases of what appear to be viral respiratory tract infections with negative molecular results. With no formal surveillance system currently in place, sentinel laboratories with culture and high-throughput sequencing capabilities would be one solution for monitoring the emergence of sequence variants not detectable by standard molecular assays.

Reporting of Rhinovirus/Enterovirus Results

Before the availability of sequence data, rhinoviruses and enteroviruses were classified in separate genera of the family Picornaviridae. Sequencing of the majority of the genomes in both groups revealed that they were so closely related that both genera have now been combined into the single genus *Enterovirus*.[49] The close genomic similarity between the enteroviruses and rhinoviruses has made it difficult to design PCR assays that can reliably discriminate between the 2 groups, with most multiplex assays reporting specimens positive for "rhinovirus/enterovirus," a situation that can cause confusion for people receiving the results who may be thinking in terms of rhinoviruses classically causing common-cold–like infections and enteroviruses causing aseptic meningitis and other systemic illnesses. Unpublished data from the authors' own laboratory, where more than 100 positive "rhinovirus/enterovirus" from multiplex PCR testing of upper and lower respiratory tract specimens were subjected to sequencing, revealed all the positives to be rhinovirus types, with one exception. This exception was an isolate of enterovirus 68, an enterovirus type known to be a cause of respiratory tract infections.[50–52] Furthermore, other enterovirus types have also been implicated as causes of respiratory tract illness.[49] Therefore, in most cases where a "rhinovirus/enterovirus" result is reported from a patient suffering from a viral respiratory-like illness, it is likely to be due to a rhinovirus or an enterovirus capable of causing a respiratory tract infection, although the presence of an asymptomatically shed enterovirus cannot be ruled out. Virus-testing laboratories will play an important role in educating other health care workers about the changes in picornavirus taxonomy and the interpretation of results reported as positive for "rhinovirus/enterovirus."

Detection of Viral Nucleic Acids in Specimens from Asymptomatic Individuals

With the advent of molecular testing assays for respiratory virus, the paradigm of considering viral agents of respiratory disease to always be pathogenic when detected in specimens has changed. There are now numerous examples of the ability to detect respiratory virus nucleic acids in specimens from asymptomatic individuals. The primary viruses detected in asymptomatic patients are rhinoviruses/enteroviruses, which have been detected in normal children and adults, as well as immunocompromised patients.[53–60] Other viruses such as parainfluenza viruses, coronaviruses, adenoviruses, and human metapneumoviruses have been less commonly found in asymptomatic individuals.[61–68] Other studies have found viruses such as RSV, influenza, and metapneumovirus to be only rarely detected in asymptomatic individuals.[55,61,65,69] Jansen and colleagues[55] speculated that detection of virus in asymptomatic people could be due to 3 reasons: (1) detection of the virus during the acute phase of infection before the development of symptoms; (2) detection of virus still being shed after resolution of symptoms; and (3) detection of virus in specimens from individuals experiencing a subclinical infection. The same investigators also quantified the level of viral nucleic acid in specimens, and found that that in general there were higher levels of virus in cases relative to asymptomatic controls.[55] However, it should be noted that none of the currently available FDA-cleared assays have the ability to quantify virus in specimens. In addition, there are issues with standardizing collection methods for respiratory specimens to produce meaningful quantitative results.

The detection of viruses in asymptomatic persons is of concern, especially when rhinovirus/enteroviruses are detected in patients for whom other causes of their symptoms are being considered or in cases where coinfections are detected (see next section). It is suggested that laboratorians familiarize themselves with the issue of viral detection in asymptomatic people so as to be able to provide guidance to other health care workers.

Detection of Coinfections

It is well established that once multiplex molecular testing is used for the detection of respiratory viruses, specimens containing more than 1 virus (coinfections) are encountered at frequencies from approximately 10% to 30%.[70-76] Ascribing significance to coinfections with respect to causing more severe illness is complicated, because researchers have studied different patient populations using assays capable of detecting different sets of viruses. Some studies have found certain combinations of viruses to be associated with more severe illness,[73] whereas others have reported that infection with some viruses may interfere with infection with other viruses.[77] It is beyond the scope of this review to go into this topic in depth, so the reader is referred to the article by Paranhos-Baccala and colleagues[74] for a more detailed discussion.

There are likely several methods by which a patient could become infected by more than 1 respiratory virus, and these in turn could affect the outcome. If a patient is unfortunate enough to become acutely infected with 2 or more viruses at the same time, depending on the host and the virus(es), the outcome could be a more severe illness. If, on the other hand, an individual had a previous infection with a virus such as a rhinovirus and was still asymptomatically shedding virus and then became acutely superinfected with a second virus, such a scenario likely would not produce a more significant illness despite the fact that 2 viruses would be detected. In any event, laboratories instituting multiplex molecular testing for respiratory viruses can expect to see an increase in the incidence of multiple viral infections, and they should be prepared to answer questions from clinicians using the tests.

SUMMARY

Over the past several years the market has gone from virtually no FDA-cleared molecular assays for the detection of respiratory viruses to the wide variety discussed in this review. It should be mentioned that in addition to the tests listed in this article there are a number of other tests available outside the United States or within the United States that are sold in research-use-only or other non-cleared formats. The tests described here range from kits containing primers and probes detecting specific groups of viruses to self-contained systems requiring specialized instruments that extract nucleic acids and perform PCR with little operator input. Some of the tests target just the viruses involved in large yearly epidemics such as RSV and influenza or specific groups of viruses such as the adenoviruses or parainfluenza viruses, while others can detect most of the known respiratory viruses as well as some bacterial agents. Some systems utilize 96-well plate formats with the corresponding high through-put as compared to others which have much more limited throughput. All of these things represent factors that have to be taken into account when deciding to use one of these assays. It is expected that there will be more cleared tests for more analytes reaching the market in the future thereby increasing competition and the options available. We are also likely to see the more complicated tests requiring trained technologists replaced by easy-to-perform sample-in-answer-out format tests. Some of these tests will be so simple that they may be granted waived status and will therefore be found in provider offices and other point-of-care situations where individuals such as microbiologists and infectious disease physicians may not be overseeing their use. While this will bring the ability to rapidly and sensitively detect respiratory viruses to places where it was not previously possible to do so, it is hoped that this simplification of molecular tests will not cause those using them to lose sight of some of the important issues associated with these tests such as false negative results due to sequence variants, the ability to detection of viruses in individuals not exhibiting symptoms and the significance of the detection of co-infections.

REFERENCES

1. Monto AS. Epidemiology of viral respiratory infections. Am J Med 2002; 112(Suppl 6A):4S–12S.
2. van Gageldonk-Lafeber AB, Heijnen ML, Bartelds AI, et al. A case-control study of acute respiratory tract infection in general practice patients in The Netherlands. Clin Infect Dis 2005;41(4):490–7.
3. Greenberg SB. Respiratory viral infections in adults. Curr Opin Pulm Med 2002; 8(3):201–8.
4. Greenberg SB. Viral respiratory infections in elderly patients and patients with chronic obstructive pulmonary disease. Am J Med 2002;112(Suppl 6A): 28S–32S.
5. Renaud C, Campbell AP. Changing epidemiology of respiratory viral infections in hematopoietic cell transplant recipients and solid organ transplant recipients. Curr Opin Infect Dis 2011;24(4):333–43.
6. Weigt SS, Gregson AL, Deng JC, et al. Respiratory viral infections in hematopoietic stem cell and solid organ transplant recipients. Semin Respir Crit Care Med 2011;32(4):471–93.
7. Sethi S. Molecular diagnosis of respiratory tract infection in acute exacerbations of chronic obstructive pulmonary disease. Clin Infect Dis 2011;52(Suppl 4): S290–5.
8. Gern JE. Viral respiratory infection and the link to asthma. Pediatr Infect Dis J 2004;23(Suppl 1):S78–86.
9. Tan WC. Viruses in asthma exacerbations. Curr Opin Pulm Med 2005;11(1):21–6.
10. Shetty AK, Treynor E, Hill DW, et al. Comparison of conventional viral cultures with direct fluorescent antibody stains for diagnosis of community-acquired respiratory virus infections in hospitalized children. Pediatr Infect Dis J 2003;22(9): 789–94.
11. LaSala PR, Bufton KK, Ismail N, et al. Prospective comparison of R-mix shell vial system with direct antigen tests and conventional cell culture for respiratory virus detection. J Clin Virol 2007;38(3):210–6.
12. Saiki RK, Gelfand DH, Stoffel S, et al. Primer-directed enzymatic amplification of DNA with a thermostable DNA polymerase. Science 1988;239(4839):487–91.
13. Wittwer CT, Kusukawa N. Real-time PCR and melting analysis. In: Persing DH, editor. Molecular microbiology. Washington, DC: ASM Press; 2011. p. 63–82.
14. Buller RS, Arens MQ. Molecular detection of respiratory viruses. In: Persing DH, editor. Molecular microbiology. 2nd edition. Washington, DC: ASM Press; 2011. p. 605–30.
15. Mahony JB. Detection of respiratory viruses by molecular methods. Clin Microbiol Rev 2008;21(4):716–47.
16. Loeffelholz MJ, Pong DL, Pyles RB, et al. Comparison of the FilmArray respiratory panel and Prodesse real-time PCR assays for detection of respiratory pathogens. J Clin Microbiol 2011;49(12):4083–8.
17. Tang YW, Lowery KS, Valsamakis A, et al. Validation of a PLEX-ID Flu device for simultaneous detection and identification of influenza viruses A and B. J Clin Microbiol 2012;51:40–5.

18. Selvaraju SB, Selvarangan R. Evaluation of three influenza A and B real-time reverse transcription-PCR assays and a new 2009 H1N1 assay for detection of influenza viruses. J Clin Microbiol 2010;48(11):3870–5.
19. Available at: http://www.quidel.com/molecular/documents/us.php. Accessed January 28, 2013.
20. Popowitch EB, Rogers E, Miller MB. Retrospective and prospective verification of the Cepheid Xpert influenza virus assay. J Clin Microbiol 2011;49(9): 3368–9.
21. Jenny SL, Hu Y, Overduin P, et al. Evaluation of the Xpert Flu A Panel nucleic acid amplification-based point-of-care test for influenza A virus detection and pandemic H1 subtyping. J Clin Virol 2010;49(2):85–9.
22. Miller S, Moayeri M, Wright C, et al. Comparison of GeneXpert FluA PCR to direct fluorescent antibody and respiratory viral panel PCR assays for detection of 2009 novel H1N1 influenza virus. J Clin Microbiol 2010;48(12):4684–5.
23. Sambol AR, Iwen PC, Pieretti M, et al. Validation of the Cepheid Xpert Flu A real time RT-PCR detection panel for emergency use authorization. J Clin Virol 2010; 48(4):234–8.
24. Dimaio MA, Sahoo MK, Waggoner J, et al. Comparison of Xpert Flu rapid nucleic acid testing with rapid antigen testing for the diagnosis of influenza A and B. J Virol Methods 2012;186(1–2):137–40.
25. Novak-Weekley SM, Marlowe EM, Poulter M, et al. Evaluation of the Cepheid Xpert Flu Assay for rapid identification and differentiation of influenza A, influenza A 2009 H1N1, and influenza B viruses. J Clin Microbiol 2012;50(5):1704–10.
26. Available at: http://www.iquum.com/products/faba.shtml. Accessed January 24, 2013.
27. Alby K, Popowitch EB, Miller MB. Comparative evaluation of the Nanosphere Verigene RV+ Assay with the Simplexa Flu A/B & RSV Kit for the detection of influenza and respiratory syncytial viruses. J Clin Microbiol 2013;51:352–3.
28. Available at: http://www.focusdx.com/pdfs/pi/US/MOL2650.pdf. Accessed January 24, 2013.
29. Thaxton CS, Georganopoulou DG, Mirkin CA. Gold nanoparticle probes for the detection of nucleic acid targets. Clin Chim Acta 2006;363(1–2):120–6.
30. Pierce VM, Hodinka RL. Comparison of the GenMark diagnostics eSensor respiratory viral panel to real-time PCR for detection of respiratory viruses in children. J Clin Microbiol 2012;50(11):3458–65.
31. Babady NE, Mead P, Stiles J, et al. Comparison of the Luminex xTAG RVP Fast assay and the Idaho Technology FilmArray RP assay for detection of respiratory viruses in pediatric patients at a cancer hospital. J Clin Microbiol 2012;50(7): 2282–8.
32. Krunic N, Merante F, Yaghoubian S, et al. Advances in the diagnosis of respiratory tract infections: role of the Luminex xTAG respiratory viral panel. Ann N Y Acad Sci 2011;1222:6–13.
33. Balada-Llasat JM, LaRue H, Kelly C, et al. Evaluation of commercial ResPlex II v2.0, MultiCode-PLx, and xTAG respiratory viral panels for the diagnosis of respiratory viral infections in adults. J Clin Virol 2011;50(1):42–5.
34. Mahony J, Chong S, Merante F, et al. Development of a respiratory virus panel test for detection of twenty human respiratory viruses by use of multiplex PCR and a fluid microbead-based assay. J Clin Microbiol 2007;45(9):2965–70.
35. Pabbaraju K, Tokaryk KL, Wong S, et al. Comparison of the Luminex xTAG respiratory viral panel with in-house nucleic acid amplification tests for diagnosis of respiratory virus infections. J Clin Microbiol 2008;46(9):3056–62.

36. Wong S, Pabbaraju K, Lee BE, et al. Enhanced viral etiological diagnosis of respiratory system infection outbreaks by use of a multitarget nucleic acid amplification assay. J Clin Microbiol 2009;47(12):3839–45.

37. Dundas NE, Ziadie MS, Revell PA, et al. A lean laboratory: operational simplicity and cost effectiveness of the Luminex xTAG respiratory viral panel. J Mol Diagn 2011;13(2):175–9.

38. Mahony JB, Blackhouse G, Babwah J, et al. Cost analysis of multiplex PCR testing for diagnosing respiratory virus infections. J Clin Microbiol 2009;47(9):2812–7.

39. Gharabaghi F, Hawan A, Drews SJ, et al. Evaluation of multiple commercial molecular and conventional diagnostic assays for the detection of respiratory viruses in children. Clin Microbiol Infect 2011;17(12):1900–6.

40. Rand KH, Rampersaud H, Houck HJ. Comparison of two multiplex methods for detection of respiratory viruses: FilmArray RP and xTAG RVP. J Clin Microbiol 2011;49(7):2449–53.

41. Gadsby NJ, Hardie A, Claas EC, et al. Comparison of the Luminex Respiratory Virus Panel fast assay with in-house real-time PCR for respiratory viral infection diagnosis. J Clin Microbiol 2010;48(6):2213–6.

42. Poritz MA, Blaschke AJ, Byington CL, et al. FilmArray, an automated nested multiplex PCR system for multi-pathogen detection: development and application to respiratory tract infection. PloS One 2011;6(10):e26047.

43. Hayden RT, Gu Z, Rodriguez A, et al. Comparison of two broadly multiplexed PCR systems for viral detection in clinical respiratory tract specimens from immunocompromised children. J Clin Virol 2012;53(4):308–13.

44. Pierce VM, Elkan M, Leet M, et al. Comparison of the Idaho Technology FilmArray system to real-time PCR for detection of respiratory pathogens in children. J Clin Microbiol 2012;50(2):364–71.

45. Renaud C, Crowley J, Jerome KR, et al. Comparison of FilmArray Respiratory Panel and laboratory-developed real-time reverse transcription-polymerase chain reaction assays for respiratory virus detection. Diagn Microbiol Infect Dis 2012;74(4):379–83.

46. Beck ET, He J, Nelson MI, et al. Genome sequencing and phylogenetic analysis of 39 human parainfluenza virus type 1 strains isolated from 1997-2010. PloS One 2012;7(9):e46048.

47. Rebuffo-Scheer C, Bose M, He J, et al. Whole genome sequencing and evolutionary analysis of human respiratory syncytial virus A and B from Milwaukee, WI 1998-2010. PloS One 2011;6(10):e25468.

48. Ripa T, Nilsson PA. A *Chlamydia trachomatis* strain with a 377-bp deletion in the cryptic plasmid causing false-negative nucleic acid amplification tests. Sex Transm Dis 2007;34(5):255–6.

49. Tapparel C, Siegrist F, Petty TJ, et al. Picornavirus and enterovirus diversity with associated human diseases. Infect Genet Evol 2013;14:282–93.

50. Jacobson LM, Redd JT, Schneider E, et al. Outbreak of lower respiratory tract illness associated with human enterovirus 68 among American Indian children. Pediatr Infect Dis J 2012;31(3):309–12.

51. Renois F, Bouin A, Andreoletti L. Enterovirus 68 in pediatric patients hospitalized for acute airway diseases. J Clin Microbiol 2013;51:640–3.

52. Tokarz R, Firth C, Madhi SA, et al. Worldwide emergence of multiple clades of enterovirus 68. J Gen Virol 2012;93(Pt 9):1952–8.

53. Fry AM, Lu X, Olsen SJ, et al. Human rhinovirus infections in rural Thailand: epidemiological evidence for rhinovirus as both pathogen and bystander. PloS One 2011;6(3):e17780.

54. Graat JM, Schouten EG, Heijnen ML, et al. A prospective, community-based study on virologic assessment among elderly people with and without symptoms of acute respiratory infection. J Clin Epidemiol 2003;56(12):1218–23.

55. Jansen RR, Wieringa J, Koekkoek SM, et al. Frequent detection of respiratory viruses without symptoms: toward defining clinically relevant cutoff values. J Clin Microbiol 2011;49(7):2631–6.

56. Nokso-Koivisto J, Kinnari TJ, Lindahl P, et al. Human picornavirus and coronavirus RNA in nasopharynx of children without concurrent respiratory symptoms. J Med Virol 2002;66(3):417–20.

57. Peltola V, Waris M, Osterback R, et al. Rhinovirus transmission within families with children: incidence of symptomatic and asymptomatic infections. J Infect Dis 2008;197(3):382–9.

58. Srinivasan A, Flynn P, Gu Z, et al. Detection of respiratory viruses in asymptomatic children undergoing allogeneic hematopoietic cell transplantation. Pediatr Blood Cancer 2013;60(1):149–51.

59. van Benten I, Koopman L, Niesters B, et al. Predominance of rhinovirus in the nose of symptomatic and asymptomatic infants. Pediatr Allergy Immunol 2003; 14(5):363–70.

60. Wright PF, Deatly AM, Karron RA, et al. Comparison of results of detection of rhinovirus by PCR and viral culture in human nasal wash specimens from subjects with and without clinical symptoms of respiratory illness. J Clin Microbiol 2007;45(7):2126–9.

61. Advani S, Sengupta A, Forman M, et al. Detecting respiratory viruses in asymptomatic children. Pediatr Infect Dis J 2012;31(12):1221–6.

62. Debiaggi M, Canducci F, Sampaolo M, et al. Persistent symptomless human metapneumovirus infection in hematopoietic stem cell transplant recipients. J Infect Dis 2006;194(4):474–8.

63. Jartti T, Jartti L, Peltola V, et al. Identification of respiratory viruses in asymptomatic subjects: asymptomatic respiratory viral infections. Pediatr Infect Dis J 2008;27(12):1103–7.

64. Kalu SU, Loeffelholz M, Beck E, et al. Persistence of adenovirus nucleic acids in nasopharyngeal secretions: a diagnostic conundrum. Pediatr Infect Dis J 2010; 29(8):746–50.

65. Peck AJ, Englund JA, Kuypers J, et al. Respiratory virus infection among hematopoietic cell transplant recipients: evidence for asymptomatic parainfluenza virus infection. Blood 2007;110(5):1681–8.

66. Prill MM, Iwane MK, Edwards KM, et al. Human coronavirus in young children hospitalized for acute respiratory illness and asymptomatic controls. Pediatr Infect Dis J 2012;31(3):235–40.

67. Singleton RJ, Bulkow LR, Miernyk K, et al. Viral respiratory infections in hospitalized and community control children in Alaska. J Med Virol 2010;82(7):1282–90.

68. Walsh EE, Peterson DR, Falsey AR. Human metapneumovirus infections in adults: another piece of the puzzle. Arch Intern Med 2008;168(22):2489–96.

69. Falsey AR, Criddle MC, Walsh EE. Detection of respiratory syncytial virus and human metapneumovirus by reverse transcription polymerase chain reaction in adults with and without respiratory illness. J Clin Virol 2006;35(1):46–50.

70. Aberle JH, Aberle SW, Pracher E, et al. Single versus dual respiratory virus infections in hospitalized infants: impact on clinical course of disease and interferon-gamma response. Pediatr Infect Dis J 2005;24(7):605–10.

71. Canducci F, Debiaggi M, Sampaolo M, et al. Two-year prospective study of single infections and co-infections by respiratory syncytial virus and viruses

identified recently in infants with acute respiratory disease. J Med Virol 2008; 80(4):716–23.

72. Franz A, Adams O, Willems R, et al. Correlation of viral load of respiratory pathogens and co-infections with disease severity in children hospitalized for lower respiratory tract infection. J Clin Virol 2010;48(4):239–45.

73. Kouni S, Karakitsos P, Chranioti A, et al. Evaluation of viral co-infections in hospitalized and non-hospitalized children with respiratory infections using microarrays. Clin Microbiol Infect 2012. [Epub ahead of print].

74. Paranhos-Baccala G, Komurian-Pradel F, Richard N, et al. Mixed respiratory virus infections. J Clin Virol 2008;43(4):407–10.

75. Tanner H, Boxall E, Osman H. Respiratory viral infections during the 2009-2010 winter season in Central England, UK: incidence and patterns of multiple virus co-infections. Eur J Clin Microbiol Infect Dis 2012;31(11):3001–6.

76. Zhang G, Hu Y, Wang H, et al. High incidence of multiple viral infections identified in upper respiratory tract infected children under three years of age in Shanghai, China. PloS One 2012;7(9):e44568.

77. Greer RM, McErlean P, Arden KE, et al. Do rhinoviruses reduce the probability of viral co-detection during acute respiratory tract infections? J Clin Virol 2009; 45(1):10–5.

Molecular Diagnostics and Parasitic Disease

Shawn Vasoo, MBBS, MRCP, Bobbi S. Pritt, MD*

KEYWORDS

- Malaria • PCR • *Trichomonas* • Leishmaniasis • Babesiosis • Trypanosomiasis
- Amebiasis • NAAT

KEY POINTS

- Molecular tests play a growing role as adjuncts to traditional parasitology diagnostics, and in select situations, may replace traditional methods.
- Benefits of molecular methods may include increased sensitivity and specificity, but standardization of assays and paucity of commercial platforms are major limitations.
- Instrumentation and work flow requirements pose significant challenges for many parasite-endemic, resource-poor settings, although new applications of isothermal methods show significant promise for wider implementation.

INTRODUCTION

Despite advances in medical knowledge and practice, parasitic diseases remain a significant global health burden. Malaria alone is estimated to have caused 216 million infections in 2010.[1] In addition to malaria, 11 of the 17 'neglected tropical diseases' identified by the World Health Organization (WHO), which affect 1 billion persons overall, are parasitic in origin.[2] Although often thought of as an affliction of residents of tropical and developing countries and travelers, these parasitic diseases cause significant morbidity in developed countries too. In the United States, for example, the Centers for Disease Control and Prevention (CDC) has identified 5 parasitic diseases (Chagas disease, neurocysticercosis, toxocariasis, toxoplasmosis, and trichomoniasis) that require public health action based on their substantial national disease burden.

Diagnostics in parasitology have traditionally centered on morphology using light microscopy and various histochemical stains. Although this is a time-honored and valuable technique, morphologic interpretation is subjective and requires significant expertise. With the advent of polymerase chain reaction (PCR) testing in the 1980s, molecular assays have been developed for most parasitic human infections, including

Department of Laboratory Medicine and Pathology, Division of Clinical Microbiology, Mayo Clinic, 200 1st Street Southwest, Rochester, MN 55905, USA
* Corresponding author.
E-mail address: pritt.bobbi@mayo.edu

Clin Lab Med 33 (2013) 461–503
http://dx.doi.org/10.1016/j.cll.2013.03.008
0272-2712/13/$ – see front matter © 2013 Elsevier Inc. All rights reserved.

labmed.theclinics.com

infections with significant worldwide morbidity and mortality, such as malaria and leishmaniasis. Since then, developments in postamplification techniques (eg, microarrays, DNA sequencing), and also recent advances in mass spectrometry (MS) and proteomics, have shown promise for the laboratory diagnosis of parasitic infections. Regardless of these advances, most molecular tests are not well suited for widespread adoption in resource-poor/field settings, in which many of these diseases are endemic. Testing systems are often complex and expensive, requiring sophisticated instrumentation, molecular grade reagents, highly skilled operators, consistent electricity sources, temperature and humidity controls, and highly regulated transportation and storage capabilities for patient specimens and reagents (ie, maintenance of a cold chain). New applications of isothermal nucleic acid amplification tests (NAAT) such as loop-mediated isothermal amplification (LAMP) and nucleic acid sequence based amplification (NASBA) show promise for future widespread implementation in resource-poor settings because need for a thermocycler is obviated, although additional challenges remain.

The paucity of commercially available and US Food and Drug Administration (FDA)-approved/CE-marked molecular parasitology tests is also problematic. Most molecular tests are based on nonstandardized, laboratory-developed methods, requiring significant maintenance demands and quality control measures to ensure optimal assay performance. As a result, the use of laboratory-developed tests is generally limited to centralized reference laboratories, public health laboratories such as the CDC, and specialized research facilities. Several new methods are under development and are expected to be commercially available in the future.

As the use of molecular methods become more widespread, clinicians and laboratorians need to address important questions such as how the tests should be incorporated into the work flow of the parasitology laboratory, the role of traditional diagnostics as supplemental or confirmatory methods, and the interpretation of positive results with respect to clinical infection. In particular, molecular testing is often more sensitive than traditional microscopy, and nucleic acid may be detectable long after the patient has been successfully treated. In these situations, it is not well understood if individuals with positive molecular tests invariably progress to clinical disease or experience a relapse after treatment.

Despite these uncertainties, we believe that in the near future, molecular diagnostics for parasitology will become more accessible and standardized for use, both in the field and in clinical laboratories for screening diagnosis of parasitic infections. In this review, the available molecular assays for the diagnosis of the major and more common human parasites are examined (see also **Table 1**). These assays include the few that have been approved or cleared by the FDA, as well as the more widespread laboratory-developed tests. Newer technologies such as isothermal amplification techniques and MS as applied to diagnostic molecular parasitology are also briefly reviewed.

BLOOD PARASITES
Malaria

Background
Malaria is a potentially deadly infection caused by protozoan parasites in the *Plasmodium* genus. Infection is transmitted by the bite of an infected female *Anopheles* sp mosquito, resulting in erythrocyte infection and destruction. Although once widespread, disease is now mostly limited to the tropics and subtropics worldwide, including many poor nations with limited resources and health care infrastructure.

The 5 primary species that infect humans are *P falciparum, P vivax, P ovale, P malariae,* and *P knowlesi.* Light microscopic examination of thick and thin blood films is considered the gold standard for diagnosis of acute or relapsing disease. This time-honored technique is dependent on the availability of skilled and experienced microscopists, good-quality reagents, and well-maintained microscopes. Malaria rapid diagnostic tests (RDTs), which detect *Plasmodium* antigens (histidine-rich protein [HRP], lactate dehydrogenase, or aldolase) have also been developed, and have been shown to be useful in both endemic and nonendemic settings.[72–75] In general, malaria RDTs perform almost as well as microscopy for *P falciparum*[73]; however, they do not fare so well for other species such *P vivax or P malariae,*[75] especially when PCR is used as a comparator,[10] and false-negatives may result from a prozone phenomenon with high levels of parasitemia[76,77] or a lack of production of the target antigen (HRP 2 and 3 in certain *P falciparum* variants).[78] Molecular tests do not suffer from these limitations and therefore offer a viable diagnostic alternative in certain settings.[79]

Design and performance of molecular diagnostics

Most NAATs target the genes encoding the malarial 18S small subunit ribosomal RNA (ssu rRNA). PCR-based assays have adopted a variety of detection chemistries including hydrolysis (TaqMan)[6] or hybridization (fluorescent resonance energy transfer [FRET])[7] probes. More recently, reverse transcriptase real-time PCR assays have been described that amplify total nucleic acid (RNA and DNA) of the 18S rRNA genes, which have an even higher sensitivity (limit of detection [LOD] as low as 0.000362 parasites/µL).[8] None of these assays have been approved or cleared by the FDA. Multiple studies have shown PCR-based assays to be superior to microscopy for the detection of malaria. The lower LOD of microscopy for malaria in the best of hands has been estimated to be as low as 0.0001% to 0.0004% parasitemia ($\sim$5–20 parasites/µL),[80] whereas for PCR it is estimated to be $\sim$1 log lower (0.7–4 parasites/µL in 1 study).[5]

In addition to *Plasmodium* detection, many PCR assays are capable of speciation. A variety of strategies have been used to distinguish between species, including the use of multiple different primers/probes for each species[3,9] and species differentiation by melting temperature analysis using hybridization probes[7] (**Fig. 1**) or other formats. Some assays allow for differentiation of the newly described *P ovale* subspecies, *P ovale curtisi,* and *P ovale wallikeri.*[11,12]

Some molecular methods have also been described for detection of single-nucleotide polymorphisms associated with parasite resistance to various antimalarials, such as *Pfcrt* (chloroquine), *pfmdr* (chloroquine/mefloquine), *dhps/dhft* (sulfadoxine/pyrimethamine), cytochrome b (atovaquone), and *pfATPase6/pfmdr* (artemisinin). These polymorphisms can be detected via real-time PCR[81] or in a high-throughput DNA microarray format.[82] It is anticipated that genetic markers will be more widely used for detecting and monitoring antimalarial resistance at a population level, and possibly at the individual level in the future. However, more work is needed in furthering our understanding of the contribution of these markers to resistance and treatment failure, which is often multifactorial. These issues have been thoroughly addressed in several recent articles.[83–85]

Clinical usefulness of molecular diagnostics

PCR-based tests can play an important role for initial testing of suspected malaria cases, provided that testing can be performed on site, and expeditiously. Positive results still require a review of peripheral blood smears to ascertain percentage parasitemia, because this is used to guide therapy. In addition to primary testing, molecular

Table 1
Overview of select diagnostic tests

Disease	Molecular Method	Target	Notes	Reference(s)
Malaria	Nested conventional PCR	18S small subunit ribosomal RNA genes (18S rDNA)	LOD of at least 6 parasites/µL of blood using DNA from blood spots with in vitro cultured Plasmodium falciparum on filter paper[3]; better for detecting mixed infections than nonnested PCR, especially with low-level parasitemia[4]	3,4
	Real-time PCR Multiplex TaqMan probe		LOD of 0.7, 4.0, and 1.5 parasites/µL for P falciparum, P vivax, and P ovale, respectively.[5] Specificity and sensitivity for single infections of 100% compared with nested PCR[6]	5,6
	Multiplex real-time PCR, FRET hybridization probes		Comprises 1 primer set and 2 probe sets. Able to distinguish all 5 malarial species based on melting temperature analysis	7
	Reverse transcriptase quantitative real-time PCR		Amplification of total nucleic acids (RNA and DNA) LOD 0.002 parasite/µL for Plasmodium genus level identification; 1.22 parasite/µL for P falciparum identification	8
	Real-time PCR with 4 primers		Higher analytical sensitivity with 4 primer PCR (LOD of 0.02, 0.004, and 0.006 for parasites/µL of P falciparum/P vivax, P ovale, and P malariae respectively); detection of 15 additional mixed infections compared with panprimer PCR with 4 probes	9
	SYBR Green-based real-time PCR		In a study of 338 febrile patients in Bangladesh with suspected malaria, RDTs and microscopy gave low sensitivity (76.9%, 95% CI 56.4–91) in detecting of P vivax when compared with real-time PCR	10

Real-time PCR	rbp2 gene	Assay distinguishes between P ovale curtisi and P ovale wallikeri by melting temperature analysis	11
TaqMan probe Real-time PCR	18S small subunit ribosomal RNA genes (18S rDNA)	Distinguishes P ovale wallikeri and P ovale curtisi	12
Real-time quantitative NASBA with molecular beacon probes	18S small subunit ribosomal RNA (18S rRNA)	LOD of 0.01–0.1 Plasmodium spp parasites per diagnostic sample (50 µL of blood). Isothermal method; detects rRNA that are present in more copies than rDNA, and is therefore believed to be more sensitive	13
LAMP	18S small subunit ribosomal RNA genes (18S rDNA)	Sensitivity of 98.3% and specificity of 100% when testing 110 blood samples (60 positive for malaria)[14]	14,15
PCR-based ELISA microplate hybridization assay	18S small subunit ribosomal RNA genes (18S rDNA)	PCR amplicons are hybridized with species-specific probes for P falciparum, P vivax, P malariae, and P ovale immobilized in microtiter plate wells and detected by colorimetric assay with a microplate reader. Sensitivity 91.4% for P falciparum, 94.2% for P vivax. Semiquantitative and able to detect mixed infections	16
PCR-NALFIA		Pan-Plasmodium PCR products detected by NALFIA, LOD 0.3–3 parasites/µL[17]	17
LDMS	P falciparum hemozoin	LDMS sensitivity was 52% when compared with PCR, possibly because of suboptimal volumes of blood analyzed (1 µL vs 20–30 µL). Further studies needed	18

(continued on next page)

Table 1
(continued)

Disease	Molecular Method	Target	Notes	Reference(s)
Babesiosis	Real-time PCR, conventional PCR	18S small subunit ribosomal RNA genes	LOD of 3 parasites (merozoites)/50 μL reaction,[19] 100 gene copies in 5 μL of blood[20]	19,20
Chagas disease	TaqMan probe real-time PCR	18S rRNA gene, kinetoplastic DNA (kDNA), nuclear DNA (nDNA/minisatellite TCZ region)	CDC study. LOD ranges from 0.1 fg/μL to 10 fg/μL for discrete typing units (DTU) I and II for the 3 assays. kDNA PCR is sensitive, but less specific, and TCZ PCR is less sensitive and more specific than kDNA PCR, and 18S PCR is the most specific, but least sensitive. 2 or more real-time PCR assays are suggested for diagnosis of Chagas disease, and PCR of buffy coat allows earlier detection of increasing parasitemia	21
	Conventional PCR[22] Nested PCR[23]	kDNA,[22] nDNA[23]	In chronic disease, kDNA PCR was found to have only 70% sensitivity when compared with an immunoblot assay, and is therefore recommended only as an adjunct to diagnosis in this setting.[22] A nested PCR approach may be helpful in chronic disease with equivocal serology test results[23]	22,23

African trypanosomiasis Genus level identification	SYBR Green-based real-time PCR	177-bp satellite repeat	Performed on blood samples collected on Whatman FTA cards, extracted with Chleex 100 resin, LOD 100 trypanosomes/mL of blood (0.1 genomic equivalents) [24]
	Conventional PCR	ITS1 rDNA	Detects both human-pathogenic and animal-pathogenic African trypanosomes [25]
	PCR-oligochromatography	18S rDNA	LOD of 5 fg of pure *Trypanosoma brucei* DNA; able to detect 1 parasite/180 µL of blood. Visualization of results in dipstick format within 5 min after PCR step [26]
	LAMP	PFRA	One of the primer sets for LAMP studied was found to be 100 times more sensitive than PCR (LOD 1pg vs 100 pg) [27]
	LAMP	RIME	Real-time detection with SYTO-9 fluorescence dye added, or via agarose gel electrophoresis. LOD of RIME LAMP assay is 0.001 trypanosomes/mL compared with 0.1–1000 trypanosomes/mL for PCR [28]
	NASBA-OC (oligochromatography)	18S rRNA	LOD of 1–10 parasites/mL from nucleic acid extracts of parasite culture; LOD of 10 parasites/mL in spiked blood [29]
	PNA-FISH	18S rDNA	LOD of 500 trypanosomes/mL of blood (100 times more sensitive than the conventional counting chamber detection limit), improved to 5 trypanosomes/mL after cytospin, thus approaching sensitivity of molecular amplification approaches [30]
	SELDI-TOF	206 protein clusters	Sensitivity of 100% and specificity of 98.6%, in a study of a 109 patients. Requires further studies [31]

(continued on next page)

Table 1
(continued)

Disease	Molecular Method	Target	Notes	Reference(s)
African trypanosomiasis Species level identification	LAMP	SRA gene	Identifies *Trypanosoma brucei rhodesiense*. LOD of 1 pg of purified DNA (equivalent to 10 trypanosomes/mL) and 0.1 pg (1 trypanosome/mL) with heat-treated buffy coat, superior to conventional SRA PCR (LOD 1000 trypanosomes/mL)	32
	Conventional PCR	Expression-site-associated gene 6 and 7 (ESAG6/7)	Identifies *Trypanosoma brucei gambiense*. Sensitivity of 87% and specificity of 97% for microscopically positive cases. With an estimate of 20 copies of target/cell, the LOD was ~40 trypanosomes/mL blood[33]	33
Filariasis				
Wuchereria bancrofti	PCR	188 bp DNA sequence Ssp-I	Sensitivity of 0.1 pg *Wuchereria bancrofti* genomic DNA; 1 microfilaria in 100 μL human blood	34
	TaqMan probe real-time PCR	Long DNA repeat (LDR)	Found to be more sensitive than a PCR assay based on the bacterial endosymbiont *Wolbachia* 16S rDNA; PCR was not positive in microfilaremic patients with samples drawn in the day, implying that intact microfilaria DNA was detected rather than residual circulating DNA.[35] Can be multiplexed with other assays (eg, to detect malaria)[36]	35,36
Brugia malayi	TaqMan probe real-time PCR	Hha I repeat region	The Eclipse MGB real-time PCR was found to have a LOD of 0.1 fg, or approximately 22 Hha I copies	37
Loa loa	TaqMan probe real-time PCR	Expressed sequence tags (LLMF72 and LLMF269)	LOD of 0.1 pg genomic DNA (1% of DNA extracted from blood spiked with a single *Loa loa* microfilaria)	38

Leishmaniasis	Conventional PCR	kDNA	Best overall sensitivity in New World cutaneous leishmaniasis compared with culture/smears/skin test[39] kDNA PCR was the most sensitive (96.6%) diagnostic assay compared with smear/culture/ITS1 PCR in a study of 32 clinical samples of Old World cutaneous leishmaniasis caused by *Leishmania tropica*.[40] A *Viannia* subgenus PCR detected 86.4% of patients with confirmed mucosal leishmaniasis vs only 16.7% by microscopy[41]	39–41
	Hybridization probes, real-time PCR assay, Smart Leish	16S rDNA – *Leishmania* genus identification Glucose phosphate isomerase–*Leishmania major* detection	FDA approved for use in the US military on the Cepheid SmartCycler system. Sensitivity and specificity for *Leishmania* genus are 99.1%/67%; for *Leishmania major*, 95.8%/91.2%	42,43
	TaqMan real-time PCR assay	Glucose phosphate isomerase	Detects *Leishmania (Viannia)* spp, *Leishmania mexicana*, *Leishmania donovani/infantum*, and *Leishmania major* with identification to the complex level. Highly specific, LOD of 5.6 pg of genomic DNA (approximately 165.4 genome copies)	44
	SYBR Green–based real-time PCR and TaqMan real-time PCR assay	Glucose-6-phosphate dehydrogenase	SYBR Green assay with 2 independent primers identify both cutaneous leishmaniasis subgenera, *Leishmania (Viannia)* and *Leishmania (Leishmania)* in the Americas. TaqMan probes enable distinction between *Leishmania (Viannia) peruviana* or *Leishmania (Viannia) braziliensis* from other *Leishmania (Viannia)* species	45
	LAMP	kDNA	Detected 1 fg of *Leishmania donovani* DNA, 10-fold more sensitive than conventional PCR	46

(continued on next page)

Table 1
(continued)

Disease	Molecular Method	Target	Notes	Reference(s)
Toxoplasma gondii	Conventional PCR	B1 gene	Multicopy target, which is believed to increase sensitivity of assay	47
	PCR	REP-52	Multicopy target, but was found to be absent in 4.8% of *Toxoplasma gondii*-positive blood samples from HIV-infected patients in 1 study	48
	LAMP	SAG-1, SAG-2, B1 gene	More sensitive than nested PCR against the B1 gene, LOD 0.1 tachyzoite	49
Free-living amoebae	Multiplex, TaqMan probe real-time PCR	18S rDNA	CDC assay detecting *Acanthamoeba* spp, *Naegleria fowleri*, and *Balamuthia mandrillaris*. LOD 1 amoeba per sample processed. It is estimated that *Acanthamoeba* has approximately 600 copies of the ribosomal repeat unit; *Naegleria* spp several thousand copies	50
Entamoeba histolytica/dispar	Conventional PCR	18S rDNA - small subunit (ssu) rRNA genes	LOD of 1 trophozoite per reaction, in contrast to both of the stool antigen kits tested (*Entamoeba* CELISA PATH kit and TechLab *Entamoeba histolytica* II kit), which were estimated to require 1000–10,000 trophozoites/well for detection	51
	Conventional PCR	p30 (30 kDa) antigen genes	Of 19 patients with suspected amoebic liver abscesses, 100% were confirmed by PCR on abscess material, but only 2 were positive by microscopy	52
	Conventional PCR	Hemolysin gene	This study found that PCR targeting the hemolysin gene was more sensitive than the ssu rRNA and p30 gene PCR. In amoebic liver abscess material, sensitivity was 89% (18/23) compared with 77% and 28%, respectively	53

Disease	Method	Target	Comments	Ref
Giardiasis	TaqMan probe real-time PCR	18S rDNA ssu rRNA genes	As sensitive as antigen assay in this study (98%) vs microscopy (89%), and was able to detect infection earlier than microscopy or antigen testing in 2 patients who submitted multiple samples	54
	Conventional PCR,[55] TaqMan probe real-time PCR[56]	β-Giardin gene	LOD of a single cyst of Giardia intestinalis.[56] Can be coupled to restriction length polymorphism assay for genotyping[55]	55,56
Cryptosporidiosis	TaqMan probe real-time PCR	Cryptosporidium parvum- specific 452-bp fragment	Identified a 138-bp segment within 452-bp fragment. LOD of 6 Cryptosporidium parvum oocysts	57
	TaqMan probe real-time PCR	Cryptosporidium oocyte wall protein (COWP)	LOD 1 oocyst of Cryptosporidium parvum	56
Dientamoeba fragilis infection	Conventional PCR	ssu ribosomal RNA gene	Sensitivity of 93.5% (detected 29/31 samples) and specificity of 100% when compared with microscopy	58
	Conventional PCR	5.8S ribosomal RNA gene	PCR was positive in 93% and 84% in specimens for which microscopy was positive in 2 and 1 specimen, respectively	59

(continued on next page)

Table 1
(continued)

Disease	Molecular Method	Target	Notes	Reference(s)
Infection with intestinal protozoa/helminth multiplex	TaqMan probe real-time PCR	18S rRNA gene (*Entamoeba histolytica/Giardia lamblia*), COWP (*Cryptosporidium parvum*)	Multiplex detecting *Entamoeba histolytica*, *Giardia intestinalis*, and *Cryptosporidium parvum* on extracted stool (100 µL). LOD and sensitivity were 1 trophozoite/86%, 10 trophozoites/89%, and 100 oocysts/90%, respectively. Singleplex versions of individual assays showed slight increase in sensitivity	60
	Luminex bead based multiplex real-time PCR	18S rRNA gene (*Entamoeba. histolytica*, *Giardia lamblia*, and *Strongyloides stercoralis*) COWP (*Cryptosporidium parvum*), ITS1 (*Ascaris lumbricoides*) ITS2 (*Ascaris duodenale* and *Necator americanus*)	2 multiplex PCR assays (protozoa and helminth) with subsequent detection of amplicons on the Luminex platform. Compared with parent multiplex real-time PCR, Luminex assay had 83% sensitivity and 100% specificity	61
	TaqMan Array Card (TAC) in 384 well singleplex real-time PCR	19 enteropathogens: including viruses (5), bacteria (9), protozoa (*Cryptosporidium* spp., *Giardia intestinalis*, *Entamoeba histolytica*), and helminths (*Ascaris lumbricoides*, *Trichuris trichiura*)	Average sensitivity and specificity of 85% and 77% compared with conventional methods (including culture, immunoassay, and microscopy) and 98% and 96% compared with laboratory-developed PCR-Luminex	62
	Pentaplex TaqMan probe real-time PCR	ITS1 (*Ascaris lumbricoides*), ITS2 (*Ancylostoma duodenale*, *Necator americanus*), 18S rRNA gene (*Strongyloides stercoralis*)	Positivity rates of 62.3% (48 of 77 specimens) vs 7.8% (6 specimens) for microscopy. gB gene of phocine herpesvirus 1 used as an internal control	63
	xTAG Gastrointestinal Pathogen Panel (xTAG GPP, Luminex) Luminex bead based multiplex real-time PCR	15 diarrheagenic pathogens, including 9 bacterial, 3 viral, and 3 parasitic targets (*Giardia intestinalis*, *Entamoeba histolytica*, and *Cryptosporidium* spp)	No published data. One multicenter study reported sensitivities for protozoal targets between 97.5% and 99%, when compared with conventional methods. Seeking status as an FDA cleared IVD by 2013	64

	Platform/Assay	Target	Comments	Reference
	FilmArray GI (BioFire Diagnostics) Nested PCR	23 diarrheagenic pathogens (including Giardia intestinalis, Entamoeba histolytica, Cryptosporidium spp, and Cyclospora cayetanensis)	No published data. Limited data on performance characteristics for parasitic component of assay. Seeking status as an FDA cleared IVD by 2014	65
Schistosomiasis	PCR-ELISA	Highly repeated short 0.64-kb DNA sequence	LOD of 1.3 fg of Schistosoma mansoni genomic DNA; ~0.15 Schistosoma mansoni eggs per gram of feces (fractions of an egg). Sensitivity and specificity 97.4% and 85.1%, when compared with Kato-Katz method	66
	Multiplex real-time PCR	Cytochrome c oxidase gene	84.1% PCR detection rate similar to 79.5% in microscopy (when microscopy was performed in duplicate stool specimens)	67
Trichomoniasis	Transcription-mediated amplification Aptima Trichomonas vaginalis (ATV) assay (Gen-Probe, San Diego, CA)	16S rRNA	FDA cleared. In this study involving specimens from 766 patients, ATV found to be more sensitive than the Affirm assay for Trichomonas vaginalis (sensitivity 100% vs 63.4%)	68
	BD Affirm VPIII (Affirm) assay (Becton Dickinson, Sparks, MD)	RNA probe		
Microsporidiosis	Real-time PCR (in SYBR Green,[69] TaqMan,[70] hybridization probes[71])	rRNA ssu or ITS regions	Panmicrosporidial and species-specific targets available Real-time PCR approach with 2-log unit–4-log unit increase in sensitivity over routine stool smears[71]	69–71

Abbreviations: CDC, Centers for Disease Control and Prevention; CI, confidence interval; ELISA, enzyme-linked immunosorbent assay; FRET, fluorescence resonance energy transfer; ITS1, internal transcribed spacer 1; kDNA, kinetoplastic (mitochondrial) DNA; LDMS, laser desorption mass spectrometry; LOD, (lower) limit of detection; NALFIA, nucleic acid lateral flow immunoassay; PCR, polymerase chain reaction; PFRA, paraflagellar rod protein A gene; rbp2, reticulocyte binding protein 2; RDT, rapid diagnostic test; SELDI-TOF MS, surface-enhanced laser desorption/ionization time-of-flight mass spectrometry.

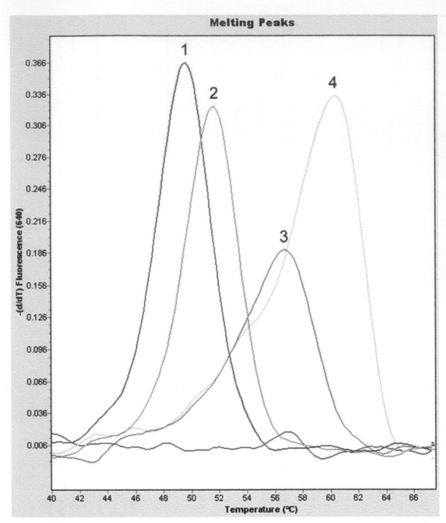

Fig. 1. Malaria PCR using hybridization probes and melting temperature analysis to distinguish *P ovale* (1), *P vivax* (2), *P malariae* (3), and *P falciparum* (4). *Plasmodium knowlesi* is detected on a different fluorescent channel using a separate probe set.

methods may be useful for confirming cases in which there is diagnostic uncertainty (eg, malaria vs babesiosis or artifacts) or for determining the infecting species when the morphology is not clear. Given their superior sensitivity, molecular assays like PCR are also useful for the detection of low-level parasitemia, mixed infections, and congenital infections (PCR on placental tissue). For mixed infections with a low parasite density, a nested PCR strategy seems to offer the best sensitivity and ability to detect and identify the infecting species.[4]

Emerging technologies
Despite the advantages of molecular malaria diagnostics, implementation in endemic, often resource-limited settings, poses many challenges. Fortunately, NAAT techniques using isothermal techniques such as NASBA and LAMP have emerged. These

techniques show promise for use in endemic settings, especially when run on platforms that do not require electrical power.[13–15,86] One innovative prototype described recently is the NINA (noninstrumented nucleic acid) platform: a cheap, electricity-free heater consisting of an improvised thermos container with calcium oxide generating heat via an exothermic chemical reaction to support LAMP.[86] Other potential strategies for malaria diagnosis in resource-limited settings include coupling NAATs to enzyme-linked immunosorbent assay (ELISA) (PCR-ELISA)[16] or RDTs (nucleic acid lateral flow immunoassay [NALFIA]).[17]

MS may also hold promise for malaria diagnosis. In 1 study, Laser desorption MS (LDMS) detected *P falciparum* hemozoin in 15 of 45 pregnant Zambian women who were asymptomatic and smear negative, but had a sensitivity of 52% when compared with PCR, possibly because of a suboptimal volume of blood used.[18] It is possible that further refinements in assay protocol will allow MS to emerge as a potential alternative method for malaria diagnosis.

Babesiosis

Background

Apicomplexan parasites of the *Babesia* genus (including *Babesia microti*, *Babesia duncani* and a strain currently designated MO-1 [Missouri-01] in the United States, and *Babesia divergens* in Europe and elsewhere) cause human babesiosis, a tick-borne illness the geographic distribution which seems to be underappreciated and the incidence of which is rising.[20,87–89] It is also the most commonly reported transfusion-transmitted parasitic infection in the United States.[90,91] Like malaria, babesiosis diagnosis is traditionally performed through examination of thick and thin blood films. Although microscopy is a cheap and acceptable standard for *Babesia* diagnosis, the clinical manifestations of malaria and babesiosis overlap and there is potential difficulty in distinguishing the ring forms of *Babesia* morphologically from those of *P falciparum* on blood smears. Therefore, diagnosis may be difficult or underappreciated in areas in which *Plasmodium* and *Babesia* parasites cocirculate[88,92] or in travelers who have been exposed to both malarious and *Babesia*-endemic areas. Serologic methods are also available and may be used for population and blood donor screening. However, these tests are insensitive during acute disease and are unable to distinguish between previous exposure and active infection (titers have been reported to be increased up to 6 years after infection).[87] Molecular methods, available mainly in reference laboratories as laboratory-developed PCR tests, therefore have potential usefulness in several clinical scenarios.

Design and performance of molecular diagnostics

PCR assays, based on detection of the ssu rDNA, have been developed for both *Babesia microti*[19,20] and *Babesia divergens*[92] and offer superior sensitivity compared with standard microscopy (LOD ~100 gene copies or ~0.0001% parasitemia).[20]

Clinical usefulness of molecular diagnostics

Testing can be offered individually or incorporated into a tick-borne diseases panel for entities with similar clinical presentations. For example, an acute tick-borne disease panel may include serologic testing for Lyme disease and PCR testing for agents of ehrlichiosis and anaplasmosis. The CDC is working with partners to develop a potential screening test for babesiosis, and studies are under way to evaluate PCR for blood product screening to prevent transfusion-associated babesiosis.[93] A potential role for NAAT for the prevention of transfusion-transmitted *Babesia* is seasonal NAAT screening of blood supplies as a complement to serologic screening, during periods when ticks are active (~May to September).[94] PCR may also be useful in the evaluation of congenital babesiosis, in which PCR is performed on placental tissue or newborn blood.[95] When requesting PCR testing for *Babesia*, it is important for clinicians to understand which species are detected with the assay and if cross-reaction with other *Babesia* species or even other parasites (eg, malaria) may be seen.

Emerging technologies

A variation on *Babesia* PCR is used by the PLEX-ID system by Abbott Ibis Biosciences (Abbott Park, IIL). This system uses conventional PCR followed by electrospray ionization MS (ESI-MS) for broad-ranged microbial identification from clinical specimens. Multiplex PCR reactions first take place in microtiter plate using broad-range and target specific primers directed against various classes of microorganisms (bacteria, fungi, parasites, viruses). Identification and speciation are then performed by ESI-MS from the amplified DNA. The manufacturers of this platform offer a vector-borne panel with a small parasite library detecting *Babesia microti*, *Babesia divergens*, the nonhuman pathogens *Babesia bovis*, *Babesia gibsoni*, and *Babesia canis*, and the filarial nematode *Dirofilaria immitis*.[96] However, this system is currently classified as a research-use only device, with limited availability.

Chagas Disease

Background

Chagas disease (American trypanosomiasis) is a potentially life-threatening illness caused by the protozoan hemoflagellate, *Trypanosoma cruzi*. Disease is prevalent throughout parts of South and Central America where infection most commonly occurs through the bite of an infected blood-feeding triatomine reduviid bug. Unlike most vector-borne diseases, transmission does not occur through the bug's saliva, but instead through the bug's feces, which contain infective metacyclic trypomastigotes and enter the bite wound. Other, less common, means of infection include blood transfusion, organ transplantation, transplacental spread, and ingestion of food or beverages (eg, Açaí juice) containing reduviid bug feces. In nonendemic areas that receive migrants from Latin America, transmission of disease from serologically positive, asymptomatic blood or organ donors is a growing concern. Subsequent disease in recipients of organ transplant may occur either from reactivation of latent/chronic disease during immunosuppression or by acquisition from an infected organ donor. In the United States, autochthonous (locally acquired) transmission has also been reported in South Texas and Louisiana[97,98] Infection may manifest acutely, or with chronic sequelae involving cardiac (heart failure and arrhythmias) and gastrointestinal (megacolon, megaesophagus) abnormalities. Diagnosis is traditionally performed by blood smear microscopy (for identification of circulating trypomastigote forms), serology (for later stage disease) and cardiac biopsy (for identification of nonmotile amastigote forms).

Design and performance of molecular diagnostics

PCR assays, either in real-time or conventional format[99] generally target the kinetoplastic (mitochondrial) DNA (kDNA, also known as the minicircle) or nuclear DNA (nDNA, also known as the minisatellite TCZ region), which are present in multiple copies (repeated ~100,000 times in each parasite). The presence of multiple target copies significantly increases assay sensitivity.[21,100] Recent efforts have been directed to international validation and standardization of PCR procedures for the best detection of *Trypanosoma cruzi* in human blood samples.[21,99] Preanalytical factors such as heating of blood after addition of guanidine hydrochloride,[101] or extracting DNA from the blood specimen's buffy coat,[21] increase the sensitivity of PCR. In a recent study by Qvanstrom and colleagues,[21] PCR of the buffy coat extract allowed diagnosis of reactivation of Chagas disease as much as 2 weeks earlier than whole blood analysis and increased yield of diagnosis by 26%.

Clinical usefulness of molecular diagnostics

PCR-based molecular assays show the most promise for diagnosis of Chagas disease in the following scenarios[100,102]: detection during acute disease,[102–104] early identification of reactivated Chagas disease in immunosuppressed hosts (eg, after transplant, human immunodeficiency virus [HIV] infection),[105–107] diagnosis of congenital infection,[108] and assessing response to therapy.[109]

In acute infection, peripheral blood smears have traditionally been the mainstay of diagnosis. Concentration techniques (eg, with a microhematocrit tube) can improve the LOD to ~40 parasites/mL.[110] Parasitemia subsequently decreases, usually within 90 days of infection.[102] PCR, which is considered to be more sensitive than the traditional peripheral smear in the early stages, can be used as an adjunct to microscopy if acute Chagas disease is suspected but initial slides are negative.

For chronic infection, serology is the mainstay of diagnosis, and is also method of choice for blood donor screening. Peripheral blood PCR is not so sensitive in chronic infection, although it may be a complementary tool when serologic testing is equivocal.[22,23,102,111] However, PCR of tissue (eg, cardiac, esophageal) in chronic chagasic disease may prove useful, and sensitivity has been shown to be increased if targeted PCR is performed on tissue biopsies showing inflammatory changes.[112]

For congenital disease, PCR of peripheral blood of the neonate has a higher sensitivity than the microhematocrit concentration method[108] and seems to be most sensitive when performed on the infant's peripheral blood near the second month after birth.[113] If PCR is positive shortly (days to weeks) after birth, it is recommended that a second sample be tested 1 to 3 months after birth to confirm infection, because nonviable, lysed parasites might cause false-positive results in infants born to mothers who are chronically infected.[100] In cases of proven congenital infection, PCR may be useful for following treatment response.[108] Placental PCR positivity does not seem to be useful for predicting congenital transmission or maternal bloodstream PCR positivity.[114] Serology may complement the diagnosis of congenital infection for older infants 6 months and older after maternal antibodies are cleared.

Molecular testing in the United States is available via the CDC. (Consultations for known/suspected *Trypanosoma cruzi* infections and testing can be directed to Dr Frank Steurer at the Parasitic Diseases Branch, CDC (email: fsteurer@cdc.gov; telephone: 404-718-4175.) Because of the current variable sensitivities/specificities of the various PCR assays, the CDC uses a multitarget approach comprising 3 real-time PCR assays performed in tandem on kDNA, nDNA/TCZ, and 18S targets.[21]

Human African Trypanosomiasis

Background

Human African trypanosomiasis (HAT) is caused by the protozoan hemoflagellates, *Trypanosoma brucei* subspecies *gambiense* (west/central sub-Saharan Africa) and *rhodesiense* (east sub-Saharan Africa). Clinical illness may be acute or chronic. Acute illness (stage I) may be associated with a chancre at the inoculation site of the tsetse fly vector, followed by a hemolymphatic phase (fever, lymphadenopathy). Chronic illness (stage II, sleeping sickness or the meningoencephalitic stage) results from invasion of the central nervous system (CNS) by the parasite and is fatal if untreated.[115,116] Both subspecies can cause stage II disease, although *Trypanosoma b gambiense* tends to have a lower parasite count compared with *Trypanosoma b rhodesiense*.[115] Diagnosis is traditionally performed by identification of trypomastigotes in peripheral blood films, cerebrospinal fluid (CSF), and lymph node aspirates. The preferred treatment differs according to the infecting subspecies and disease stage.[117] Therefore, determining the infecting subspecies and extent of dissemination are important components for determining treatment. The 2 subspecies are morphologically identical, and subspeciation is instead based on the patient's geographic location. Uganda is the 1 country where both species circulate (Gambian HAT in the northwest, and Rhodesian HAT in the southeast). Although transmission is still within geographically separate regions of Uganda, the gap has narrowed in recent years, thus raising concerns for the convergence and cotransmission of both subspecies.[118,119] The infected traveler who visits multiple African countries may also pose a diagnostic dilemma when attempting subspeciation. In these situations, accurate diagnostics that allow for clear subspeciation are needed.

In addition to microscopy, the card agglutination test for trypanosomiasis (which detects the LiTat 1.3 surface glycoprotein) is widely used for field screening for *Trypanosoma b gambiense*. Although sensitivities are good at 87% to 98%, the test has been reported to be falsely negative as a result of LiTat 1.3 variants, and may also be falsely positive in cases in which there is a cross-reaction with other parasites or nonpathogenic trypanosomes, especially if end titers are not obtained. Therefore, microscopic examination for parasites is still needed for confirmation of disease. However, standard microscopy, being imperfect, is estimated to still miss 20% to 30% of cases.[120] Furthermore, for *Trypanosoma b rhodesiense*, there is still no good field serologic test, and screening is mostly still based on parasitic examination (blood, lymph node aspirates). Given the limitations of conventional diagnostics, there is an important potential role for sensitive tests capable of subspeciation.

Design and performance of molecular diagnostics

Various NAATs have been developed for HAT. Early assays were mostly based on conventional PCR,[121,122] whereas newer assays have used real-time PCR technologies.[24] Multiplexed PCR assays have also been developed for subspecies differentiation.[123] Other NAATs that have been developed include LAMP[27,28,32,124] and NASBA-based assays.[29,125] The genetic targets used include the 177 bp satellite DNA (~thousands of copies/parasite)[121] or expression-site-associated genes 6/7 (*ESAG6/7*) (~20 copies/parasite),[33] which identify the subgenus *Trypanozoon* (thus detecting *Trypanosoma brucei* as well as nonhuman *Trypanosoma* species). Theoretically, assays with multicopy targets are more sensitive. Other targets include the internal transcribed spacer region of the ribosomal RNA gene cluster (ITS1 rDNA)[25] and 18S rDNA.[26] LAMP assays have been described targeting the paraflagellar rod protein A gene (PFRA),[27] repetitive insertion mobile element (RIME),[28] and also NASBA targeting 18S rRNA.[29]

For distinguishing the 2 pathogenic human subspecies, differential assays directed against specific single-copy genes have been described, in PCR or LAMP format: the serum resistance-associated gene for *Trypanosoma b rhodesiense*,[32,123,126] a 5.8S rRNA-ITS2 gene[127] and *Trypanosoma b gambiense*-specific glycoprotein (TgsGP) gene for *Trypanosoma b gambiense*.[124,128] LAMP especially seems to be a promising and attractive strategy for both field diagnosis and subspeciation. In 1 study,[124] the analytical sensitivity of TgsGP LAMP was found to be 1 to 10 trypanosomes/mL, whereas PCR ranged from 10 to 10^3 trypanosomes/mL.

LAMP can be performed without a thermocycler, and results can be inspected visually (for turbidity).[124]

Clinical usefulness of molecular diagnostics

Molecular tests can be used for diagnosis of acute cases, confirmation of disease in serologically positive cases, subspeciation of positive cases, and for HAT staging (eg, in patients with suspected CNS involvement but equivocal/negative CSF findings). For HAT staging, caution should be exercised when interpreting a positive CSF result, because a positive test does not necessarily indicate the presence of viable organisms or disease. This distinction is important, because the treatment for stage II disease is potentially toxic.

NAATs can be performed directly on peripheral whole blood or from eluates of blood collected onto filter paper devices designed for nucleic acid amplification. Filter paper collection is especially convenient in the field setting; furthermore, nucleic acid eluates can be amplified and then coupled with oligochromatography (OC) for detection, (ie, LAMP-OC, NASBA-OC, PCR-OC) with amplified products detected in a convenient dipstick format[26,29] possibly coupled with labeled fluorescent probes,[129] or microfluidic chips.[130]

Emerging technologies

It is envisaged that NAAT strategies like LAMP will soon become available for more widespread use in endemic areas, where resources are often limited. WHO and the Foundation for Innovative New Diagnostics (http://www.finddiagnostics.org/) are collaborating to develop diagnostic tools for the control of HAT that are easy and ready for use, require minimal training, are stable at room temperature, and are affordable. Fluorescent in situ hybridization with peptide nucleic acid probes,[30] coupled with a concentration procedure (eg, cytospin or microhematocrit or minianion-exchange centrifugation), and possibly light-emitting diode–powered fluorescent microscopy, show promise as an amplification-independent procedure for the field diagnosis of HAT. For a more detailed discussion of HAT molecular assays, readers are referred to 2 recent reviews.[115,131]

Papadopoulos and colleagues[31] recently described surface-enhanced laser desorption/ionization time-of-flight MS for diagnosis of HAT on the Ciphergen Protein-Chip System Series PBS II (now Bio-Rad Laboratories, Hercules, CA), with reported sensitivities of 100%. This is a variation of matrix-assisted laser desorption/ionization time-of-flight (MALDI-TOF) MS in which the sample bearing surface has intrinsic laser desorption ionization matrix properties and bioaffinity interaction capability. Further validation is required, and this technology requires complex instrumentation and computed interpretive algorithms, which are not feasible in the field setting.

Filariasis

Background

Eight filarial nematodes commonly infect humans (not including *Dirofilaria* spp.), but 4 are responsible for most infections (*Wuchereria bancrofti, Brugia malayi, Loa loa*, and *Onchocerca volvulus*).[132] All are transmitted by insect vectors, and disease manifestation varies by species. Traditional diagnosis entails microscopic examination of blood samples (*Wuchereria bancrofti, Brugia* spp, *Loa loa, Mansonella perstans*, and *M ozzardi*.) or skin snips (*O volvulus* and *Mansonella streptocerca*). Sensitivity of parasitologic examination of blood samples can be increased with concentration methods such as Knott concentration or filtration using a Nuclepore™ filter (Whatman Inc, Florham Park, NJ). Problems with traditional methods include the need for considerable technical expertise in microfilarial identification and speciation and the requirement for timed blood draws to match the circadian periodicity of certain species.[34]

Design and performance of molecular diagnostics

Initial molecular techniques in the 1980s and 1990s saw the development of DNA probes for detection of microfilaria with or without PCR amplification.[133,134] For *Wuchereria bancrofti*, the commonly used targets include the repeated 188 bp DNA sequence Ssp-I[34] or the long DNA repeat[35]; for *Brugia malayi*, the Hha I repeat region has been used.[37]

In a recent study of 200 patients with suspected filariasis referred to the National Institutes of Health, PCR was shown to be as sensitive to blood filtration examination for *Wuchereria bancrofti*, and *Loa loa*, and significantly more sensitive for detection of *O volvulus* microfiladermia, when compared with skin snip microscopy after incubation in saline for 24 hours (PCR detected all 12 cases compared with only 2 detected by microscopy).[135] Similarly, Rao and colleagues[37] developed and compared 2 PCR assays for *Brugia* spp and found that an assay using a minor groove binder probe showed sensitivity that was comparable with night blood membrane filtration.

PCR may also be used for sensitive detection of *Loa loa-O volvulus* coinfection. This is a potentially important clinical scenario, because fatal reactions can occur when coinfected patients with dense microfilaremia receive ivermectin (a commonly used antifilarial drug). To meet this clinical need, a quantitative PCR assay based on expressed sequence tags was developed that had a lower LOD of ~50 microfilariae/mL or 1 pg of genomic DNA. This assay was also able to detect low-level *Loa loa* microfilaremia in 5 of 16 patients who were deemed to be amicrofilaremic by microscopy.[38] Multiplex PCR assays have been described that simultaneously detect *Wuchereria bancrofti* and the 4 main *Plasmodium* spp,[36] which may be useful in clinical settings in which many of these pathogens are endemic.

Overall, from the available data, it does seem that PCR is at least as sensitive or more sensitive in some instances compared with traditional microscopy with concentration techniques, although expert opinions differ.[132,136] Based on limited data, it appears that the sensitivity of NAATs may vary with the time of blood draw, as is true for light microscopy, depending on circadian rhythmicity of the microfiliariae.[37] There are few data comparing NAATs with antigen-based assays. However, in a recent large multicenter study to evaluate the best screening modality to define an end point for mass drug administration for bancroftian filariasis, positivity rates for an immunochromatographic test for filarial antigen (Binax ICT) and an ELISA test (Og4C3 antigen) were noted to be substantially higher than both PCR (using pooled blood specimens) or traditional microscopy,[137] underscoring the difficulty in defining what constitutes a gold standard for comparative studies.

Clinical usefulness of molecular diagnostics

Although molecular testing may be used for detection of active disease, PCR has been especially useful for epidemiologic purposes. It has been used for monitoring vector infection rates in filaria control programs, with material often tested in a pooled fashion.[138] Furthermore, specialized techniques like random amplified polymorphic DNA PCR (DNA fingerprinting) have been used, for example, to monitor the resurgence of *Wuchereria bancrofti* in Thailand, believed to be imported in by Myanmese migrants.[139] Highly sensitive techniques such as these may prove to be critical in monitoring for cases of low microfilaremia as countries worldwide come closer to their goal of eradicating lymphatic filariasis.

TISSUE PARASITES
Leishmaniasis

Background
There are approximately 21 *Leishmania* species that infect humans, and these are morphologically indistinguishable by light microscopy.[140] The infective stage is the flagellated promastigote, which is transmitted by sandflies, whereas the form seen in humans is the nonmotile amastigote. The disease has 2 main forms: cutaneous or visceral, depending on the infecting species, geographic location, and the host immune response. Visceral leishmaniasis (VL) is usually caused by *Leishmania donovani* (Indian subcontinent and Asia, Africa) and *Leishmania infantum/Leishmania chagasi* (Southwest and Central Asia, South America Mediterranean),[141] whereas cutaneous leishmaniasis (CL) is usually secondary to *Leishmania major, Leishmania tropica, Leishmania aethiopica* (Old World leishmaniasis), *Leishmania chagasi* and *Leishmania infantum* (Caspian sea regions and Mediterranean), *Leishmania mexicana, Leishmania amazonensis, Leishmania braziliensis, Leishmania (Viannia) panamensis, Leishmania (Viannia) peruviana*, and *Leishmania (Viannia) guyanensis* (New World leishmaniasis).[140,141] A potentially severe complication of cutaneous infection is mucocutaneous leishmaniasis (MCL), in which parasites disseminate from the skin to the oral and nasal mucosa and cause destructive, recalcitrant disease. MCL is caused by *Leishmania braziliensis, Leishmania (Viannia) panamensis*, and *Leishmania (Viannia) guyanensis* and should always be treated aggressively, because it can become life-threatening when there is severe inflammation and mucosal destruction.[141] Similarly, cutaneous disease by species that can cause MCL should also be treated aggressively.

Diagnosis is traditionally accomplished by microscopic and culture-based methods. Culture allows for propagation of the infective promastigote form and subsequent isoenzyme analysis for speciation (important for cases at risk of MCL). However, this method requires technical expertise and special culture media and is usually performed only at facilities with reference laboratories like the CDC. A variety of serodiagnostic methods (eg, rapid rK39 strip dipstick test) are also commonly used in endemic settings for detection of VL, with varying sensitivities and specificities.

Design and performance of molecular diagnostics
Molecular targets for PCR-based assays have included DNA polymerase, kDNA, and rDNA. ITS1-PCR restriction fragment length polymorphism (RFLP) and real-time PCR assays targeting glucose phosphate isomerase and glucose-6-phosphate dehydrogenase have also been described, which enable speciation.[40,44,45]

In general, NAAT techniques seem to be more sensitive than conventional methods. A recent meta-analysis[142] found that in HIV-infected patients with VL in Europe, PCR-based tests had the highest diagnostic odds ratio (compared with ELISA, immunoblotting, direct agglutination, and immunofluorescence antibody testing). Similarly, in a Peruvian study by Boggild and colleagues[39] involving 145 patients with 202 CL lesions, conventional PCR directed against the kDNA was found to have the best overall sensitivity (96.9%) compared with traditional culture (57.8%), a microculture technique (78.3%), smears (71.4%), and the leishmanin skin test (LST) (78.2%) when a composite gold standard was used (a true-positive result was deemed to be a case in which 2 of the 4 tests were positive). Also, PCR was positive in an additional 14 lesions not detected by the other methods. In a subanalysis, for chronic lesions (>1 year), the LST performed as well as PCR, whereas traditional culture and smears had poor sensitivities for chronic (24% culture, 44% smear) and nonulcerative lesions (34.5% culture; 65.5% smear). Based on their data, the investigators suggest an algorithmic approach to diagnosis, favoring PCR or LST for patients with chronic or nodular lesions (sensitivity of 88% and 93.1%, respectively, for PCR in these 2 clinical settings; 93.3% and 71.4% for LST). LAMP for VL caused by *Leishmania donovani* has been described recently,[46] which was able to detect 1 fg of DNA and was found to be 10-fold more sensitive than conventional PCR. This isothermal NAAT can be applied to other specimen sources, and be more easily applied for use in the field.

Clinical usefulness of molecular diagnostics

PCR-based assays may be used for diagnosis, *Leishmania* speciation, and monitoring for resolution or recurrence of disease. Molecular methods may be especially helpful for detecting cases of mucosal disease, in which the parasite load is low and sensitivity of smear (10%–45%) and cultures (less than 50%) are poor.[41] PCR of dermal lesions and blood has also been shown to be useful in cases of VL or post–kala-azar dermal leishmaniasis in the unusual circumstance in which the disease is suspected clinically but screening with the rK39 strip test is negative.[143] Real-time quantitative PCR has been used to follow up parasite loads in patients treated for VL and this might help avert invasive procedures and aid in detecting treatment failure.[144,145] However, *Leishmania* DNA can be detected in the blood in asymptomatic persons, probably because of a lack of complete parasite clearance by specific cell-mediated immunity. The significance of this finding and the potential of this group of persons to transmit infection requires further study.[146] In the United States, diagnosis of leishmaniasis via culture and PCR should be performed with prior consultation with the CDC, and individualized to each patient (contact Dr Frank Steurer at the CDC's Parasitic Diseases Branch; telephone: 404-718-4175; email: fsteurer@cdc.gov).

Emerging technologies

The Smart Leish real-time PCR assay (run on the Smart cycler II), codeveloped by the Walter Reed Army Institute of Research, the US Army Medical Material Development Activity and Cepheid (Sunnyvale, CA), was recently cleared by the FDA.[42] The assay is designed for the diagnosis of CL and contains genus-specific *Leishmania* probes and species-specific probes for *Leishmania major*. However, its use is restricted to Department of Defense Laboratories.[42,43]

Toxoplasmosis

Background

Toxoplasmosis is caused by the apicomplexan parasite *Toxoplasma gondii*, for which there are 3 predominant lineages: types I, II, and III, as defined by PCR-RFLP or multilocus enzyme electrophoresis.[147] Infection is acquired in 3 main ways: (1) consumption of undercooked meat, water, or foods contaminated with *Toxoplasma gondii* oocysts shed in cat's feces, (2) transplacentally from mother to unborn child, and (3) blood transfusion/organ transplantation. Clinical syndromes include acute toxoplasmosis, which can manifest as a mononucleosislike illness, reactivation disease in an immunocompromised host (eg, toxoplasma encephalitis), congenital toxoplasmosis, and ocular toxoplasmosis (which can occur in acute disease or manifest later in life from congenitally acquired disease). Serology and NAAT are the main diagnostic modalities, and less commonly, direct observation of the parasite via histopathology/microscopy.

Evaluation of toxoplasmosis can be challenging in that a myriad of serologic tests are available and may be difficult to interpret. Test results by different methods or by different laboratories may not be quantitatively compared.[148] Positive IgM results (with a negative IgG) may indicate acute infection versus a false-positive IgM. If both IgM and IgG are positive, this might indicate a recent infection within the past 12 months. In either scenario, repeat testing is recommended, preferably at an experienced reference laboratory.[148] PCR assays may also vary widely in performance, depending on the DNA target used and preanalytical considerations like the method of extraction.[149–152] An accurate diagnosis is important, especially in the case of congenital disease, because it determines therapeutic and monitoring decisions for both mother and fetus/infant, including the option to terminate the pregnancy.

Design and performance of molecular diagnostics

Various multicopy targets have been used for PCR-based *Toxoplasma gondii* assays, including the B1 gene, the REP-52 repeated sequence (AF146527), and the ITS1 or 18S rDNA gene.[47,153,154] REP-52 is present in higher copy numbers than the B1 gene and is believed to be a more sensitive target. However, previous estimates that suggested that B1 is present at ~35 repeated copies[47] and REP-52 at 200 to 300 copies[153] may be lower by 5 to 12 and 4 to 8 times, respectively,[155] possibly because of the subjectivity of older methods in estimating target copy numbers (blotting following conventional PCR). Also, the REP-52 gene was found to be absent in 4.8% of *Toxoplasma gondii*-positive blood samples from HIV-infected patients in a Swedish study (although the B1 assay was positive in these), suggesting that in some parasite strains, the REP-52 element may be deleted.[48]

Clinical usefulness of molecular diagnostics

The use of PCR in the diagnosis of toxoplasmosis lends itself to 3 main areas: (1) diagnosis of congenital toxoplasmosis prenatally or in the newborn by testing amniotic fluid, placenta, or cord blood; (2) reactivation disease in the immunocompromised host (ie, cerebral, pulmonary, or disseminated toxoplasmosis; specimen sources include blood, CSF, bronchoalveolar lavage fluid, and tissue); and (3) ocular toxoplasmosis (retinochoroiditis) by testing aqueous or vitreous humor.[156] These applications are described in greater detail later.

Routine screening for toxoplasmosis in pregnancy has been adopted by some European countries (eg, France, Austria) that historically have high rates of congenital toxoplasmosis. Screening is not routine in the United States, although a recent study has suggested that prematurity and severity of illness is associated with certain *Toxoplasma gondii* alleles (designated nonexclusively II) in the United States, and these are more prevalent with particular demographics (rural residence, Hispanic ethnicity, lower social economic status),[157] thus suggesting a potential role for screening in certain US populations. Because congenital infection is a concern only when toxoplasmosis is acquired during pregnancy, initial testing usually begins in the intrapartum period, with maternal serologic screening. When serology is suspicious for recent infection (eg, IgG±, IgM+ with increasing IgG titers, or low IgG avidity, indicating recent infection[158]), amniotic fluid can be tested by PCR (at ~>16 weeks' gestation, preferably >4 weeks after estimated time of maternal infection) and appropriate treatment with spiramycin or pyrimethamine/sulfonamide begun.[156] PCR on amniotic fluid is reported to have a nearly 100% negative and positive predictive value for maternal infection in the first or second trimester of pregnancy.[156] This technique has largely replaced cordocentesis for culture and fetal serologic testing in the prenatal period. However, a negative amniotic fluid evaluation does not completely preclude congenital toxoplasmosis, because infection can still be caused by low concentrations of tachyzoites in amniotic fluid samples (<5–10 *Toxoplasma gondii* cells/ml),[152,159] and postnatal evaluation should be attempted when maternal infection during pregnancy is suspected.

Postnatal diagnosis can be facilitated by IgM or IgA testing (most sensitively using an immunosorbent agglutination assay [ISAGA]) of cord blood or neonate-specific IgG/IgM Western blots, and also PCR on placental tissue (sensitivity 42%–71%, specificity 92%–100%).[156] An isolated positive PCR result on placenta may not be fully reliable, and an attempt with a second corroborative method (serology, pathology, mouse inoculation) should be attempted to confirm congenital infection.[156,160]

In immunocompromised patients, seropositive allogeneic stem cell transplant patients[161] and patients with AIDS seem to be at the highest risk of reactivation of toxoplasmosis. Older studies based on conventional PCR estimate the sensitivities of CSF and blood PCR to be between 33% and 65% and 16% and 23%, respectively, for the diagnosis of cerebral toxoplasmosis[156] and have suggested that blood PCR in patients with AIDS with cerebral toxoplasmosis is probably unfruitful except in disseminated disease.[162] However, more recent studies have suggested otherwise, with reported sensitivities of up to 80% to 97.2% for blood PCR for patients with cerebral toxoplasmosis and AIDS,[163,164] and 78.6% to 100% for CSF PCR,[164] although these findings have not been replicated in other studies.[165] A recently developed novel duplex reverse transcriptase PCR assay targeting tachyzoite (SAG1) genes and bradyzoite (BAG1) performed well in blood specimens in patients with advanced HIV and cerebral toxoplasmosis (87.5% sensitivity; 100% specificity), but did not detect parasite in CSF samples.[166] Clearly, there is wide variation in the performance of these assays; differences in PCR targets, technical aspects of the assay, study setting, patient characteristics, and previous antiparasitic therapy probably all contribute to the heterogeneity of observed study results.

Toxoplasma retinochoroiditis is a diagnosis primarily made on the ophthalmologic examination, in which focal, white retinal lesions and a vitreous inflammatory reaction are characteristic. However, testing of the aqueous or vitreous humor may be useful when the diagnosis is uncertain or in cases in which there is a failure of response to therapy. Sensitivity is estimated to be 16% to 55%.[156]

Emerging technologies

LAMP seems to be a promising new strategy for detection of toxoplasmosis. LAMP assays targeting the SAG-1, SAG-2, and B1 gene have been described in 1 human study analyzing blood samples in the setting of acute toxoplasmosis. All 3 LAMP targets were found to be more sensitive (80%–87.5%) than a nested PCR targeting the B1 gene (62.5%), with a detection limit of 0.1 tachyzoite.[49]

Free-Living Amoebae

Background

Naegleria fowleri, *Acanthamoeba* spp, and *Balamuthia mandrillaris* are free-living amoebae found in water (eg, lakes, tap water) and are opportunistic human pathogens. *Naegleria fowleri* causes acute and often fatal primary amoebic meningoencephalitis, whereas *Acanthamoeba* spp and *Balamuthia mandrillaris* cause granulomatous amoebic encephalitis affecting both immunocompromised and immunocompetent persons. *Acanthamoeba* spp also cause amoebic keratitis, which is associated with corneal trauma or contact lens use. Another free-living amoebae, *Sappinia* (now believed to be *Sappinia pedata* after further molecular testing, rather than *Sappinia diploidea*) has been described in 1 case of primary amoebic meningoencephalitis in 2001.[167]

Diagnosis of primary amoebic meningoencephalitis and granulomatous amoebic encephalitis can be difficult, given the rarity of disease and lack of expertise pathologic diagnosis. Morphologic examination of ocular (for amoebic keratitis) and CNS specimens (for primary amoebic meningoencephalitis/granulomatous amoebic encephalitis) are routinely used for diagnosis, although organisms may be few in certain clinical specimens and identification of partly degenerated trophozoites in CSF may be particularly challenging. Culture techniques are also available and provided additional sensitivity over microscopic examination; *Acanthamoeba* spp and *Naegleria fowleri* can be cultured on nonnutrient agar overlain with bacteria as a food source for the amoebae, whereas *Balamuthia mandrillaris* requires specimen cell culture. However, culture methods are not widely available and can take a week or more to become positive. Molecular methods are thus a welcome tool, and can help expedite accurate diagnosis and treatment.

Design and performance of molecular diagnostics

Most PCR assays for amoebae in the literature have been singleplex and based on conventional PCR.[168–170] More recently a multiplex, TaqMan probe-based, real-time PCR targeting the nuclear small subunit ribosomal (18S rRNA) gene was developed by the CDC. This assay allows the simultaneous detection and differentiation of *Naegleria fowleri*, *Acanthamoeba* and *Balamuthia mandrillaris*, with a detection limit of ~1 amoebae per processed sample,[50] and was initially validated for CSF and brain tissue with a turn-around time of 5 hours or less (2–3 hours for CSF specimens). Processed samples comprised CSF sediment resuspended in 50 μL of sample supernatant or 50 mg of brain tissue. Samples were then subjected to extraction before PCR. The *Acanthamoeba* portion of this multiplex can also be adapted to a singleplex assay for the sole evaluation of amoebic keratitis. Recently, Khairnar and colleagues[171] compared the *Acanthamoeba* component of the CDC assay with another real-time PCR assay,[172] 2 gel-based conventional PCR assays, and direct microscopy or culture as a gold standard and found that the real-time PCR assays outperformed the conventional PCR assays (sensitivity 82.1%–89.3% compared with 50%–53.6%).

Clinical usefulness of molecular diagnostics

Molecular assays for free-living amoebae offer significant potential advantages over less sensitive microscopic methods and time-consuming cultures. Given that CNS infection with any of these amoebae is often fatal, the availability of rapid and sensitive diagnostics is of utmost clinical importance. However, when using or developing PCR assays, a point to be considered is whether the target region is able to detect the clinically genotypes desired. For example, the Rivere assay, although it also targets 18S rRNA, detects only genotypes T1 and T4, which cause amoebic keratitis (AK), and not genotypes T7 and T10, which cause granulomatous amoebic encephalitis (GAE).[168,172] Clinicians should fully understand the design and potential limitations of these laboratory-developed tests, because performance characteristics likely vary by assay.

INTESTINAL AND UROGENITAL PARASITES
Intestinal Protozoal Infections

Background

Diarrhea remains 1 of the top 5 causes of morbidity and mortality in children worldwide, to which the protozoa *Cryptosporidium* spp, *Giardia intestinalis* (also known as *Giardia lamblia* and *Giardia duodenalis*) and *Entamoeba histolytica* contribute significantly, particularly in endemic regions such as sub-Saharan Africa.[173] *Giardia* and *Cryptosporidium* also cause periodic outbreaks in developed countries (typically waterborne in nature) and significant and sometimes life-threatening diarrhea in persons with immunocompromising conditions (eg, HIV/AIDS). Diagnosis is challenging because viral and bacterial causes present similarly, and traditional stool microscopy lacks sensitivity and specificity. This complication is because of intermittent parasite shedding (requiring the submission of multiple stool specimens), variability in technical expertise, and inherent limitations of stool concentration and staining techniques. In addition, *Entamoeba histolytica* cannot be distinguished morphologically from the nonpathogenic *Entamoeba dispar*,[174] and the more recently described *Entamoeba moshkovskii*[175] and *Entamoeba bangladeshi*,[176] which may be pathogenic to humans. *Entamoeba histolytica* may also be confused with other nonpathogenic intestinal protozoa (such as *Entamoeba coli*, *Entamoeba hartmanni*, *Entamoeba gingivalis*, *Endolimax nana*, and *Iodamoeba buetschlii*) in the hands of less experienced microscopists. WHO recommends that "optimally, *Entamoeba histolytica* should be *specifically* identified and, if present, treated."[177]

Design and performance of molecular diagnostics
Singleplex NAATs have been developed for the detection of the major intestinal protozoa: *Entamoeba histolytica*/*Entamoeba dispar* with various targets such as ssu-RNA,[51,178] p30,[52] and the hemolysin gene[53]; *Giardia intestinalis* targeting ssu rRNA,[54,179] glutamate dehydrogenase,[180] elongation factor 1-α,[181] triosephosphate isomerase,[182] and β-giardin genes,[55,56] and *Cryptosporidium* targeting *Cryptosporidium parvum*-specific 452-bp fragment[57] and the *Cryptosporidium* oocyte wall protein.[56] PCR for *Entamoeba histolytica* was shown to have similar sensitivities to antigen testing in some early studies in endemic areas[178]; later studies have shown PCR to be more sensitive and specific.[51] All assays are laboratory developed and likely have different performance characteristics. Assays for *Giardia intestinalis* and *Cryptosporidium* spp also show increased sensitivity when compared with conventional methods (see **Table 1**).

Multiplex laboratory-developed assays have also been developed for these parasites, including a triplex PCR for *Cryptosporidium* spp, *Giardia intestinalis*, and *Entamoeba histolytica*,[60] a heptaplex PCR based on Luminex technology (Luminex, Austin, TX) for 7 intestinal parasites,[61] and more recently, a multiplex assay in a Taq-Man Array Card format detecting 19 enteropathogens, (including 5 viruses, 7 bacterial targets, *Cryptosporidium* spp, *Giardia intestinalis*, *Entamoeba histolytica*, and the helminths *Ascaris lumbricoides* and *Trichuris trichiura*).[62] The TaqMan Array Card assay was reported to have a sensitivity and specificity of 85% and 77% compared with conventional methods (including microscopy, immunoassays, and culture).

Clinical usefulness of molecular diagnostics
Given that antigen tests for *Giardia intestinalis*, *Cryptosporidium* spp, and *Entamoeba histolytica* are relatively sensitive and commercially available, it may be difficult to justify the additional expense of PCR methods for these organisms. Situations in which PCR may be particularly useful are for detection of species not covered by antigen tests (eg, *Entamoeba moshkovskii* and *Entamoeba bangladeshi*), and in multiplex assays for multiple pathogens (see also later discussion).

Emerging technologies
Commercial multiplex PCR-based assays for multiple gastrointestinal pathogens should make NAATs for some parasites more accessible for routine clinical use. The xTAG Gastrointestinal Pathogen Panel (xTAG GPP) (Luminex, Austin, TX) was CE-IVD (in vitro diagnostics) marked in 2011 and received FDA clearance in January, 2013. This is a qualitative molecular assay multiplex PCR assay based on xMAP technology (which detects analytes with reagent-coated microspheres and color-coded reporter dyes) that detects 15 total gastrointestinal pathogens (9 bacterial, 3 viral

targets along with *Giardia*, *Entamoeba histolytica*, and *Cryptosporidium* spp), with a turn-around time of 5 hours. The reported sensitivities of the xTAG GPP for the proto-zoal targets were 97.5% to 99% in a multicenter study.[64] Another similar commercial assay, the FilmArray GI (BioFire Diagnostics, Salt Lake City, UT), is seeking to achieve status as an FDA cleared IVD in 2014. This is a nested PCR assay (1 specimen per pouch) targeting 23 diarrheagenic pathogens (including *Giardia intestinalis*, *Entamoeba histolytica*, *Cryptosporidium* spp, and *Cyclospora cayetanensis*), which is reported to have a hands-on time of 5 minutes and a turn-around time of 1 hour.[65] There is no peer-reviewed literature for either platform at the time of writing.

Other common protozoa that may be associated with diarrheal disease include *Dientamoeba fragilis* and possibly *Blastocystis hominis*. PCR assays have been devel-oped for both of these organisms[58,59,183,184]; however, they are not included in the commercial multiplex assays seeking FDA approval and are not discussed further here.

Intestinal Helminths

Background
The intestinal helminths encompass a vast array of genetically diverse parasites, including cestodes (tapeworms), trematodes (flukes), and nematodes (round worms). Diagnosis is most commonly performed through microscopic examination of stool us-ing the time-honored ova and parasite examination, which typically includes a concentrated stool preparation and a permanently stained, unconcentrated prepara-tion. Microscopy is advantageous, because patients are often coinfected with multiple different helminths and it is impractical to perform separate assays for each that may be present. In this setting, microscopy serves as a true multiplex examination, which can detect all infecting species in the same preparation. Examination of at least 3 stool specimens is required for sensitive detection of helminths,[185] and in some cases, 6 or more separate specimens may be necessary.[186] This process is burdensome on both the patient and the laboratory. In addition, expertise for differentiating the large num-ber of helminth eggs that may be seen in stool is declining in nonendemic settings. Serologic tests for many helminths are also available, but many suffer from cross-reactivity between different helminths, and performance characteristics may vary greatly. Given these limitations of traditional methods, there is a need for an affordable and sensitive multiplex assay for the simultaneous detection of numerous gastrointes-tinal helminths.

Design and performance of molecular diagnostics
A variety of laboratory-developed NAATs have been described for the many intestinal helminths, although the described assays are sometimes more applicable to research settings rather than to routine clinical use. A detailed discussion is beyond the scope of this review. However, some design techniques for important helminths are high-lighted and possible scenarios are described in which molecular testing might be clin-ically useful as these assays become more widely available.

Several studies have examined the sensitivity of PCR assays for soil-borne hel-minths, and have observed favorable results compared with traditional techniques. In a study by Basuni and colleagues,[63] a multiplex real-time PCR was found to be more sensitive than conventional microscopy for soil-borne helminths (*Ascaris lumbri-coides*, *Strongyloides stercoralis*, *Ancylostoma* spp, *Necator americanus*); PCR was positive in 62.3% of 77 samples for soil-borne helminths, whereas microscopy was positive in only 7.8%. In a similar study, real-time PCR detected an additional 18 cases of *Strongyloides stercoralis* (vs 3 detected by microscopy; an 85% increased yield), along with increase rates of detection of *Entamoeba histolytica*, *Giardia intestinalis*, and *Cryptosporidium*. However, microscopy identified an additional 10 pathogenic parasitic species (0.5% overall prevalence) that were not included on the PCR assay, thus highlighting the limitations of organism-specific assays.[187] However, the significance of this finding may vary depending on patient population and geography.

Genus-specific and species-specific PCR assays have also been developed to screen for schistosomiasis in fecal and urine specimens of residents from endemic areas as well as returning travelers.[66,67,188,189] Studies have shown these PCR assays to be more sensitive than stool/urine microscopy, thus decreasing the number of samples that need to be submitted. In addition, these assays may help overcome the issue of nonspecificity seen with the widely used serologic methods for this organism.

Clinical usefulness of molecular diagnostics

No FDA approved or cleared molecular assays exist for detection of gastrointestinal helminths, and thus performance characteristics of available methods vary widely. Despite this disclaimer, certain NAATs may be useful in the screening and diagnosis of the common helminthic infections that cause substantial morbidity, preferably as part of a multiplex assay (for eg, the soil-transmitted helminths *Ancylostoma duodenale*, *Ancylostoma lumbricoides*, *Necator americanus*, *Trichuris trichiura* and *Strongyloides stercoralis*).[61,63,187] Specifically, real-time PCR could be used as a sensitive tool for detecting most intestinal parasites in returning travelers in conjunction with microscopy.

NAATs can also aid in speciation in which diagnosis has clinical and public health/ infection control implications, or in cases that pose a diagnostic dilemma (eg, from paraffin-embedded specimens in which pathologic findings are not conclusive or different species are morphologically indistinguishable). For example, molecular tests can be helpful in differentiating between *Taenia solium* versus *Taenia saginata*. This differentiation is important because the former can cause cysticercosis and accurate identification would help interrupt transmission. Differentiation is not possible from examination of helminth eggs, and proglottid segments or scoleces may not be available.[190–192]

PCR can been applied to specific cases in which the diagnosis is in question, such as a case of cerebral schistosomiasis caused by *Schistosoma hematobium* in a patient in whom cerebral sparganosis was initially suspected because of cross-reacting *Spirometra erinacei* antibodies.[193] PCR has also been used for detection of *Ancylostoma lumbricoides* and *Clonorchis sinensis* 18S and 28S rDNA sequences, respectively, in biliary duct stones when a parasitic cause was suspected.[194]

Urogenital Protozoa: Trichomonas vaginalis

Background

Trichomonas vaginalis, the most common protozoal infection in industrialized countries,[195] is transmitted sexually and causes vaginitis and cervicitis in women. In men, it can cause urethritis, epididymitis, and prostatitis. It is also associated with adverse pregnancy outcomes[196] and increased shedding of HIV and potential increased risk of transmission.[197] Traditional diagnosis is through wet-mount microscopic identification of motile parasites from vaginal secretions, or by culture methods. *Trichomonas vaginalis* can also be identified in Papanicolaou-stained endocervical preparations. Although these methods are widely used, they suffer from poor sensitivity.[198–200]

Design and performance of molecular diagnostics

Two commercial molecular assays have now been approved by the FDA for detection of *Trichomonas vaginalis*, representing an important step forward in parasitology diagnostics. The BD Affirm VPIII (Affirm) assay (Becton Dickinson, Sparks, MD) is an RNA-probe–based direct-specimen test for bacterial vaginosis/vaginitis that detects nucleic acid of *Gardnerella vaginalis*, *Trichomonas vaginalis*, and *Candida* species). More recently, the transcription-mediated amplification (TMA) based Aptima *Trichomonas vaginalis* (ATV) assay (Gen-Probe, San Diego, CA) (performed on the TIGRIS DTS System or the more recently approved PANTHER platform) has been cleared for use on female urine, endocervical, and vaginal specimens. In a recent head-to-head comparison, the ATV assay outperformed the Affirm assay for detection of *Trichomonas vaginalis* with a sensitivity of 100% versus 63.4% respectively, thus identifying 36.6% more positive patients.[68] TMA is also decidedly superior to traditional wet-mount microscopy,[199,200] and when compared with rapid antigen testing (OSOM TV, Genzyme Diagnostics) had a better overall sensitivity (98.4% vs 82%, composite gold standard comprising TMA, wet mount, culture, and rapid antigen testing).[199] LDTs based on PCR have also been described for *Trichomonas vaginalis*.[201,202]

Clinical usefulness of molecular diagnostics
Given that molecular methods, specifically TMA, outperform traditional methods such as the wet mount, it is reasonable to state that microscopy alone is insufficient as a stand-alone test for the diagnosis of *Trichomonas vaginalis* infection. Instead, consideration should be given to use of molecular techniques for front-line diagnosis of trichomoniasis. Although current FDA cleared assays are for use in women only, men may also be infected, and it therefore may be of value to validate the tests for use on male urine, urethral swabs, or prostate secretions.

Microsporidia

Background
Although microsporidia taxonomically belong to the kingdom Fungi, their detection has traditionally taken place in the parasitology laboratory. Of more than 1200 species, at least 15 have been identified as human pathogens[203,204] and have been associated with ocular infections like keratoconjunctivitis (eg, *Encephalitozoon cuniculi*, *Encephalitozoon hellem*, *Nosema* spp, *Vittaforma corneae*), gastrointestinal infection (eg, *Enterocytozoon bieneusi* in patients with AIDS) and disseminated infection in immunocompromised hosts (AIDS, transplant recipients, eg, with *Encephalitozoon intestinalis*). Diagnosis is traditionally by microscopic examination of various specimens using chromotrope or chemofluorescent stains. Despite these semispecific stains, interpretation is still challenging given the small size of the spores (0.8–4.0 μm in greatest dimension) and the presence of similar appearing, faintly staining objects such as yeasts. These stains do not allow for speciation, which may have important treatment and prognostic considerations and be useful in epidemiologic studies. Instead, speciation is typically performed by electron microscopy, which requires special expertise and equipment.

Design and performance of molecular diagnostics
Panmicrosporidial and species-specific targets have been mostly based on the ssu rRNA or ITS regions.[203,205,206] NAATs offer greater sensitivity compared with microscopy in both studies with spiked stool[71,207,208] and clinical isolates.[209] More recently, real-time PCR approaches have been developed with different chemistries (SYBR green,[69] TaqMan,[70] hybridization probes[71]). In our experience, a real-time PCR approach saw a 2-log unit to 4-log unit increase in sensitivity over routine stool smears for detection of *Encephalitozoon* species.[71]

Clinical usefulness of molecular diagnostics

Given the increased reported sensitivity of various assays over routine microscopy, PCR may become the test of choice in the near future for diagnosis of microsporidiosis. Samples that can be tested with PCR are broad and include corneal scrapings,[205] tissue biopsies,[206] urine, duodenal aspirates, stool (fresh or formalin fixed),[70,210–212] and trichrome-stained clinical slides.[213] Another benefit of PCR is that described assays have been designed to discriminate between clinically important species. Despite these potential advantages, there are no FDA approved or cleared assays for microsporidia and most PCR testing is limited to large-reference centers and research facilities. Of the described PCR assays, there are significant differences in preanalytical and analytical components, which can lead to wide interlaboratory variation in performance.[207]

SUMMARY

Molecular methods are a welcome addition to the diagnostic armamentarium for parasitic diseases (see **Table 1**; **Table 2**), and in select situations and disease states, they may replace traditional methods. Benefits include increased sensitivity and specificity in general; however, standardization of assays and paucity of approved platforms are major current limitations. With increased sensitivity, a positive molecular test may not always indicate viable organism, and results must be interpreted in conjunction with the

Table 2
General benefits and limitations of molecular based versus traditional tests for parasites[a]

Potential Benefits of Molecular Tests	Potential Benefits of Traditional Tests
1. Increased sensitivity, specificity and speed of diagnosis 2. Detection of coinfections 3. Differentiation of morphologically similar parasites (*Leishmania* spp, human African trypanosomes (HAT) subspecies, *P falciparum* vs *Babesia* spp)	1. Truly multiplex in that preselection of specific targets not required 2. Easier to implement in resource-poor settings with simple equipment and reagents 3. Time-honored methods
Potential Limitations of Molecular Tests	**Potential Limitations of Traditional Tests**

1. Lack of standardization and variability in performance characteristics. NAAT assays may vary by:
  a. Extraction method
  b. Choice of genetic targets and primer sequences
  c. Amplification technique (traditional, nested, real-time PCR)
  d. Type of detection system (probes, MS)
2. Lack of FDA cleared assays
3. Potential for contamination of specimens with environmental DNA
4. Possible amplification inhibitors
5. Equipment and reagent costs
6. Possibly too sensitive to meet the clinical need (eg, low-level asymptomatic malaria parasitemia may mask an alternate diagnosis, DNA may persist despite successful treatment)
	1. Labor and time intensive
	2. Dwindling expertise available in nonendemic settings
	3. Lower sensitivity, requiring multiple samples or concentration techniques to increase sensitivity

[a] Performance and requirements of individual assays may vary greatly.

clinical picture and other supplementary tests, when available. Technical complexity and instrumentation provide specific challenges to endemic, often resource-limited settings, but isothermal methods (eg, LAMP) show promise for wider implementation.

REFERENCES

1. World Health Organization. World malaria report 2011. WHO; 2011. Available at: http://apps.who.int/iris/bitstream/10665/44792/2/9789241564403_eng_full.pdf. Accessed December 8, 2012.
2. World Health Organization. Neglected tropical diseases 2012. WHO; 2012. Available at: http://www.who.int/neglected_diseases/diseases/en/. Accessed December 8, 2012.
3. Singh B, Bobogare A, Cox-Singh J, et al. A genus- and species-specific nested polymerase chain reaction malaria detection assay for epidemiologic studies. Am J Trop Med Hyg 1999;60:687–92.
4. Mixson-Hayden T, Lucchi NW, Udhayakumar V. Evaluation of three PCR-based diagnostic assays for detecting mixed Plasmodium infection. BMC Res Notes 2010;3:88.
5. Perandin F, Manca N, Calderaro A, et al. Development of a real-time PCR assay for detection of Plasmodium falciparum, Plasmodium vivax, and Plasmodium ovale for routine clinical diagnosis. J Clin Microbiol 2004;42:1214–9.
6. Shokoples SE, Ndao M, Kowalewska-Grochowska K, et al. Multiplexed real-time PCR assay for discrimination of Plasmodium species with improved sensitivity for mixed infections. J Clin Microbiol 2009;47:975–80.
7. Babady NE, Sloan LM, Rosenblatt JE, et al. Detection of Plasmodium knowlesi by real-time polymerase chain reaction. Am J Trop Med Hyg 2009;81:516–8.
8. Kamau E, Tolbert LS, Kortepeter L, et al. Development of a highly sensitive genus-specific quantitative reverse transcriptase real-time PCR assay for detection and quantitation of plasmodium by amplifying RNA and DNA of the 18S rRNA genes. J Clin Microbiol 2011;49:2946–53.
9. Cnops L, Jacobs J, Van Esbroeck M. Validation of a four-primer real-time PCR as a diagnostic tool for single and mixed Plasmodium infections. Clin Microbiol Infect 2011;17:1101–7.
10. Alam MS, Mohon AN, Mustafa S, et al. Real-time PCR assay and rapid diagnostic tests for the diagnosis of clinically suspected malaria patients in Bangladesh. Malar J 2011;10:175.
11. Oguike MC, Betson M, Burke M, et al. Plasmodium ovale curtisi and Plasmodium ovale wallikeri circulate simultaneously in African communities. Int J Parasitol 2011;41:677–83.
12. Calderaro A, Piccolo G, Gorrini C, et al. A new real-time PCR for the detection of Plasmodium ovale wallikeri. PLoS One 2012;7:e48033.
13. Mens PF, Schoone GJ, Kager PA, et al. Detection and identification of human Plasmodium species with real-time quantitative nucleic acid sequence-based amplification. Malar J 2006;5:80.
14. Sirichaisinthop J, Buates S, Watanabe R, et al. Evaluation of loop-mediated isothermal amplification (LAMP) for malaria diagnosis in a field setting. Am J Trop Med Hyg 2011;85:594–6.
15. Foundation for Innovative New Diagnostics. Loop mediated isothermal amplification (LAMP) for malaria. In: Diseases and Projects. 2012. Available at: http://www.finddiagnostics.org/programs/malaria-afs/malaria/product_development/lamp-for-malaria.html. Accessed December 8, 2012.

16. Laoboonchai A, Kawamoto F, Thanoosingha N, et al. PCR-based ELISA technique for malaria diagnosis of specimens from Thailand. Trop Med Int Health 2001;6:458–62.

17. Mens PF, van Amerongen A, Sawa P, et al. Molecular diagnosis of malaria in the field: development of a novel 1-step nucleic acid lateral flow immunoassay for the detection of all 4 human *Plasmodium* spp. and its evaluation in Mbita, Kenya. Diagn Microbiol Infect Dis 2008;61:421–7.

18. Nyunt M, Pisciotta J, Feldman AB, et al. Detection of *Plasmodium falciparum* in pregnancy by laser desorption mass spectrometry. Am J Trop Med Hyg 2005;73:485–90.

19. Persing DH, Mathiesen D, Marshall WF, et al. Detection of *Babesia microti* by polymerase chain reaction. J Clin Microbiol 1992;30:2097–103.

20. Teal AE, Habura A, Ennis J, et al. A new real-time PCR assay for improved detection of the parasite *Babesia microti*. J Clin Microbiol 2012;50:903–8.

21. Qvarnstrom Y, Schijman AG, Veron V, et al. Sensitive and specific detection of *Trypanosoma cruzi* DNA in clinical specimens using a multi-target real-time PCR approach. PLoS Negl Trop Dis 2012;6:e1689.

22. Ramirez JD, Guhl F, Umezawa ES, et al. Evaluation of adult chronic Chagas' heart disease diagnosis by molecular and serological methods. J Clin Microbiol 2009;47:3945–51.

23. Marcon GE, Andrade PD, de Albuquerque DM, et al. Use of a nested polymerase chain reaction (N-PCR) to detect *Trypanosoma cruzi* in blood samples from chronic chagasic patients and patients with doubtful serologies. Diagn Microbiol Infect Dis 2002;43:39–43.

24. Becker S, Franco JR, Simarro PP, et al. Real-time PCR for detection of *Trypanosoma brucei* in human blood samples. Diagn Microbiol Infect Dis 2004;50:193–9.

25. Njiru ZK, Constantine CC, Guya S, et al. The use of ITS1 rDNA PCR in detecting pathogenic African trypanosomes. Parasitol Res 2005;95:186–92.

26. Deborggraeve S, Claes F, Laurent T, et al. Molecular dipstick test for diagnosis of sleeping sickness. J Clin Microbiol 2006;44:2884–9.

27. Kuboki N, Inoue N, Sakurai T, et al. Loop-mediated isothermal amplification for detection of African trypanosomes. J Clin Microbiol 2003;41:5517–24.

28. Njiru ZK, Mikosza AS, Matovu E, et al. African trypanosomiasis: sensitive and rapid detection of the sub-genus *Trypanozoon* by loop-mediated isothermal amplification (LAMP) of parasite DNA. Int J Parasitol 2008;38:589–99.

29. Mugasa CM, Laurent T, Schoone GJ, et al. Nucleic acid sequence-based amplification with oligochromatography for detection of *Trypanosoma brucei* in clinical samples. J Clin Microbiol 2009;47:630–5.

30. Radwanska M, Magez S, Perry-O'Keefe H, et al. Direct detection and identification of African trypanosomes by fluorescence in situ hybridization with peptide nucleic acid probes. J Clin Microbiol 2002;40:4295–7.

31. Papadopoulos MC, Abel PM, Agranoff D, et al. A novel and accurate diagnostic test for human African trypanosomiasis. Lancet 2004;363:1358–63.

32. Njiru ZK, Mikosza AS, Armstrong T, et al. Loop-mediated isothermal amplification (LAMP) method for rapid detection of *Trypanosoma brucei rhodesiense*. PLoS Negl Trop Dis 2008;2:e147.

33. Kabiri M, Franco JR, Simarro PP, et al. Detection of *Trypanosoma brucei gambiense* in sleeping sickness suspects by PCR amplification of expression-site-associated genes 6 and 7. Trop Med Int Health 1999;4:658–61.

34. Ramzy RM. Recent advances in molecular diagnostic techniques for human lymphatic filariasis and their use in epidemiological research. Trans R Soc Trop Med Hyg 2002;96(Suppl 1):S225–9.

35. Rao RU, Atkinson LJ, Ramzy RM, et al. A real-time PCR-based assay for detection of *Wuchereria bancrofti* DNA in blood and mosquitoes. Am J Trop Med Hyg 2006;74:826–32.
36. Mehlotra RK, Gray LR, Blood-Zikursh MJ, et al. Molecular-based assay for simultaneous detection of four *Plasmodium* spp. and *Wuchereria bancrofti* infections. Am J Trop Med Hyg 2010;82:1030–3.
37. Rao RU, Weil GJ, Fischer K, et al. Detection of *Brugia* parasite DNA in human blood by real-time PCR. J Clin Microbiol 2006;44:3887–93.
38. Fink DL, Kamgno J, Nutman TB. Rapid molecular assays for specific detection and quantitation of *Loa loa* microfilaremia. PLoS Negl Trop Dis 2011;5:e1299.
39. Boggild AK, Ramos AP, Espinosa D, et al. Clinical and demographic stratification of test performance: a pooled analysis of five laboratory diagnostic methods for American cutaneous leishmaniasis. Am J Trop Med Hyg 2010;83:345–50.
40. Kumar R, Bumb RA, Ansari NA, et al. Cutaneous leishmaniasis caused by *Leishmania tropica* in Bikaner, India: parasite identification and characterization using molecular and immunologic tools. Am J Trop Med Hyg 2007;76:896–901.
41. Disch J, Pedras MJ, Orsini M, et al. *Leishmania (Viannia)* subgenus kDNA amplification for the diagnosis of mucosal leishmaniasis. Diagn Microbiol Infect Dis 2005;51:185–90.
42. Food and Drug Administration. 510 (k) Summary - k081868 (Smart Leish). 2011. Available at: http://www.accessdata.fda.gov/cdrh_docs/pdf8/K081868.pdf. Accessed December 8, 2012.
43. US Army Medical Department. Medical Research and Materiel Command. US Army Medical Materiel Development Activity. FDA Approves the SMART Leish PCR assay for Diagnosing Leishmania in Individuals with Signs and Symptoms of Leishmaniasis. 2011. Available at: http://www.usammda.army.mil/SMART_Leish_PCR.html. Accessed December 8, 2012.
44. Wortmann G, Hochberg L, Houng HH, et al. Rapid identification of *Leishmania* complexes by a real-time PCR assay. Am J Trop Med Hyg 2005;73:999–1004.
45. Castilho TM, Camargo LM, McMahon-Pratt D, et al. A real-time polymerase chain reaction assay for the identification and quantification of American *Leishmania* species on the basis of glucose-6-phosphate dehydrogenase. Am J Trop Med Hyg 2008;78:122–32.
46. Takagi H, Itoh M, Islam MZ, et al. Sensitive, specific, and rapid detection of *Leishmania donovani* DNA by loop-mediated isothermal amplification. Am J Trop Med Hyg 2009;81:578–82.
47. Burg JL, Grover CM, Pouletty P, et al. Direct and sensitive detection of a pathogenic protozoan, *Toxoplasma gondii*, by polymerase chain reaction. J Clin Microbiol 1989;27:1787–92.
48. Wahab T, Edvinsson B, Palm D, et al. Comparison of the AF146527 and B1 repeated elements, two real-time PCR targets used for detection of *Toxoplasma gondii*. J Clin Microbiol 2010;48:591–2.
49. Lau YL, Meganathan P, Sonaimuthu P, et al. Specific, sensitive, and rapid diagnosis of active toxoplasmosis by a loop-mediated isothermal amplification method using blood samples from patients. J Clin Microbiol 2010;48:3698–702.
50. Qvarnstrom Y, Visvesvara GS, Sriram R, et al. Multiplex real-time PCR assay for simultaneous detection of *Acanthamoeba* spp., *Balamuthia mandrillaris*, and *Naegleria fowleri*. J Clin Microbiol 2006;44:3589–95.
51. Stark D, van Hal S, Fotedar R, et al. Comparison of stool antigen detection kits to PCR for diagnosis of amebiasis. J Clin Microbiol 2008;46:1678–81.

52. Tachibana H, Kobayashi S, Okuzawa E, et al. Detection of pathogenic *Entamoeba histolytica* DNA in liver abscess fluid by polymerase chain reaction. Int J Parasitol 1992;22:1193–6.

53. Zindrou S, Orozco E, Linder E, et al. Specific detection of *Entamoeba histolytica* DNA by hemolysin gene targeted PCR. Acta Trop 2001;78:117–25.

54. Verweij JJ, Schinkel J, Laeijendecker D, et al. Real-time PCR for the detection of *Giardia lamblia*. Mol Cell Probes 2003;17:223–5.

55. Caccio SM, De Giacomo M, Pozio E. Sequence analysis of the beta-giardin gene and development of a polymerase chain reaction-restriction fragment length polymorphism assay to genotype *Giardia duodenalis* cysts from human faecal samples. Int J Parasitol 2002;32:1023–30.

56. Guy RA, Payment P, Krull UJ, et al. Real-time PCR for quantification of *Giardia* and *Cryptosporidium* in environmental water samples and sewage. Appl Environ Microbiol 2003;69:5178–85.

57. Fontaine M, Guillot E. Development of a TaqMan quantitative PCR assay specific for *Cryptosporidium parvum*. FEMS Microbiol Lett 2002;214:13–7.

58. Stark D, Beebe N, Marriott D, et al. Detection of *Dientamoeba fragilis* in fresh stool specimens using PCR. Int J Parasitol 2005;35:57–62.

59. Verweij JJ, Mulder B, Poell B, et al. Real-time PCR for the detection of *Dientamoeba fragilis* in fecal samples. Mol Cell Probes 2007;21:400–4.

60. Haque R, Roy S, Siddique A, et al. Multiplex real-time PCR assay for detection of *Entamoeba histolytica*, *Giardia intestinalis*, and *Cryptosporidium* spp. Am J Trop Med Hyg 2007;76:713–7.

61. Taniuchi M, Verweij JJ, Noor Z, et al. High throughput multiplex PCR and probe-based detection with Luminex beads for seven intestinal parasites. Am J Trop Med Hyg 2011;84:332–7.

62. Liu J, Gratz J, Amour C, et al. A laboratory developed TaqMan array card for simultaneous detection of nineteen enteropathogens. J Clin Microbiol 2013; 51:472–80.

63. Basuni M, Muhi J, Othman N, et al. A pentaplex real-time polymerase chain reaction assay for detection of four species of soil-transmitted helminths. Am J Trop Med Hyg 2011;84:338–43.

64. Wessels E, Zlateva KT, Rusman L, et al. Prospective application of the Luminex xTAG® GPP multiplex PCR in diagnosing infectious gastroenteritis [abstract P-080]. In: Program and abstracts of the 15th Annual meeting of the European Society for Clinical Virology. September 4–7, 2012, Madrid, Spain.

65. Vaughn MG, Harrell B, Wallace R, et al. Evaluation of the FilmArray ® gastrointestinal pathogen detection system for infectious diarrhea [abstract 1716]. In: Program and abstracts of the 112th General Meeting of the American Society for Microbiology. June 16–19, 2012, San Francisco, CA, USA. p. 169.

66. Gomes LI, Dos Santos Marques LH, Enk MJ, et al. Development and evaluation of a sensitive PCR-ELISA system for detection of schistosoma infection in feces. PLoS Negl Trop Dis 2010;4(4):e664.

67. ten Hove RJ, Verweij JJ, Vereecken K, et al. Multiplex real-time PCR for the detection and quantification of *Schistosoma mansoni* and *S. haematobium* infection in stool samples collected in northern Senegal. Trans R Soc Trop Med Hyg 2008;102:179–85.

68. Andrea SB, Chapin KC. Comparison of Aptima *Trichomonas vaginalis* transcription-mediated amplification assay and BD affirm VPIII for detection of *T. vaginalis* in symptomatic women: performance parameters and epidemiological implications. J Clin Microbiol 2011;49:866–9.

69. Polley SD, Boadi S, Watson J, et al. Detection and species identification of microsporidial infections using SYBR Green real-time PCR. J Med Microbiol 2011; 60:459–66.

70. Menotti J, Cassinat B, Porcher R, et al. Development of a real-time polymerase-chain-reaction assay for quantitative detection of *Enterocytozoon bieneusi* DNA in stool specimens from immunocompromised patients with intestinal microsporidiosis. J Infect Dis 2003;187:1469–74.

71. Wolk DM, Schneider SK, Wengenack NL, et al. Real-time PCR method for detection of *Encephalitozoon intestinalis* from stool specimens. J Clin Microbiol 2002; 40:3922–8.

72. Stauffer WM, Cartwright CP, Olson DA, et al. Diagnostic performance of rapid diagnostic tests versus blood smears for malaria in US clinical practice. Clin Infect Dis 2009;49:908–13.

73. Wilson ML. Malaria rapid diagnostic tests. Clin Infect Dis 2012;54:1637–41.

74. Dimaio MA, Pereira IT, George TI, et al. Performance of BinaxNOW for diagnosis of malaria in a U.S. hospital. J Clin Microbiol 2012;50:2877–80.

75. Bobenchik A, Shimizu-Cohen R, Humphries RM. Use of rapid diagnostic tests for diagnosis of malaria in the United States. J Clin Microbiol 2013;51:379.

76. Luchavez J, Baker J, Alcantara S, et al. Laboratory demonstration of a prozone-like effect in HRP2-detecting malaria rapid diagnostic tests: implications for clinical management. Malar J 2011;10:286.

77. Gillet P, Scheirlinck A, Stokx J, et al. Prozone in malaria rapid diagnostics tests: how many cases are missed? Malar J 2011;10:166.

78. Gamboa D, Ho MF, Bendezu J, et al. A large proportion of *P. falciparum* isolates in the Amazon region of Peru lack pfhrp2 and pfhrp3: implications for malaria rapid diagnostic tests. PLoS One 2010;5:e8091.

79. Cordray MS, Richards-Kortum RR. Emerging nucleic acid-based tests for point-of-care detection of malaria. Am J Trop Med Hyg 2012;87:223–30.

80. Garcia LS. Malaria. Clin Lab Med 2010;30:93–129.

81. Farcas GA, Soeller R, Zhong K, et al. Real-time polymerase chain reaction assay for the rapid detection and characterization of chloroquine-resistant *Plasmodium falciparum* malaria in returned travelers. Clin Infect Dis 2006;42: 622–7.

82. Steenkeste N, Dillies MA, Khim N, et al. FlexiChip package: an universal microarray with a dedicated analysis software for high-throughput SNPs detection linked to anti-malarial drug resistance. Malar J 2009;8:229.

83. Erdman LK, Hawkes M, Kain KC. Molecular approaches for diagnosis of malaria and characterization of genetic markers of drug resistance. In: Persing DH, Tenover FC, Tang YW, et al, editors. Molecular microbiology: diagnostic principles and practice. 2nd edition. Washington, DC: ASM Press; 2011. p. 691–711.

84. Vestergaard LS, Ringwald P. Responding to the challenge of antimalarial drug resistance by routine monitoring to update national malaria treatment policies. Am J Trop Med Hyg 2007;77:153–9.

85. Picot S, Olliaro P, de Monbrison F, et al. A systematic review and meta-analysis of evidence for correlation between molecular markers of parasite resistance and treatment outcome in falciparum malaria. Malar J 2009;8:89.

86. LaBarre P, Hawkins KR, Gerlach J, et al. A simple, inexpensive device for nucleic acid amplification without electricity-toward instrument-free molecular diagnostics in low-resource settings. PLoS One 2011;6:e19738.

87. Homer MJ, Aguilar-Delfin I, Telford SR 3rd, et al. Babesiosis. Clin Microbiol Rev 2000;13:451–69.

88. Kjemtrup AM, Conrad PA. Human babesiosis: an emerging tick-borne disease. Int J Parasitol 2000;30:1323–37.
89. Qi C, Zhou D, Liu J, et al. Detection of *Babesia divergens* using molecular methods in anemic patients in Shandong Province, China. Parasitol Res 2011; 109:241–5.
90. Herwaldt BL, Linden JV, Bosserman E, et al. Transfusion-associated babesiosis in the United States: a description of cases. Ann Intern Med 2011;155:509–19.
91. Centers for Disease Control and Prevention. Babesiosis and the U.S. blood supply. Available at: www.cdc.gov/parasites/babesiosis/./babesiosis_policy_brief. pdf. Accessed February 7, 2013.
92. Olmeda AS, Armstrong PM, Rosenthal BM, et al. A subtropical case of human babesiosis. Acta Trop 1997;67:229–34.
93. Young C, Chawla A, Berardi V, et al. Preventing transfusion-transmitted babesiosis: preliminary experience of the first laboratory-based blood donor screening program. Transfusion 2012;52:1523–9.
94. Leiby DA. Transfusion-transmitted *Babesia* spp.: bull's-eye on *Babesia microti*. Clin Microbiol Rev 2011;24:14–28.
95. Joseph JT, Purtill K, Wong SJ, et al. Vertical transmission of *Babesia microti*, United States. Emerg Infect Dis 2012;18:1318–21.
96. Wolk DM, Kaleta EJ, Wysocki VH. PCR-electrospray ionization mass spectrometry: the potential to change infectious disease diagnostics in clinical and public health laboratories. J Mol Diagn 2012;14:295–304.
97. Beard CB, Pye G, Steurer FJ, et al. Chagas disease in a domestic transmission cycle, southern Texas, USA. Emerg Infect Dis 2003;9:103–5.
98. Dorn PL, Perniciaro L, Yabsley MJ, et al. Autochthonous transmission of *Trypanosoma cruzi*, Louisiana. Emerg Infect Dis 2007;13:605–7.
99. Schijman AG, Bisio M, Orellana L, et al. International study to evaluate PCR methods for detection of *Trypanosoma cruzi* DNA in blood samples from Chagas disease patients. PLoS Negl Trop Dis 2011;5:e931.
100. Svoboda M, Virreira M, Truyens C, et al. Molecular approaches for diagnosis of Chagas' disease and genotyping of *Trypanosoma cruzi*. In: Persing DH, Tenover FC, Tang YW, et al, editors. Molecular microbiology: diagnostic principles and practice. 2nd edition. Washington, DC: ASM Press; 2011. p. 713–25.
101. Britto C, Cardoso MA, Wincker P, et al. A simple protocol for the physical cleavage of *Trypanosoma cruzi* kinetoplast DNA present in blood samples and its use in polymerase chain reaction (PCR)-based diagnosis of chronic Chagas disease. Mem Inst Oswaldo Cruz 1993;88:171–2.
102. Bern C, Montgomery SP, Herwaldt BL, et al. Evaluation and treatment of Chagas disease in the United States: a systematic review. JAMA 2007;298:2171–81.
103. Kirchhoff LV, Votava JR, Ochs DE, et al. Comparison of PCR and microscopic methods for detecting *Trypanosoma cruzi*. J Clin Microbiol 1996;34:1171–5.
104. Noya BA, Diaz-Bello Z, Colmenares C, et al. The performance of laboratory tests in the management of a large outbreak of orally transmitted Chagas disease. Mem Inst Oswaldo Cruz 2012;107:893–8.
105. Schijman AG, Vigliano C, Burgos J, et al. Early diagnosis of recurrence of *Trypanosoma cruzi* infection by polymerase chain reaction after heart transplantation of a chronic Chagas' heart disease patient. J Heart Lung Transplant 2000; 19:1114–7.
106. Pavia PX, Roa NL, Uribe AM, et al. Using S35-S36 and TcH2AF-R primer-based PCR tests to follow-up a Chagas disease patient who had undergone a heart transplant. Biomedica 2011;31:178–84.

107. de Freitas VL, da Silva SC, Sartori AM, et al. Real-time PCR in HIV/*Trypanosoma cruzi* coinfection with and without Chagas disease reactivation: association with HIV viral load and CD4 level. PLoS Negl Trop Dis 2011;5:e1277.

108. Schijman AG, Altcheh J, Burgos JM, et al. Aetiological treatment of congenital Chagas' disease diagnosed and monitored by the polymerase chain reaction. J Antimicrob Chemother 2003;52:441–9.

109. Duffy T, Bisio M, Altcheh J, et al. Accurate real-time PCR strategy for monitoring bloodstream parasitic loads in Chagas disease patients. PLoS Negl Trop Dis 2009;3:e419.

110. Torrico MC, Solano M, Guzman JM, et al. Estimation of the parasitemia in *Trypanosoma cruzi* human infection: high parasitemias are associated with severe and fatal congenital Chagas disease. Rev Soc Bras Med Trop 2005;38(Suppl 2): 58–61 [in Spanish].

111. Brasil PE, De Castro L, Hasslocher-Moreno AM, et al. ELISA versus PCR for diagnosis of chronic Chagas disease: systematic review and meta-analysis. BMC Infect Dis 2010;10:337.

112. Lages-Silva E, Crema E, Ramirez LE, et al. Relationship between *Trypanosoma cruzi* and human chagasic megaesophagus: blood and tissue parasitism. Am J Trop Med Hyg 2001;65:435–41.

113. Diez CN, Manattini S, Zanuttini JC, et al. The value of molecular studies for the diagnosis of congenital Chagas disease in northeastern Argentina. Am J Trop Med Hyg 2008;78:624–7.

114. Bisio M, Seidenstein ME, Burgos JM, et al. Urbanization of congenital transmission of *Trypanosoma cruzi*: prospective polymerase chain reaction study in pregnancy. Trans R Soc Trop Med Hyg 2011;105:543–9.

115. Mugasa CM, Adams ER, Boer KR, et al. Diagnostic accuracy of molecular amplification tests for human African trypanosomiasis–systematic review. PLoS Negl Trop Dis 2012;6:e1438.

116. Centers for Disease Control and Prevention. Tryapanosomiasis, African. In: DPDx. Available at: http://www.dpd.cdc.gov/dpdx/HTML/TrypanosomiasisAfrican.htm. Accessed January 12, 2013.

117. Legros D, Ollivier G, Gastellu-Etchegorry M, et al. Treatment of human African trypanosomiasis–present situation and needs for research and development. Lancet Infect Dis 2002;2:437–40.

118. Picozzi K, Fevre EM, Odiit M, et al. Sleeping sickness in Uganda: a thin line between two fatal diseases. BMJ 2005;331:1238–41.

119. Batchelor NA, Atkinson PM, Gething PW, et al. Spatial predictions of Rhodesian human African trypanosomiasis (sleeping sickness) prevalence in Kaberamaido and Dokolo, two newly affected districts of Uganda. PLoS Negl Trop Dis 2009;3. e563.

120. Chappuis F, Loutan L, Simarro P, et al. Options for field diagnosis of human African trypanosomiasis. Clin Microbiol Rev 2005;18:133–46.

121. Moser DR, Cook GA, Ochs DE, et al. Detection of *Trypanosoma congolense* and *Trypanosoma brucei* subspecies by DNA amplification using the polymerase chain reaction. Parasitology 1989;99:57–66.

122. Kyambadde JW, Enyaru JC, Matovu E, et al. Detection of trypanosomes in suspected sleeping sickness patients in Uganda using the polymerase chain reaction. Bull World Health Organ 2000;78:119–24.

123. Picozzi K, Carrington M, Welburn SC. A multiplex PCR that discriminates between *Trypanosoma brucei brucei* and zoonotic *T. b. rhodesiense*. Exp Parasitol 2008;118:41–6.

124. Njiru ZK, Traub R, Ouma JO, et al. Detection of Group 1 *Trypanosoma brucei gambiense* by loop-mediated isothermal amplification. J Clin Microbiol 2011; 49:1530–6.

125. Matovu E, Mugasa CM, Ekangu RA, et al. Phase II evaluation of sensitivity and specificity of PCR and NASBA followed by oligochromatography for diagnosis of human African trypanosomiasis in clinical samples from D.R. Congo and Uganda. PLoS Negl Trop Dis 2010;4:e737.

126. Radwanska M, Chamekh M, Vanhamme L, et al. The serum resistance-associated gene as a diagnostic tool for the detection of *Trypanosoma brucei rhodesiense*. Am J Trop Med Hyg 2002;67:684–90.

127. Thekisoe OM, Kuboki N, Nambota A, et al. Species-specific loop-mediated isothermal amplification (LAMP) for diagnosis of trypanosomosis. Acta Trop 2007;102:182–9.

128. Radwanska M, Claes F, Magez S, et al. Novel primer sequences for polymerase chain reaction-based detection of *Trypanosoma brucei gambiense*. Am J Trop Med Hyg 2002;67:289–95.

129. Njiru ZK. Rapid and sensitive detection of human African trypanosomiasis by loop-mediated isothermal amplification combined with a lateral-flow dipstick. Diagn Microbiol Infect Dis 2011;69:205–9.

130. Fang X, Liu Y, Kong J, et al. Loop-mediated isothermal amplification integrated on microfluidic chips for point-of-care quantitative detection of pathogens. Anal Chem 2010;82:3002–6.

131. Deborggraeve S, Buscher P. Molecular diagnostics for sleeping sickness: what is the benefit for the patient? Lancet Infect Dis 2010;10:433–9.

132. Fink DL, Nutman TB. Filarial nematodes. In: Versalovic J, Carroll KC, Funke G, et al, editors. Manual of clinical microbiology,, vol. 2, 10th edition. Washington, DC: ASM Press; 2011. p. 2212–21.

133. Poole CB, Williams SA. A rapid DNA assay for the species-specific detection and quantification of *Brugia* in blood samples. Mol Biochem Parasitol 1990; 40:129–36.

134. Dissanayake S, Min X, Piessens WF. Detection of amplified *Wuchereria bancrofti* DNA in mosquitoes with a nonradioactive probe. Mol Biochem Parasitol 1991; 45:49–56.

135. Fink DL, Fahle GA, Fischer S, et al. Toward molecular parasitologic diagnosis: enhanced diagnostic sensitivity for filarial infections in mobile populations. J Clin Microbiol 2011;49:42–7.

136. Simonsen P. Filariases. In: Cook GC, Zumla AI, editors. Manson's tropical diseases. 22nd edition. Philadelphia: Saunders, Elsevier; 2009. p. 1477–513.

137. Gass K, Beau de Rochars MV, Boakye D, et al. A multicenter evaluation of diagnostic tools to define endpoints for programs to eliminate bancroftian filariasis. PLoS Negl Trop Dis 2012;6:e1479.

138. Farid HA, Hammad RE, Hassan MM, et al. Detection of *Wuchereria bancrofti* in mosquitoes by the polymerase chain reaction: a potentially useful tool for large-scale control programmes. Trans R Soc Trop Med Hyg 2001;95:29–32.

139. Nuchprayoon S, Junpee A, Poovorawan Y. Random amplified polymorphic DNA (RAPD) for differentiation between Thai and Myanmar strains of *Wuchereria bancrofti*. Filaria J 2007;6:6.

140. Centers for Disease Control and Prevention. Leishmaniasis. In: DPDx. Available at: http://www.dpd.cdc.gov/dpdx/HTML/Leishmaniasis.htm. Accessed December 8, 2012.

141. Murray HW, Berman JD, Davies CR, et al. Advances in leishmaniasis. Lancet 2005;366:1561–77.
142. Cota GF, de Sousa MR, Demarqui FN, et al. The diagnostic accuracy of serologic and molecular methods for detecting visceral leishmaniasis in HIV infected patients: meta-analysis. PLoS Negl Trop Dis 2012;6:e1665.
143. Das NK, Singh SK, Ghosh S, et al. Case series of misdiagnosis with rK39 strip test in Indian leishmaniasis. Am J Trop Med Hyg 2011;84:688–91.
144. Sudarshan M, Weirather JL, Wilson ME, et al. Study of parasite kinetics with antileishmanial drugs using real-time quantitative PCR in Indian visceral leishmaniasis. J Antimicrob Chemother 2011;66:1751–5.
145. Aoun K, Chouihi E, Amri F, et al. Short report: contribution of quantitative real-time polymerase chain reaction to follow-up of visceral leishmaniasis patients treated with meglumine antimoniate. Am J Trop Med Hyg 2009;81: 1004–6.
146. Martin-Sanchez J, Pineda JA, Morillas-Marquez F, et al. Detection of *Leishmania infantum* kinetoplast DNA in peripheral blood from asymptomatic individuals at risk for parenterally transmitted infections: relationship between polymerase chain reaction results and other *Leishmania* infection markers. Am J Trop Med Hyg 2004;70:545–8.
147. Su C, Shwab EK, Zhou P, et al. Moving towards an integrated approach to molecular detection and identification of *Toxoplasma gondii*. Parasitology 2010; 137:1–11.
148. McAuley JB, Jones JL, Singh K. Toxoplasma. In: Versalovic J, Carroll KC, Funke G, et al, editors. Manual of clinical microbiology, vol. 2, 10th edition. Washington, DC: ASM Press; 2011. p. 2127–38.
149. Pelloux H, Guy E, Angelici MC, et al. A second European collaborative study on polymerase chain reaction for *Toxoplasma gondii*, involving 15 teams. FEMS Microbiol Lett 1998;165:231–7.
150. Sterkers Y, Varlet-Marie E, Marty P, et al. Diversity and evolution of methods and practices for the molecular diagnosis of congenital toxoplasmosis in France: a 4-year survey. Clin Microbiol Infect 2010;16:1594–602.
151. Edvinsson B, Jalal S, Nord CE, et al. DNA extraction and PCR assays for detection of *Toxoplasma gondii*. APMIS 2004;112:342–8.
152. Yera H, Filisetti D, Bastien P, et al. Multicenter comparative evaluation of five commercial methods for toxoplasma DNA extraction from amniotic fluid. J Clin Microbiol 2009;47:3881–6.
153. Homan WL, Vercammen M, De Braekeleer J, et al. Identification of a 200- to 300-fold repetitive 529 bp DNA fragment in *Toxoplasma gondii*, and its use for diagnostic and quantitative PCR. Int J Parasitol 2000;30:69–75.
154. Hurtado A, Aduriz G, Moreno B, et al. Single tube nested PCR for the detection of *Toxoplasma gondii* in fetal tissues from naturally aborted ewes. Vet Parasitol 2001;102:17–27.
155. Costa JM, Bretagne S. Variation of B1 gene and AF146527 repeat element copy numbers according to *Toxoplasma gondii* strains assessed using real-time quantitative PCR. J Clin Microbiol 2012;50:1452–4.
156. Robert-Gangneux F, Darde ML. Epidemiology of and diagnostic strategies for toxoplasmosis. Clin Microbiol Rev 2012;25:264–96.
157. McLeod R, Boyer KM, Lee D, et al. Prematurity and severity are associated with *Toxoplasma gondii* alleles (NCCCTS, 1981-2009). Clin Infect Dis 2012;54: 1595–605.

158. Lappalainen M, Koskela P, Koskiniemi M, et al. Toxoplasmosis acquired during pregnancy: improved serodiagnosis based on avidity of IgG. J Infect Dis 1993; 167:691–7.
159. Bastien P, Jumas-Bilak E, Varlet-Marie E, et al. Three years of multi-laboratory external quality control for the molecular detection of *Toxoplasma gondii* in amniotic fluid in France. Clin Microbiol Infect 2007;13:430–3.
160. Fricker-Hidalgo H, Pelloux H, Racinet C, et al. Detection of *Toxoplasma gondii* in 94 placentae from infected women by polymerase chain reaction, in vivo, and in vitro cultures. Placenta 1998;19:545–9.
161. Edvinsson B, Lundquist J, Ljungman P, et al. A prospective study of diagnosis of *Toxoplasma gondii* infection after bone marrow transplantation. APMIS 2008; 116:345–51.
162. Lamoril J, Molina JM, de Gouvello A, et al. Detection by PCR of *Toxoplasma gondii* in blood in the diagnosis of cerebral toxoplasmosis in patients with AIDS. J Clin Pathol 1996;49:89–92.
163. Colombo FA, Vidal JE, Penalva de Oliveira AC, et al. Diagnosis of cerebral toxoplasmosis in AIDS patients in Brazil: importance of molecular and immunological methods using peripheral blood samples. J Clin Microbiol 2005;43:5044–7.
164. Mesquita RT, Ziegler AP, Hiramoto RM, et al. Real-time quantitative PCR in cerebral toxoplasmosis diagnosis of Brazilian human immunodeficiency virus-infected patients. J Med Microbiol 2010;59:641–7.
165. Correia CC, Melo HR, Costa VM. Influence of neurotoxoplasmosis characteristics on real-time PCR sensitivity among AIDS patients in Brazil. Trans R Soc Trop Med Hyg 2010;104:24–8.
166. Sukthana Y, Mahittikorn A, Wickert H, et al. A promising diagnostic tool for toxoplasmic encephalitis: tachyzoite/bradyzoite stage-specific RT-PCR. Int J Infect Dis 2012;16:e279–84.
167. Qvarnstrom Y, da Silva AJ, Schuster FL, et al. Molecular confirmation of *Sappinia pedata* as a causative agent of amoebic encephalitis. J Infect Dis 2009;199: 1139–42.
168. Visvesvara GS, Moura H, Schuster FL. Pathogenic and opportunistic free-living amoebae: *Acanthamoeba* spp., *Balamuthia mandrillaris, Naegleria fowleri*, and *Sappinia diploidea*. FEMS Immunol Med Microbiol 2007;50:1–26.
169. Yagi S, Booton GC, Visvesvara GS, et al. Detection of *Balamuthia* mitochondrial 16S rRNA gene DNA in clinical specimens by PCR. J Clin Microbiol 2005;43: 3192–7.
170. Booton GC, Visvesvara GS, Byers TJ, et al. Identification and distribution of *Acanthamoeba* species genotypes associated with nonkeratitis infections. J Clin Microbiol 2005;43:1689–93.
171. Khairnar K, Tamber GS, Ralevski F, et al. Comparison of molecular diagnostic methods for the detection of *Acanthamoeba* spp. from clinical specimens submitted for keratitis. Diagn Microbiol Infect Dis 2011;70:499–506.
172. Riviere D, Szczebara FM, Berjeaud JM, et al. Development of a real-time PCR assay for quantification of *Acanthamoeba trophozoites* and cysts. J Microbiol Methods 2006;64:78–83.
173. Boschi-Pinto C, Lanata CF, Mendoza W, et al. Diarrheal diseases. In: Jamison DT, Feachem RG, Makgoba MW, et al, editors. Disease and mortality in Sub-Saharan Africa. 2nd edition. Washington, DC: The International Bank for Reconstruction and Development/The World Bank; 2006. Available at: http://www.ncbi.nlm.nih.gov/books/NBK2302. Accessed January 12, 2013.

174. Kebede A, Verweij JJ, Petros B, et al. Short communication: misleading microscopy in amoebiasis. Trop Med Int Health 2004;9:651–2.
175. Clark CG, Diamond LS. The Laredo strain and other '*Entamoeba histolytica*-like' amoebae are *Entamoeba moshkovskii*. Mol Biochem Parasitol 1991;46:11–8.
176. Royer TL, Gilchrist C, Kabir M, et al. *Entamoeba bangladeshi* nov. sp., Bangladesh. Emerg Infect Dis 2012;18:1543–5.
177. World Health Organization. Amebiasis. Wkly Epidemiol Rec 1997;72:97–100. Available at: http://whqlibdoc.who.int/bulletin/1997/Vol75-No3/bulletin_1997_75(3)_291-292.pdf. Accessed December 8, 2012.
178. Haque R, Ali IK, Akther S, et al. Comparison of PCR, isoenzyme analysis, and antigen detection for diagnosis of *Entamoeba histolytica* infection. J Clin Microbiol 1998;36:449–52.
179. Hopkins RM, Meloni BP, Groth DM, et al. Ribosomal RNA sequencing reveals differences between the genotypes of *Giardia* isolates recovered from humans and dogs living in the same locality. J Parasitol 1997;83:44–51.
180. Read CM, Monis PT, Thompson RC. Discrimination of all genotypes of *Giardia duodenalis* at the glutamate dehydrogenase locus using PCR-RFLP. Infect Genet Evol 2004;4:125–30.
181. Monis PT, Andrews RH, Mayrhofer G, et al. Molecular systematics of the parasitic protozoan *Giardia intestinalis*. Mol Biol Evol 1999;16:1135–44.
182. Sulaiman IM, Fayer R, Bern C, et al. Triosephosphate isomerase gene characterization and potential zoonotic transmission of *Giardia duodenalis*. Emerg Infect Dis 2003;9:1444–52.
183. Eroglu F, Genc A, Elgun G, et al. Identification of *Blastocystis hominis* isolates from asymptomatic and symptomatic patients by PCR. Parasitol Res 2009;105:1589–92.
184. Santin M, Gomez-Munoz MT, Solano-Aguilar G, et al. Development of a new PCR protocol to detect and subtype *Blastocystis* spp. from humans and animals. Parasitol Res 2011;109:205–12.
185. Thomson RB Jr, Haas RA, Thompson JH Jr. Intestinal parasites: the necessity of examining multiple stool specimens. Mayo Clin Proc 1984;59:641–2.
186. Siddiqui AA, Berk SL. Diagnosis of *Strongyloides stercoralis* infection. Clin Infect Dis 2001;33:1040–7.
187. ten Hove RJ, van Esbroeck M, Vervoort T, et al. Molecular diagnostics of intestinal parasites in returning travellers. Eur J Clin Microbiol Infect Dis 2009;28(9):1045–53.
188. Cnops L, Tannich E, Polman K, et al. Schistosoma real-time PCR as diagnostic tool for international travellers and migrants. Trop Med Int Health 2012. http://dx.doi.org/10.1111/j.1365-3156.2012.03060.x.
189. Pontes LA, Oliveira MC, Katz N, et al. Comparison of a polymerase chain reaction and the Kato-Katz technique for diagnosing infection with *Schistosoma mansoni*. Am J Trop Med Hyg 2003;68:652–6.
190. Gonzalez LM, Montero E, Harrison LJ, et al. Differential diagnosis of *Taenia saginata* and *Taenia solium* infection by PCR. J Clin Microbiol 2000;38:737–44.
191. Mayta H, Talley A, Gilman RH, et al. Differentiating *Taenia solium* and *Taenia saginata* infections by simple hematoxylin-eosin staining and PCR-restriction enzyme analysis. J Clin Microbiol 2000;38:133–7.
192. Yamasaki H, Sato MO, Sako Y, et al. Cysticercosis/taeniasis: recent advances in serological and molecular diagnoses. Southeast Asian J Trop Med Public Health 2003;34(Suppl 2):98–102.

193. Imai K, Koibuchi T, Kumagai T, et al. Cerebral schistosomiasis due to *Schistosoma haematobium* confirmed by PCR analysis of brain specimen. J Clin Microbiol 2011;49:3703–6.

194. Jang JS, Kim KH, Yu JR, et al. Identification of parasite DNA in common bile duct stones by PCR and DNA sequencing. Korean J Parasitol 2007;45:301–6.

195. Centers for Disease Control and Prevention. Trichomoniasis. In: DPDx. Available at: http://www.dpd.cdc.gov/dpdx/HTML/Trichomoniasis.htm. Accessed January 12, 2013.

196. Soper D. Trichomoniasis: under control or undercontrolled? Am J Obstet Gynecol 2004;190:281–90.

197. Wang CC, McClelland RS, Reilly M, et al. The effect of treatment of vaginal infections on shedding of human immunodeficiency virus type 1. J Infect Dis 2001;183:1017–22.

198. Leber AL, Novak-Weekley S. Intestinal and urogenital amebae, flagellates, and ciliates. In: Versalovic J, Carroll KC, Funke G, et al, editors. Manual of clinical microbiology, vol. 2, 10th edition. Washington, DC: ASM Press; 2011. p. 2149–71.

199. Huppert JS, Mortensen JE, Reed JL, et al. Rapid antigen testing compares favorably with transcription-mediated amplification assay for the detection of *Trichomonas vaginalis* in young women. Clin Infect Dis 2007;45:194–8.

200. Nye MB, Schwebke JR, Body BA. Comparison of APTIMA *Trichomonas vaginalis* transcription-mediated amplification to wet mount microscopy, culture, and polymerase chain reaction for diagnosis of trichomoniasis in men and women. Am J Obstet Gynecol 2009;200(188):e181–7.

201. McIver CJ, Rismanto N, Smith C, et al. Multiplex PCR testing detection of higher-than-expected rates of cervical mycoplasma, ureaplasma, and trichomonas and viral agent infections in sexually active Australian women. J Clin Microbiol 2009; 47:1358–63.

202. van Der Schee C, van Belkum A, Zwijgers L, et al. Improved diagnosis of *Trichomonas vaginalis* infection by PCR using vaginal swabs and urine specimens compared to diagnosis by wet mount microscopy, culture, and fluorescent staining. J Clin Microbiol 1999;37:4127–30.

203. Ghosh K, Weiss LM. Molecular diagnostic tests for microsporidia. Interdiscip Perspect Infect Dis 2009;2009:926521.

204. Centers for Disease Control and Prevention. Microsporidiosis. In: DPDx. Available at: http://dpd.cdc.gov/dpdx/HTML/Microsporidiosis.htm. Accessed January 12, 2013.

205. Joseph J, Sharma S, Murthy SI, et al. Microsporidial keratitis in India: 16S rRNA gene-based PCR assay for diagnosis and species identification of microsporidia in clinical samples. Invest Ophthalmol Vis Sci 2006;47:4468–73.

206. Franzen C, Muller A, Hegener P, et al. Polymerase chain reaction for microsporidian DNA in gastrointestinal biopsy specimens of HIV-infected patients. AIDS 1996;10:F23–7.

207. Rinder H, Janitschke K, Aspock H, et al. Blinded, externally controlled multicenter evaluation of light microscopy and PCR for detection of microsporidia in stool specimens. The Diagnostic Multicenter Study Group on Microsporidia. J Clin Microbiol 1998;36:1814–8.

208. Garcia LS. Laboratory identification of the microsporidia. J Clin Microbiol 2002; 40:1892–901.

209. Taniuchi M, Verweij JJ, Sethabutr O, et al. Multiplex polymerase chain reaction method to detect *Cyclospora*, *Cystoisospora*, and *Microsporidia* in stool samples. Diagn Microbiol Infect Dis 2011;71:386–90.

210. Talal AH, Kotler DP, Orenstein JM, et al. Detection of *Enterocytozoon bieneusi* in fecal specimens by polymerase chain reaction analysis with primers to the small-subunit rRNA. Clin Infect Dis 1998;26:673–5.
211. Subrungruang I, Mungthin M, Chavalitshewinkoon-Petmitr P, et al. Evaluation of DNA extraction and PCR methods for detection of *Enterocytozoon bienuesi* in stool specimens. J Clin Microbiol 2004;42:3490–4.
212. Dowd SE, Gerba CP, Enriquez FJ, et al. PCR amplification and species determination of microsporidia in formalin-fixed feces after immunomagnetic separation. Appl Environ Microbiol 1998;64(1):333–6.
213. Chan KS, Koh TH. Extraction of microsporidial DNA from modified trichrome-stained clinical slides and subsequent species identification using PCR sequencing. Parasitology 2008;135(6):701–3.

Invasive Fungal Infections
Biomarkers and Molecular Approaches to Diagnosis

Audrey N. Schuetz, MD, MPH

KEYWORDS

- Aspergillosis • Candidiasis • Invasive fungal infection • Biomarker • Galactomannan
- β-D-Glucan • Polymerase chain reaction • Molecular

KEY POINTS

- Galactomannan shows high positive predictive value and negative predictive value for the diagnosis of invasive aspergillosis.
- The utility of galactomannan from bronchoalveolar lavage fluid appears promising for the diagnosis of invasive aspergillosis, and is more sensitive in some clinical contexts than serum galactomannan.
- Two consecutively positive serum samples for galactomannan provide strong evidence for the diagnosis of invasive aspergillosis. 1,3-β-D-Glucan demonstrates high negative predictive value for invasive aspergillosis but only moderate positive predictive value.
- It is recommended to apply the use of galactomannan and 1,3-β-D-glucan together to increase the probability of correct diagnosis, and to interpret results of these tests in conjunction with clinical, microbiologic, and radiologic data.
- Molecular platforms offer promise in their ability to provide rapid results, a wide range of testable specimen types, and unique species identification.
- The real-time aspect of many of these platforms aids in early diagnosis, allowing clinicians to focus on antifungal therapy.

INTRODUCTION

Invasive fungal infections are rising in importance because of the growing population of transplant recipients and other immunosuppressed populations. Diagnosis of invasive fungal infections (IFI) is difficult due to the diverse organism population that may cause disease, as well as limits in currently available diagnostic techniques. Many medical centers have observed a changing spectrum of organisms causing disease, and such changes challenge our diagnostic testing approaches.[1] Historically, culture has reliably been the standard of care for detection of fungi, but organisms may take weeks to grow in culture and the sensitivity of culture can be low. Blood-culture

The author has no disclosures to provide.

Department of Pathology and Laboratory Medicine, Weill Cornell Medical College, New York-Presbyterian Hospital, 525 East 68th Street, Starr 737C, New York, NY 10065, USA

E-mail address: ans9112@med.cornell.edu

Clin Lab Med 33 (2013) 505–525

http://dx.doi.org/10.1016/j.cll.2013.03.009

labmed.theclinics.com

methods using the lysis centrifugation (LS) system have demonstrated moderate sensitivity. In one study, the LS system for candidemia was positive for only 43% of the autopsy-confirmed cases of *Candida*.[2] Indeed, blood cultures are negative for *Candida* species in approximately 50% of autopsy-proven cases of disseminated candidiasis.[2] In addition, tissue specimens, which are obtained more and more frequently with interventional radiology and spare more invasive excisional biopsy approaches, are often submitted in formalin and bypass the clinical microbiology laboratory for culture.[1] Therefore, alternative methods are needed for the diagnosis of IFI. Biomarkers and molecular methods are gaining in popularity as they are generally noninvasive and, in most cases, provide an earlier diagnosis than morphologic evaluation by culture.

THE ROLE OF BIOMARKERS IN THE DIAGNOSIS OF IFI
Definition

According to the Definitions Biomarkers Working Group, a biomarker, or biologic marker, is "…a characteristic that is objectively measured and evaluated as an indicator of normal biologic processes, pathogenic processes, or pharmacologic responses to a therapeutic intervention."[3] Although strictly defined as quantifiable, measurable substances produced by the human body in response to a particular infection, or a recent change in the health status of the person, biomarkers can also be defined as substances or microbial exoantigens released by organisms into a person's body. The study of biomarkers has become popular in recent years because of the rapid information that can be provided from relatively noninvasive specimen sources beyond the routine traditional clinical and laboratory data. Two fungal biomarkers have been extensively researched and published over the last 20 years: galactomannan and 1,3-β-D-glucan. The performance of these and other less studied biomarkers are reviewed here regarding their roles in the diagnosis of IFI.

Galactomannan

Galactomannan (GM) is a cell-wall polysaccharide released from growing hyphae of *Aspergillus* spp and various other fungi in serum, bronchoalveolar lavage (BAL) fluid, and other body fluids. GM is not released by conidia, which are the colonizing forms in bronchial airways; therefore, GM positivity can indicate tissue invasion in the correct clinical situation. Galactomannan is available commercially as an immunoenzymatic microplate sandwich assay (Platelia Aspergillus; BioRad Laboratories, Hercules, CA), which detects GM using a rat monoclonal antibody. The antibody reacts with the β (1→5)-linked galactofuranosyl residues of the side chains of the GM molecule.[4] Results are expressed in index values based on optical density measurements, and can be available within 3 hours. The kit has been cleared by the Food and Drug Administration (FDA) and standardized for serum and, recently, BAL samples. Galactomannan has also been used on other specimen types, such cerebrospinal fluid (CSF) and urine.

Performance characteristics of GM in serum and BAL fluid

Early animal studies demonstrated that serum GM levels in untreated rabbit models paralleled an increasing burden of disease in the animals caused by pulmonary invasive aspergillosis (IA).[5] Human studies also demonstrated a strong correlation between serum GM levels and clinical outcomes.[6,7] Early clinical studies and case reports suggested that sampling of GM in specimens other than serum could be useful, especially in culture-negative cases.[8] In guinea pig models, sensitivity of the GM assay in BAL fluid was higher than that of whole blood or serum, indicating that

BAL fluid was more suitable for the early detection of IA.[9] Studies on human subjects have demonstrated similar results. Husain and colleagues[10] reported 82% sensitivity for GM in BAL fluid (at index cutoffs of both 0.5 and 1.0) and 95.8% specificity in their solid organ transplant patients with aspergillosis. The serum GM samples of these patients were positive in only 19.4% of patients who had simultaneous BAL fluids positive for GM. Higher sensitivities for GM of BAL fluids in comparison with sera have been noted by other researchers in various other patient populations.[11,12]

Generally lower sensitivity rates have been obtained from pediatric patients when compared with adult patients in studies evaluating the utility of GM antigenemia in early diagnosis of IA.[13] The performance of GM has not been well evaluated in neonatal specimens, and may exhibit reduced sensitivity in patients with chronic granulomatous disease.[14] The sensitivity of GM is also reduced in the presence of antifungal agents in patients receiving prophylaxis. In one study, the sensitivity dropped from 80% to 20% in bone marrow transplant recipients receiving prophylaxis with fluconazole or amphotericin B.[15]

False-positive results for GM have been reported in patients receiving certain antibiotics, such as piperacillin-tazobactam and amoxicillin-clavulanate, in neonates colonized with *Bifidobacterium*, patients receiving enteral nutrition, and in BAL-fluid specimens containing Plasma-Lyte with gluconate (**Table 1**).[16–19] Cross-reactivity of GM with other fungi has been reported in patients with invasive mycoses attributable to *Histoplasma*, *Blastomyces*, *Prototheca*, and *Fusarium*, among others.[20–23] Of interest, a recent study has shown that the newer piperacillin-tazobactam formulation (Tazocin; Pfizer, New York, NY) seems to be no longer responsible for false-positive GM results.[24]

Cutoff values
Many studies have examined the utility of various optical density cutoff values for this assay, especially because the cutoff values used in the United States vary from those used in Europe. The cutoff value typically used in the European kit is an index of 1.0 for indeterminate and 1.5 for positive. However, the FDA-cleared version of the Platelia kit used in the United States, which was approved in 2003, established a cutoff index value of 0.5 (**Table 2**). In a recent study, investigators attempted to determine which cutoff values for GM from BAL fluid were useful in their mixed population of solid organ transplant patients and patients with hematologic malignancies, all of whom were at risk for invasive pulmonary aspergillosis.[25] As determined by a receiver-operator curve, there was an optimal index of at least 0.8. Very high indexes, such as 3.0 or

Table 1
Causes of false positivity or cross-reactivity in the galactomannan (GM) test

False-Positive Results Due to GM Contamination	Cross-Reactivity Caused by Similar Cell-Wall Antigens
Piperacillin-tazobactam	*Histoplasma*
Amoxicillin-clavulanate	*Blastomyces*
Other β-lactam antibiotics	*Prototheca*
Neonates colonized with *Bifidobacterium*	*Fusarium*
Enteral nutrition	*Penicillium*
Gluconate-containing Plasma-Lyte	*Geotrichum*
Other intravenous fluids containing gluconate	
Possibly cardboard or soybean protein	

Table 2
Typical cutoff index values used for the galactomannan assay

	Negative	Indeterminate	Positive
Europe	<0.5	1.0	>1.5
United States	<0.5		>0.5

greater, were more likely to indicate invasive pulmonary aspergillosis. On the other hand, indexes of less than 0.5 demonstrated 93.2% sensitivity in ruling out infection. Another analysis of GM from BAL fluid in hematology patients demonstrated that an index value of at least 1.0 for BAL fluid was preferred in identifying *Aspergillus* spp as a cause of pulmonary disease.[26] The autopsy rate for this study was 60%, allowing for a large number of proven cases of IA with which to compare the BAL GM results.

Clinical outcomes and guidelines

Galactomannan is one of the diagnostic criteria for the diagnosis of IA, as stated by the European Organization for Research and Treatment of Cancer/Invasive Fungal Infections Cooperative Group and the National Institute of Allergy and Infectious Diseases Mycoses Study Group (EORTC/MSG).[27] Another organization, the Infectious Diseases Working Party in Haematology and Oncology of the German Society for Haematology and Oncology (AGIHO), advises routine GM antigen detection in patients at risk for IA, with testing at least twice per week, because circulation of the GM antigen in serum is transient.[28] The Infectious Diseases Society of America (IDSA) guidelines for the treatment of aspergillosis, on the other hand, only state that the combined use of serum GM antigen measurement with the early use of computed tomography (CT) scans should improve detection of invasive pulmonary aspergillosis.[29]

Despite these conflicting guidelines, it is generally agreed upon that detection of positive results in 2 consecutive serum samples provides strong evidence for the diagnosis of IA.[28] Early diagnosis using GM is possible, as antigen positivity can be detected a median of 5 to 8 days (range 1–27 days) before clinical signs of infection develop.[30] Animal models have shown that GM from BAL fluid turns positive 2 days sooner than GM from serum.[31] Galactomannan testing is most useful when used for serial monitoring of patients at high risk for development of IA and if results are available within 48 hours.

In summary, GM for detection of IA shows a high positive predictive value (PPV) and negative predictive value (NPV) (**Table 3**). In an effort to determine whether GM provides an earlier assessment of treatment response, a group of researchers compared the current criteria for treatment response of IA based on EORTC/MSG guidelines to the GM index.[32] The current 6-week EORTC/MSG end point reviews a combination of factors, including clinical and radiologic findings, negative microbiologic markers including culture results, and survival at specific time points.[33] In this comparison study

Table 3
Relative negative predictive value (NPV) and positive predictive value (PPV) of galactomannan and 1,3-β-D-glucan in diagnosis of invasive aspergillosis and invasive candidiasis

		PPV	NPV
Galactomannan	Invasive aspergillosis	Excellent	Excellent
1,3-β-D-glucan	Invasive candidiasis	Low	Low
	Invasive aspergillosis	Low to moderate	Excellent

of 115 patients with cancer, treatment response was best determined using GM at a median of 21 days after treatment initiation, which was 3 weeks before the EORTC/MSG time point. The investigators concluded that GM index may shorten the time to response assessment and should be considered a primary end point in IA trials.

1,3-β-D-Glucan

Another well-studied circulating biomarker of fungal disease is 1,3-β-D-glucan (BDG). BDG is a major cell-wall component in almost all fungi, except for *Cryptococcus* spp and fungi of the order Mucorales. In addition, *Blastomyces dermatitidis* depletes BDG in its cell wall when it converts from mycelial to yeast form, limiting the utility of BDG in diagnosis, as this fungus is present as yeast in the human body.[34] The BDG Fungitell assay (Associates of Cape Cod, Inc, East Falmouth, MA) is FDA-approved for the diagnosis of invasive mycoses. The recommended positive cutoff value is 80 pg/mL. Another possible method to detect BDG is the Tachypleus or Limulus Amoebocyte Lysate pathway assay (Glucatell; Associates of Cape Cod, Inc), which is a variation of the limulus lysate assay used to detect gram-negative endotoxin.[35]

Performance characteristics of BDG

Difficulties arise when comparing data from various studies because different patient populations, cutoff values, and sites of infection (eg, deep-seated vs bloodstream) have been used in the many studies on BDG and other fungal biomarkers. However, in general the performance characteristics of BDG in the diagnosis of IFI vary but show low sensitivity. Lu and colleagues,[36] in their meta-analysis of 15 studies assessing the overall accuracy of BDG in the diagnosis of IFI, reported a high specificity in patients with hematologic disorders but low performance of the assay in solid organ transplant recipients. The investigators concluded that BDG results must be interpreted in association with clinical findings and that 2 sequential positive BDG results are needed to diagnose probable IFI. Use of a combination of BDG and GM was helpful in confirming the diagnosis of IFI in this meta-analysis. A meta-analysis from the Third European Conference on Infections in Leukemia examined the performance of BDG antigenemia for the diagnosis of IFI in hemato-oncologic patients.[37] The sensitivity of BDG was low in this meta-analysis, ranging from 50% to 85%, implying that a negative result should not be used to rule out IFI.

BDG shows a high NPV but only moderate PPV in the diagnosis of IA.[38,39] When measured serially, BDG often is positive 2 to 5 days on average before the microbiological or clinical diagnosis of IA.[39] Specific performance data on BDG in the diagnosis of invasive candidiasis (IC) are limited. Earlier studies demonstrated serum BDG sensitivities of approximately 80% to 90% in patients with candidemia.[40] However, subsequent studies have shown that the sensitivity of BDG varies by patient population (ie, adult vs pediatric; hematologic vs nonhematologic), and generally ranges from 47% to 87%.[41,42] One study compared the performance of several potential biomarkers of candidiasis in critically ill patients, including BDG, *Candida albicans* germ tube antibody (CAGTA), procalcitonin, and C-reactive protein (CRP).[43] The investigators reported that BDG in combination with CAGTA accurately differentiated *Candida* colonization from IC in patients with severe abdominal conditions, whereas procalcitonin and CRP did not. Jaijakul and colleagues[44] evaluated serial monitoring of serum BDG in predicting treatment responses in patients with proven IC. This study demonstrated that a decrease in BDG levels during therapy was associated with successful treatment, and that an initial BDG level lower than 416 pg/mL may predict successful patient outcome. More data should be gathered on the role of BDG in intensive care unit patients who are at high risk for candidemia.[45]

The presence of BDG in serum is not specific for *Candida* or *Aspergillus* spp. A recent meta-analysis of 14 studies in immunosuppressed patients showed that serum or plasma BDG demonstrated excellent sensitivity (average 94.8% [range 90.8–97.1%]) and very good specificity (average 86.3% [range 81.7–89.9%]) for the diagnosis of *Pneumocystis jirovecii* pneumonia.[46] A diagnosis of *Pneumocystis* for all patients in these studies was confirmed by alternative means, whether by conventional staining methods or molecular detection. BDG may also be positive in cases of histoplasmosis.[47] The BDG assay also suffers from issues of false positivity, as does GM. For instance, a false-positive BDG assay may result from: glucan-contaminated blood-collection tubes and surgical gauze dressings; dialysis with cellulose membranes; bacteremia due to several gram-positive organisms, particularly *Streptococcus pneumoniae*; use of products with cellulose depth filters such as albumin; gut inflammation; and antibiotics such as amoxicillin-clavulanate.[29,48]

Clinical outcomes and guidelines

According to the EORTC/MSG guidelines, there is currently no strong evidence for a correlation between BDG and outcome of IA, as opposed to GM for aspergillosis.[32] The recent EORTC/MSG guidelines list BDG detection in serum as one of the mycological criteria for the diagnosis of probable invasive fungal disease other than cryptococcosis and zygomycosis.[27] No recommendations regarding the timing and number of measurements, cutoffs, or use of different assays were offered. On the other hand, the AGIHO guidelines recommend the measurement of plasma BDG to aid in the diagnosis of IFI in high-risk hematologic patients.[28]

In summary, BDG demonstrates high NPV in ruling out IA. Both the PPV and NPV of BDG are questionable in diagnosing invasive *Candida* infection. It is important to take into account the poor specificity of BDG for IFI in general. Unnecessary treatment because of a potential false-positive test result can result in exposure of the patient to a variety of toxicities and adverse effects of some antifungals (eg, drug interactions of azoles, nephrotoxicity of polyenes, and acquired resistance during therapy). The additional costs associated with antifungal therapy, such as direct drug costs and therapeutic drug monitoring, should also be considered.

Other Biomarkers: Mannan and Arabinitol

Mannan is a polysaccharide unit of the *Candida* cell wall and is highly immunogenic.[49] Mannan antibodies and mannan antigens can increase in the serum of patients with candidiasis. The Platelia (BioRad) mannan antigen and antibody tests are available tools for the detection of mannan serum levels. The clearance of mannan antigen from the bloodstream is rapid; thus, the number of serum samples obtained affects the sensitivity of the assay.[13] Varying sensitivities and specificities have been reported in the literature, but it is generally agreed that the mannan antigen and antibody tests should be used in combination for optimal results.[41,49] Mikulska and colleagues[50] reported that the combination mannan/antimannan test sensitivity and specificity values for the diagnosis of IC were 83% and 93%, respectively. The IDSA candidiasis guidelines state that combined measurement of mannan and antimannan antibodies are worthy of further evaluation, but are not recommended for routine use.[51]

The 5-carbon sugar alcohol D-arabinitol is a metabolite of most pathogenic *Candida* spp, excluding *Candida glabrata* and *Candida krusei*.[49] The exclusion of *C glabrata* and *C krusei* limits the applicability of the D-arabinitol test, as both species are significant pathogens in the immunosuppressed population and exhibit high levels of fluconazole resistance (intrinsic 100% resistance for *C krusei*). Serum levels of D-arabinitol may be increased in patients with IC; however, abnormal renal function can also raise levels.[52] In cases of renal insufficiency, some investigators use the serum or urinary D-arabinitol/creatinine ratio. Other researchers have suggested serum or urinary D-arabinitol/L-arabinitol ratios. Routine measurement of the arabinitol levels and ratios has not yet been implemented in the clinical laboratory, although some early studies suggested relatively high sensitivity and specificity.[53] Further studies are needed to assess the role of arabinitol assays in the diagnosis of IFI.

Summary

Galactomannan demonstrates high PPV and NPV for the diagnosis of IA. The utility of GM from BAL fluid appears promising for the diagnosis of IA, and is more sensitive in some clinical contexts than serum GM. More data on the use and interpretation of GM in the pediatric population are needed. Sensitivity of the galactomannan assay is decreased in patients exposed to antifungal prophylaxis agents, and the high false-positivity rate of GM in some situations can also limit its usefulness. Cutoff values for GM differ among studies, rendering direct comparison between studies difficult. Galactomannan is included as a diagnostic criterion by some guideline-setting organizations, and 2 consecutively positive serum samples for GM provide strong evidence for the diagnosis of IA. GM antigenemia can be detected before clinical signs of infection are evident, and is most useful for serial monitoring of patients at high risk for development of IA if results are available within 48 hours. BDG, on the other hand, demonstrates good NPV for IA but moderate PPV. The role of BDG is questionable in diagnosing invasive *Candida* infection and IFI in general. BDG is recommended as a complementary tool for the diagnosis of invasive mycoses in high-risk hemato-oncologic patients, but the role of BDG in various other patient populations should be further investigated. BDG levels should be followed by serial monitoring and, similar to GM, BDG antigenemia can be detected before clinical signs of infection. Finally, more research is needed on the use of mannan, arabinitol, and other fungal biomarkers in the diagnosis of IFI. Overall, it is recommended to apply the use of these biomarkers in conjunction with each other to increase the accuracy of diagnosis, and to interpret the results of these tests in conjunction with clinical, microbiological, and radiologic data, as suggested by published clinical guidelines.

THE ROLE OF MOLECULAR TECHNIQUES IN THE DIAGNOSIS OF IFI

The success of molecular approaches to diagnosis in areas of microbiology such as virology and bacteriology has encouraged many laboratorians and clinicians to explore the role of molecular techniques in the diagnosis of IFI. Biomarkers are currently in more frequent use than molecular techniques in the care of patients with suspected IFI, but biomarkers fall short in many respects. Biomarkers cannot identify to the species level and sometimes cannot even reliably identify organisms to the genus level. In addition, biomarkers offer an earlier diagnosis than culture, but this may not be early enough to make a significant impact on patient care. Finally, performance characteristics of the most frequently used biomarkers are lacking in certain patient populations or for certain disease states.

Molecular tests for the identification of fungi have been widely published, particularly over the past 3 years. In 2009, Khot and Fredericks[54] published their review of polymerase chain reaction (PCR)-based studies for fungal diagnostics over the past decade using the Minimum Information for Publication of Quantitative Real-Time PCR Experiments (MIQE) guidelines. Khot and Fredericks reported that 68 studies qualified for analysis, and demonstrated a wide range of sensitivity and specificity, with the majority of molecular assays available in-house. More recently, there have been many publications related to molecular techniques for IFI diagnosis. Few of these have included clinical outcome data, and most have focused solely on diagnosis.

Current Commercially Available Molecular Assays for the Diagnosis of Fungal Infections

There are 6 commercially available molecular assays for the diagnosis of fungal infections (**Table 4**), namely Yeast Traffic Light PNA FISH, Multiplex xTAG Fungal ASR Luminex assay, *Aspergillus* and *Candida* Real-Time PCR Panel by Viracor, PLEX-ID Broad Fungal Assay, MycAssay *Aspergillus*, and SeptiFast. Each assay is discussed here.

The Yeast Traffic Light peptide nucleic acid fluorescence in situ hybridization assay (PNA FISH; AdvanDx, Inc, Woburn, MA) provides rapid identification within 2 to 3 hours of up to 5 different *Candida* species from blood-culture bottles flagged positive for growth. PNA FISH is a multicolor, qualitative nucleic acid hybridization assay using fluorescence microscopy. The performance characteristics are generally high, with sensitivities ranging from 94% to 100% for various *Candida* species, and specificities approaching 100%.[55,56] The grouping of *C glabrata* and *C krusei* separates these 2 fluconazole-resistant species from other species, which is helpful in guiding antifungal therapy. Hall and colleagues[55] used the 3-probe system for *C albicans/Candida parapsilosis*, *C glabrata/C krusei*, and *Candida tropicalis*, with both the 30- and 90-minute hybridization steps on 216 positive blood culture isolates, with identities confirmed by sequencing. The system correctly identified 96% of *Candida* isolates with 2 false-negative reactions (1 each for *C parapsilosis* and *C tropicalis*) and 1 misidentification of *C parapsilosis* as *C tropicalis*. The investigators also challenged the system with a wide range of other yeasts, which produced some known cross-reactivity with yeasts rarely encountered in the clinical microbiology laboratory (ie, *Candida bracarensis*). Another study of 176 blood cultures positive for yeast reported a sensitivity of 98.9% and specificity of 100% of the PNA FISH for the 5 aforementioned species.[56] The yeasts in this study were confirmed by biochemical testing at a reference laboratory, with unusual yeasts additionally confirmed by sequencing. Disadvantages of PNA FISH include the inability to distinguish among certain *Candida* species, depending on the assay, which may be problematic if fungal resistance patterns differ in various health care settings (eg, *C albicans* vs *C parapsilosis*; also *C glabrata* vs *C krusei*). Moreover, sensitivity of the PNA FISH assay depends on organism load, as this is a nonamplified assay. A recent forum of microbiologists noted that their centers largely discontinued this testing, as clinicians were reluctant to switch back to fluconazole from echinocandin therapy despite *C albicans* results on PNA FISH, owing to concerns of mixed *Candida* infection.[1] This interesting observation points to a need for improved sensitivity in detecting lower organism burden and mixed infections, as well as earlier detection of candidemia. The importance of the early treatment of candidemia was demonstrated in one study that showed a trend toward higher mortality when a delay of greater than 12 hours in reporting a blood culture positive for *Candida* was seen.[57]

The Luminex multiplex PCR xMAP (Luminex Corp, Austin, TX) bead probe fluid array with xTAG analyte-specific reagents (ASR) has performed well in *Candida* species identification in positive blood-culture bottles, and can rapidly identify other yeast-like organisms as well (*Cryptococcus* spp and dimorphic molds).[58] A recent study by Babady and colleagues[59] on the yeast and mold ASR assays demonstrated 100% sensitivity and specificity for the 7-plex *Candida* panel run on 22 positive blood-culture bottles and 43 *Candida* culture isolates. The 11-plex mold assay in their study demonstrated 58% to 100% sensitivity and 92% to 98% specificity in detecting various molds when run directly on 43 respiratory specimens (17 sputa, 16 bronchial washes, 5 lung biopsies, 2 BALs, 2 pleural fluids, 1 tracheal secretion) and 1 appendix tissue. Twenty-three of the 44 direct specimens were positive for mold, and the assay demonstrated a relatively low sensitivity of 58% to 76% for Aspergillus fumigatus and Aspergillus flavus on direct specimens. The assay also did not perform well for fungi in the order Mucorales. One advantage of this study was the wide variety of fungal isolates assessed other than A fumigatus and C albicans; however, studies should be performed to assess a larger and wider range of molds. The 11-plex mold assay is attractive for its genus differentiation among hyaline molds, such as Fusarium spp, which is often resistant. In another study, the 11-plex mold assay demonstrated good specificity when run on 58 fungal reference strains, but some cross-reactivity between Scedosporium apiospermum primers with Paecilomyces lilacinus and between Aspergillus terreus primers with S apiospermum was demonstrated.[60] Of note, the assay was unable to detect the 4 tested Mucorales isolates, similar to the study by Babady and colleagues.[59] The investigators concluded that the limit of detection may be suboptimal for performance of testing directly from patient specimens, and that further work should be done to improve sensitivity. The testing time on this platform averages 5 to 6 hours. Similarly to PNA FISH, the Luminex platform can be run on positive blood-culture bottles, but the system also has the added advantage of identifying Candida to the species level. The Luminex platform requires considerable molecular technologist expertise, and is expensive. Therefore, most clinical laboratories that run this test perform it on an as-needed basis, depending on the laboratory's staffing capabilities, which limits the clinical utility of this test.

Viracor-IBT Laboratories (Lee's Summit, MO) offers the Aspergillus PCR and Candida PCR assays, which are not available as commercial kits that laboratories can run on their own. The qualitative Aspergillus PCR panel comprises 3 real-time PCR assays: a pan-Aspergillus PCR assay, which detects all Aspergillus spp; an A fumigatus assay; and an A terreus assay, which detects this clinically important species inherently resistant to amphotericin B, a common treatment for aspergillosis. The assays can be run on BAL fluid or bronchial washings. According to a recent retrospective study, the Viracor pan-Aspergillus assay showed 100% sensitivity and 88% specificity for IA in 150 BALs from lung transplant patients (including 16 samples of proven/probable IA; 26 Aspergillus colonization; 11 non-Aspergillus colonization).[61] The 12% false-positivity rate was due primarily to Aspergillus colonization of the airways, which was defined in this study as BAL culture positivity for Aspergillus but with a normal bronchoscopic examination and chest CT scan. One limitation of this study was its retrospective nature and the gold-standard definitions of proven and probable IA relying on a positive culture and chest CT findings, respectively. Given the detection of low levels of Aspergillus with this sensitive technique, it is imperative that clinicians use information from such molecular testing when the clinical suspicion of disease is high.

The qualitative Candida real-time PCR panel (Viracor) targets various Candida spp but cannot distinguish between some of the species. The assay is capable of detecting C albicans and/or C tropicalis; C glabrata and/or C krusei; and C parapsilosis species complex. In one study of 55 patients with Candida in different locations (candidemia vs deep-seated candidiasis), the assay demonstrated 80% sensitivity and 70% specificity when run on serum and plasma for the diagnosis of IC.[62] Cases were defined based on the recovery of Candida from various body sites by culture, combined with clinical evidence of infection. Colonization controls in this study were defined as recovery of Candida from nonsterile body sites in patients without signs or symptoms of candidal disease. Therefore, it is possible that the specificity of this assay was undercalled, based on misclassification of controls owing to the

Table 4
Commercially available molecular assays for the diagnosis of fungal infections

Assay	Method	Company	Targets	Results	Specimen	TAT	FDA-Approved/Cleared
Yeast Traffic Light	PNA FISH	AdvanDx, Inc, Woburn, MA, USA	26S rRNA for *Candida* spp	Qualitative, with speciation of most *Candida* spp	Blood culture bottles positive for growth	2–3 h	Yes
Multiplex xTAG Fungal ASR Assay	Multiplex PCR and bead-based flow cytometry	Luminex Corp, Austin, TX, USA	23 clinically significant fungi (yeasts and molds)	Qualitative, with detection to the species level when possible	Respiratory specimens; blood culture bottles positive for growth	5–6 h post extraction	No
Aspergillus Real-Time PCR Panel	Real-time PCR	Viracor-IBT Laboratories, Lee's Summit, MO, USA	18S rRNA and ITS1 for *Aspergillus* spp	Qualitative, with detection of *Aspergillus* spp, *Aspergillus fumigatus*, or *Aspergillus terreus*	BAL; bronchial washing	Within 8–12 h of specimen receipt at Viracor	No

Candida Real-time PCR Panel	Real-time PCR	Viracor-IBT Laboratories, Lee's Summit, MO, USA	ITS1 for Candida spp	Qualitative, with detection of Candida albicans and/or Candida tropicalis; Candida glabrata and/or Candida krusei; and Candida parapsilosis complex	Plasma; serum	Same day of specimen receipt at Viracor	No
PLEX-ID Broad Fungal Assay	Multiplex PCR and mass spectrometer	Abbott Ibis Biosciences, Abbott Park, IL, USA	Up to 75 fungi	Qualitative, unique organism identification	BAL; blood	Within 6 h, or 1 working day	No
MycAssay Aspergillus	Real-time PCR	Myconostica Ltd, Cambridge, UK	18S rRNA for Aspergillus spp	Qualitative	Serum; BAL	3 h	No
SeptiFast	Real-time PCR	Roche Molecular Diagnostics, Pleasanton, CA, USA	5 species of Candida and A fumigatus	Qualitative	Blood	6 h	No

Abbreviations: ASR, analyte-specific reagent; BAL, bronchoalveolar lavage fluid; FDA, US Food and Drug Administration; FISH, fluorescence in situ hybridization; ITS, internal transcribed spacer; PCR, polymerase chain reaction; PNA, peptide nucleic acid; TAT, turnaround time.

microbiologic culture definition. The performance of the Viracor-IBT *Candida* real-time PCR assay was also compared with BDG. Although in this study the sensitivities of PCR and BDG were not significantly different in diagnosing candidemia, PCR was more sensitive than BDG for deep-seated candidiasis (89% vs 53%, *P* = .004). The investigators concluded that PCR and, to a lesser extent, BDG testing enhance performance of blood cultures for IC diagnosis.

The PLEX-ID Broad Fungal Assay (Abbott Ibis Biosciences, Abbott Park, IL) is a qualitative assay intended for the detection and identification of clinically relevant fungal species by nucleic acid amplification and subsequent mass spectrometry (MS) analysis. The PLEX-ID system is based on multilocus PCR and electrospray ionization MS. Gu and colleagues[63] reported 98% accuracy in identifying *Candida* to the species level from 76 reference strains and 61 clinical isolates recovered from culture, but more data are needed regarding the performance of this system on direct patient specimens for clinically relevant fungi.

The MycAssay *Aspergillus* PCR (Myconostica Ltd, Cambridge, UK) is a real-time PCR assay that uses molecular beacon technology. It detects DNA from 15 different *Aspergillus* spp, targeting the 18S rRNA. Sensitivity ranged from 60% to 70% in serum, with 90.5% to 100% specificity, depending on whether 1 or more than 1 specimen was used to define PCR positivity.[64] Although 170 clinical specimens were evaluated in this study, a limited number of patients were included, specifically 10 with proven or probable IA and 21 control patients with no evidence of IA. For BAL fluid the sensitivity in another study was 94%, with 99% specificity.[65] Sixteen of 17 (94%) patients with proven/probable IA based on EORTC/MSG guidelines (with blinding to GM results) were positive while 139 of 141 (98.6%) patients without proven/probable IA were negative by this assay. The investigators also reported performance of the MycAssay *Aspergillus* PCR comparable with that of GM in the diagnosis of IA. Results may be available within 3 hours, and this CE-marked product is approved for use on various molecular platforms.

Roche Molecular Diagnostics (Pleasanton, CA) offers a rapid SeptiFast assay for the diagnosis of sepsis, which includes qualitative diagnosis of 5 *Candida* species and *A fumigatus* directly from blood. In one pediatric study of 803 children with suspected sepsis including 1673 blood samples, Lucignano and colleagues[66] reported that the SeptiFast assay performed better than routine blood cultures, with a higher positivity rate in patients receiving antibiotics at the time of blood draw. Compared with blood cultures, SeptiFast was 85% sensitive and 93.5% specific and identified 97 additional clinically significant isolates not recovered by blood culture (24.7% of which was *Pseudomonas* spp; 14% *Klebsiella* spp; and 14% *Candida* spp). This real-time PCR assay, which is run on the LightCycler (Roche), is not available for use in the United States, but has CE-In Vitro Diagnostic Medical Devices status in Europe.

Molecular Platforms under Development for Fungal Diagnostics

Some newer commercial platforms are currently being evaluated for the diagnosis of fungal infections. An in-house multiplex-tandem PCR platform for the detection of candidemia using whole blood, serum, or plasma specimens performed well in identifying *Candida* species prior to blood-culture positivity.[67] This multiplex-tandem PCR assay uses melt-curve analysis for species identification; therefore, no specialized equipment (eg, flow cytometer) is needed. Great Basin Corporation (Salt Lake City, UT) is designing a rapid fungal assay to identify clinically significant *Candida* species; the technology combines isothermal amplification with silicon macroarray chip-based detection.[68] Another system in development, the RenDx Fungiplex panel (Renishaw Diagnostics, Hoffman Estates, IL), can detect a variety of *Candida* and *Aspergillus* spp from whole blood, plasma, or serum using the technique of surface-enhanced resonance Raman spectroscopy.[69] Finally, T2 Biosystems (Lexington, MA) is also in development, and uses nanotechnology with a magnetic biosensor platform for detection of *Candida* from whole blood.[70] Other investigators and groups are developing and testing RNA-based methods for detection of fungi from blood cultures.[71]

Matrix-assisted laser desorption ionization–time-of-flight (MALDI-TOF) MS has also been evaluated in identification of yeasts from plated isolates and directly from positive blood-culture broths.[72,73] Although detection rates from plated isolates of yeasts are high, ranging from 85% to 96%, lower detection rates have been reported for yeast isolates directly from positive blood-culture bottles. Identification of molds using MALDI-TOF MS technology remains challenging, although some investigators have made progress in the identification of dermatophytes and fungi of the order Mucorales, in particular.[74,75]

Performance Characteristics

Certain issues with molecular testing for fungal diagnosis discourage its widespread use and application, such as the lack of standardization between assays (especially preanalytical steps) and other factors, including different extraction methods, timing of testing, volume used, and type of specimen tested. The high sensitivity of many of these platforms may detect mere colonization, rather than infection or disease, which could be particularly problematic for BAL fluid owing to the presence of colonization with *Aspergillus* conidia. In addition, Sampsonas and colleagues[76] underline the importance of the standardized sample-collection technique of BAL fluid as the clinical effectiveness of newer diagnostic techniques become available. These investigators assessed the adoption of a standardized protocol for BAL collection, and reported that physician adherence to the standardized protocol was greater than 90%. Furthermore, they postulate that adoption of a standardized protocol may facilitate comparisons of biomarkers and/or molecular testing on BAL fluid across studies.

The effect of antifungal therapy on performance characteristics of molecular assays has been assessed. In the study by Nguyen and colleagues,[62] in which the Viracor-IBT *Candida* real-time PCR assay was compared with Fungitell BDG on 55 prospectively identified patients with IC, PCR sensitivity was not affected by antifungal therapy. In another study of 226 patients with hematologic malignancies at high risk for IA (48 with proven/probable IA), therapy with 2 or more antifungals before BAL sampling significantly decreased sensitivity of a nested *Aspergillus* PCR assay.[77] However, the number of days of antifungal use before BAL sampling was not recorded in this study.

A meta-analysis of the accuracy of PCR in the diagnosis of IC directly from blood samples included 54 studies with more than 4600 patients, 963 of whom were cases of proven/probable or possible IC.[78] The investigators reported 100% sensitivity and specificity for whole blood samples for detection of candidemia when the control group included patients at risk for sepsis but who did not have candidemia. Blood cultures among proven/probable IC cases showed positivity rates of only 38%. It was concluded from this meta-analysis that direct PCR of blood samples demonstrated good sensitivity and specificity overall. In addition, serial sampling increased the specificity of testing. PCR results preceded candidemia or clinical signs of IC in 7 of 54 studies, ranging from 1 day to 4 weeks.

Outcomes Data and Clinical Guidelines

Outcomes data for molecular testing for IFI are growing, but these have not yet provided enough evidence for the inclusion of molecular diagnostics in clinical guidelines.

The IDSA has not incorporated molecular testing in their guidelines; likewise, the EORTC/MSG consensus group determined that nucleic acid–based test validations have not been adequately assessed for formal inclusion.[27] However, guidelines from the AGIHO note that molecular diagnostic testing should be performed in combination with other nonculture techniques, such as antigen detection.[28] AGIHO remarks that molecular diagnostic tools are promising and display high sensitivity and specificity, but are as yet not mandatory, because of poor standardization and poor availability. Given this standardization issue, the European *Aspergillus* PCR Initiative is attempting to address methodological issues with PCR, such as optimal extraction and primer design, as well as proper specimen choice.[79]

Some outcomes studies have provided evidence for use of certain molecular testing platforms for IFI diagnosis. Forrest and colleagues[80] reported significant reduction in caspofungin use with use of the *C albicans* PNA FISH test from 31 *C albicans*–positive blood cultures, resulting in cost savings of $1729 per patient. These savings were obtained while batch testing once per day, and could presumably be larger if more frequent testing were performed. In another study, the investigators predicted a saving of $1837 per treated patient when comparing use of the *C albicans* PNA FISH test performed on blood flagged as positive with yeast, with the rapid chromogenic *C albicans* screen test usually performed 2 days after flagging of the bottle and growth of the isolate in culture.[81] Most of the savings were realized through lower costs of antifungal drugs, when antifungal therapy was narrowed because of *C albicans* diagnosis.

Clinical outcomes data are sparse. Various studies using in-house PCR tests for *Aspergillus* and/or *Candida* PCR have demonstrated no improvement in clinical outcome.[82,83] One study of 107 patients with hematologic malignancies showed some improvement in clinical outcome, probably related to earlier diagnosis, when an in-house *Aspergillus* nested PCR from BAL fluid was used.[84] The mortality rate for patients diagnosed with PCR was 35.6%, as opposed to the higher 80% mortality rate of traditionally diagnosed cases. A randomized controlled trial of in-house *Aspergillus* and *Candida* PCR performed on whole blood specimens was designed to compare survival between allogenic stem cell transplant (allo-SCT) recipients who received empiric antifungal treatment and those who received empiric plus PCR-based antifungal treatment.[85] The investigators demonstrated better survival at day 30 of the allo-SCT group, whose treatment decisions were in part based on PCR, but survival did not differ by day 100.

Summary

Molecular platforms offer promise in their ability to provide rapid results, a wide range of testable specimen types, and unique species identification. The multiplex aspect of some platforms for simultaneous detection of pathogens is especially attractive. Some platforms are designed with custom primer sets, which allow various institutions to tailor testing to their patient population. Other platforms may design targets that identify to the species level or offer broad-range targets. The real-time aspect of many of the aforementioned platforms aids in early diagnosis, allowing clinicians to narrow antifungal therapy. Future studies should assess the ability of these systems to be run directly from whole blood specimens, as opposed to blood-culture bottles that flag positive for growth, as this would narrow the time to appropriate, targeted antifungal therapy. The potential for quantitation, although not yet reached, may in future allow clinicians the opportunity to follow burden and/or progression of disease. However, certain molecular platforms are expensive, and require expertise that may not be available in general clinical microbiology laboratories.

ROLE OF BIOMARKERS AND MOLECULAR DIAGNOSTICS IN 2012 FUNGAL MENINGITIS OUTBREAK

In September 2012, a rare fungal meningitis complication associated with contaminated steroid injections for the treatment of chronic pain was reported.[86] The methylprednisolone used for injection was purchased from a single compounding pharmacy. *Exserohilum rostratum* fungal infections were noted in many patients who received this steroid. Because of the low yield of traditional diagnostic methods such as culture, molecular testing was performed by the Centers for Disease Control and Prevention (CDC) on joint fluid and CSF from 386 case patients using PCR with broad-range internal transcribed spacer fungal primers.[87] Of the case patients, 111 had evidence of fungus documented by PCR, culture, and/or histopathology. Seventy-six of 111 (68%) were diagnosed by PCR alone; 13 were diagnosed by culture alone; and 22 were documented by more than 1 technique. The broad-range PCR used in this multistate outbreak allowed for early and sensitive diagnosis, aiding in the rapid public health response and prompt recall of the contaminated product. Lyons and colleagues[88] reported their use of BDG in a recent case series of 5 patients who were potentially exposed to contaminated drugs during this outbreak. Three patients were positive for BDG in the CSF (range <39 to 2396 pg/mL), whereas all cases were negative by culture. Three cases were negative by PCR performed on CSF at the CDC; however, the PCRs were performed on previous CSF samples. The investigators concluded that BDG might be a useful adjunct to diagnosis in such cases.

MOLECULAR DIAGNOSTICS ON FORMALIN-FIXED PARAFFIN-EMBEDDED TISSUES

Development of molecular assays for use on formalin-fixed, paraffin-embedded (FFPE) tissue is also needed, because clinical microbiology laboratories sometimes do not receive fresh specimens for culture. In such cases, microbiologists and clinicians must rely on limited diagnosis of morphologic tissue from histopathology. Although special stains such as Fontana Masson may narrow the differential diagnosis in FFPE tissue, several fungal organisms closely resemble each other in tissue sections.[89] For instance, *Scedosporium* spp, *Fusarium* spp, and occasionally certain yeast such as *Candida* spp, may form hyphae that resemble *Aspergillus* hyphal forms in tissue. It is important to differentiate as much as possible among these fungi, as antifungal resistance varies widely by fungus. Molecular testing, such as quantitative real-time PCR with sequencing and ribosomal RNA FISH, is currently being developed for use on FFPE.[90] Rickerts and colleagues[91] reported on the use of FISH and broad-range PCR followed by sequencing on a collection of 40 FFPE tissue samples primarily from lung, gastrointestinal tract, and sinus from 33 patients with proven invasive fungal disease. PCR followed by sequencing identified 28 of 40 samples (70%), with the best performance for yeast and molds with septate hyphae. FISH yielded correct results in 19 of 40 samples (47.5%), with better performance for yeast than molds in general. The hybridization readings for FISH were hampered by autofluorescence of hyphae and necrotic backgrounds, which are a common problem in biopsy specimens. In addition, the study was limited by culture results being available for only 14 samples, of which 5 were culture-proven mucormycoses and were missed by sequencing. Another group of researchers evaluated 5 different commercial DNA extraction kits and 3 different panfungal PCR assays on 81 archived FFPE tissues positive by the Gomori methenamine silver (GMS) stain, and noted PCR efficiency ranging from 58% to 93%.[92] Most methods report amplification rates ranging from 60% to 80% from FFPE; therefore, more work is needed in this area.

FUTURE DIRECTIONS

As more data are gathered on the performance characteristics and effectiveness of molecular fungal testing, various organizations may in the future be able to address the appropriateness of use of such testing in their guidelines. At present, many molecular testing platforms are available only in research settings and are not applicable for use in clinical microbiology laboratories. However, there is much growth in the area of molecular diagnostics for IFI. More clinical outcome data are needed on both biomarker and molecular testing, and larger prospective comparative studies including biomarkers and molecular testing are needed. None of the biomarkers stand on their own as sole diagnostic entities, but the results should be combined with other data. Although almost all molecular assays are qualitative in nature, there may be a role for the use of quantitative molecular testing to guide diagnosis in specimens wherein colonization is possible, and to guide clinicians in patient management when considering disease progression. Given the increasing antifungal resistance of many *Candida* spp and other fungi, testing for drug-resistance markers would greatly aid clinicians in antifungal choices.

REFERENCES

1. Klutts JS, Robinson-Dunn B. A critical appraisal of the role of the clinical microbiology laboratory in diagnosis of invasive fungal infections. J Clin Microbiol 2011;49:S39–42.
2. Berenguer J, Buck M, Witebsky F, et al. Lysis-centrifugation blood cultures in the detection of tissue-proven invasive candidiasis. Diagn Microbiol Infect Dis 1993; 17:103–9.
3. Biomarkers Definitions Working Group. Biomarkers and surrogate endpoints: preferred definitions and conceptual framework. Clin Pharmacol Ther 2001;69: 89–95.
4. Stynen D, Sarfati J, Goris A, et al. Rat monoclonal antibodies against *Aspergillus* galactomannan. Infect Immun 1992;60:2237–45.
5. Petraitiene R, Petraitis V, Groll AH, et al. Antifungal activity and pharmacokinetics of posaconazole (SCH 56592) in treatment and prevention of experimental invasive pulmonary aspergillosis: correlation with galactomannan antigenemia. Antimicrob Agents Chemother 2001;45:857–69.
6. Miceli MH, Grazziutti ML, Woods G, et al. Strong correlation between serum *Aspergillus* galactomannan index and outcome of aspergillosis in patients with hematological cancer: clinical and research implications. Clin Infect Dis 2008;46:1412–22.
7. Anaissie EJ. Trial design for mold-active agents: time to break the mold—aspergillosis in neutropenic adults. Clin Infect Dis 2007;44:1298–306.
8. Klont RR, Mennink-Kersten MA, Verweij PE. Utility of *Aspergillus* antigen detection in specimens other than serum specimens. Clin Infect Dis 2004;39: 1467–74.
9. Lengerova M, Kocmanova I, Racil Z, et al. Detection and measurement of fungal burden in a guinea pig model of invasive pulmonary aspergillosis by novel quantitative nested real-time PCR compared with galactomannan and (1,3)-β-D-glucan detection. J Clin Microbiol 2012;50:602–8.
10. Husain S, Clancy CJ, Nguyen MH, et al. Performance characteristics of the Platelia *Aspergillus* enzyme immunoassay for detection of *Aspergillus* galactomannan antigen in bronchoalveolar lavage fluid. Clin Vaccine Immunol 2008; 15:1760–3.

11. Becker MJ, Lugtenburg EJ, Cornelissen JJ, et al. Galactomannan detection in computerized tomography-based broncho-alveolar lavage fluid and serum in haematological patients at risk for invasive pulmonary aspergillosis. Br J Haematol 2003;121:448–57.

12. Meersseman W, Lagrou K, Maertens J, et al. Galactomannan in bronchoalveolar lavage fluid: a tool for diagnosing pulmonary aspergillosis in intensive care unit patients. Am J Respir Crit Care Med 2008;177:27–34.

13. Oz Y, Kiraz N. Diagnostic methods for fungal infections in pediatric patients: microbiological, serological and molecular methods. Expert Rev Anti Infect Ther 2011;9:289–98.

14. Verweij PE, Weemaes CM, Curfs JH, et al. Failure to detect circulating *Aspergillus* markers in a patient with chronic granulomatous disease and invasive aspergillosis. J Clin Microbiol 2000;38:3900–1.

15. Marr KA, Balajee SA, McLaughlin L, et al. Detection of galactomannan antigenemia by enzyme immunoassay for the diagnosis of invasive aspergillosis: variables that affect performance. J Infect Dis 2004;190:641–9.

16. Sulahian A, Touratier S, Ribaud P. False positive test for *Aspergillus* antigenemia related to concomitant administration of piperacillin and tazobactam. N Engl J Med 2003;349:2366–7.

17. Mennink-Kersten MA, Klont RR, Warris A, et al. Bifidobacterium lipoteichoic acid and false ELISA reactivity in *Aspergillus* antigen detection. Lancet 2004;363: 325–7.

18. Girmenia C, Santilli S, Ballaro D, et al. Enteral nutrition may cause false-positive results of *Aspergillus* galactomannan assay in absence of gastrointestinal diseases. Mycoses 2011;54:e883–4.

19. Petraitiene R, Petraitis V, Witt JR, et al. Galactomannan antigenemia after infusion of gluconate-containing Plasma-Lyte. J Clin Microbiol 2011;49:4330–2.

20. Mikulska M, Furfaro E, Del Bono V, et al. Galactomannan testing might be useful for early diagnosis of fusariosis. Diagn Microbiol Infect Dis 2012;72:367–9.

21. Van den Bossche D, De Bel A, Hendrickx M, et al. Galactomannan enzymatic immunoassay cross-reactivity caused by *Prototheca* species. J Clin Microbiol 2012;50:3371–3.

22. Vergidis P, Walker RC, Kaul DR, et al. False-positive *Aspergillus* galactomannan assay in solid organ transplant recipients with histoplasmosis. Transpl Infect Dis 2012;4:213–7.

23. Van der Veer J, Lewis RJ, Emtiazjoo AM, et al. Cross-reactivity in the Platelia *Aspergillus* enzyme immunoassay caused by blastomycosis. Med Mycol 2012;50: 396–8.

24. Mikulska M, Furfaro E, Del Bono V, et al. Piperacillin/tazobactam (Tazocin) seems to be no longer responsible for false-positive results of the galactomannan assay. J Antimicrob Chemother 2012;67:1746–8.

25. D'Haese J, Theunissen K, Vermeulen E, et al. Detection of galactomannan in bronchoalveolar lavage fluid samples of patients at risk for invasive pulmonary aspergillosis: analytical and clinical validity. J Clin Microbiol 2012;50: 1258–63.

26. Maertens J, Maertens V, Theunissen K, et al. Bronchoalveolar lavage fluid galactomannan for the diagnosis of invasive pulmonary aspergillosis in patients with hematologic diseases. Clin Infect Dis 2009;49:1688–93.

27. De Pauw B, Walsh TJ, Donnelly JP, et al. Revised definitions of invasive fungal disease from the European Organization for Research and Treatment of Cancer/ Invasive Fungal Infections Cooperative Group and the National Institute of

Allergy and Infectious Diseases Mycoses Study Group (EORTC/MSG) Consensus Group. Clin Infect Dis 2008;46:1813–21.

28. Ruhnke M, Bohme A, Buchheidt D, et al. Diagnosis of invasive fungal infections in hematology and oncology- guidelines from the Infectious Diseases Working Party in Haematology and Oncology of the German Society for Haematology and Oncology (AGIHO). Ann Oncol 2012;23:823–33.

29. Walsh TJ, Anaissie EJ, Denning DW, et al. Treatment of aspergillosis: clinical practice guidelines of the Infectious Diseases Society of America. Clin Infect Dis 2008;46:327–60.

30. Chen SC, Kontoyiannis DP. New molecular and surrogate biomarker-based tests in the diagnosis of bacterial and fungal infection in febrile neutropenic patients. Curr Opin Infect Dis 2010;23:567–77.

31. Lengerova M, Kocmanova I, Hrncirova K, et al. Comparison of quantitative real-time PCR (Q-RT-PCR), galactomannan enzyme immunoassay (GM) and 1,3-beta-D-glucan detection (BG) in a guinea pig model of invasive aspergillosis. Abstract M-1696a. Abstracts of the 49th Interscience Conference on Antimicrobial Agents and Chemotherapy, San Francisco, CA, September, 2009. In: Patterson TF. Clinical utility and development of biomarkers in invasive aspergillosis. Trans Am Clin Climatol Assoc 2011;122:174–83.

32. Nouer SA, Nucci M, Kumar NS, et al. Earlier response assessment in invasive aspergillosis based on the kinetics of serum *Aspergillus* galactomannan: proposal for a new definition. Clin Infect Dis 2011;53:671–6.

33. Segal BH, Herbrecht R, Stevens DA, et al. Defining responses to therapy and study outcomes in clinical trials of invasive fungal diseases: Mycoses Study Group and European Organization for Research and Treatment of Cancer consensus criteria. Clin Infect Dis 2008;47:674–83.

34. Girouard G, Lachance C, Pelletier R. Observations on (1-3)-β-D-glucan detection as a diagnostic tool in endemic mycosis caused by *Histoplasma* or *Blastomyces*. J Med Microbiol 2007;56:1001–2.

35. Obayashi T, Yoshida M, Tamura H, et al. Determination of plasma $(1\rightarrow3)$ β-D-glucan: a new diagnostic aid to deep mycosis. J Med Vet Mycol 1992;30:275–80.

36. Lu Y, Chen Y, Guo Y, et al. Diagnosis of invasive fungal disease using serum $(1\rightarrow3)$-β-D-glucan: a bivariate meta-analysis. Intern Med 2011;50:2783–91.

37. Lamoth F, Cruciani M, Mengoli C, et al. β-Glucan antigenemia assay for the diagnosis of invasive fungal infections in patients with hematological malignancies: a systematic review and meta-analysis of cohort studies from the Third European Conference on Infections in Leukemia (ECIL-3). Clin Infect Dis 2012;54:633–43.

38. Fontana C, Gaziano R, Favaro M, et al. (1-3)-β-D-Glucan vs galactomannan antigen in diagnosing invasive fungal infections (IFIs). Open Microbiol J 2012;6:70–3.

39. Pazos C, Ponton J, Del Palacio A. Contribution of $(1\rightarrow3)$-β-D-glucan chromogenic assay to diagnosis and therapeutic monitoring of invasive aspergillosis in neutropenic adult patients: a comparison with serial screening for circulating galactomannan. J Clin Microbiol 2005;43:299–305.

40. Obayashi T. Reappraisal of the serum $(1\rightarrow3)$ β-D-glucan for the diagnosis of invasive fungal infections: a study based on autopsy cases from 6 years. Clin Infect Dis 2008;46:1864–70.

41. Alam FF, Mustafa AS, Khan ZU. Comparative evaluation of (1,3)-β-D-glucan, mannan and anti-mannan antibodies, and *Candida* species-specific snPCR in patients with candidemia. BMC Infect Dis 2007;7:103.

42. Mohr JF, Sims C, Paetznick V, et al. Prospective survey of (1→3) β-D-glucan and its relationship to invasive candidiasis in the surgical intensive care unit setting. J Clin Microbiol 2011;49:58–61.
43. Leon C, Ruiz-Santana S, Saavedra P, et al. Value of β-D-glucan and *Candida albicans* germ tube antibody for discriminating between *Candida* colonization and invasive candidiasis in patients with severe abdominal conditions. Intensive Care Med 2012;38:1315–25.
44. Jaijakul S, Vazquez JA, Swanson RN, et al. (1,3)-β-D-glucan as a prognostic marker of treatment response in invasive candidiasis. Clin Infect Dis 2012;55:521–6.
45. Eggimann P, Marchetti O. Is (1→3)-β-D-glucan the missing link from bedside assessment to pre-emptive therapy of invasive candidiasis? Crit Care 2011;15:1017.
46. Karageorgopoulos DE, Qu JM, Korbila IP, et al. Accuracy of β-D-glucan for the diagnosis of *Pneumocystis jirovecii* pneumonia: a meta-analysis. Clin Microbiol Infect 2013;19:39–49.
47. Egan L, Connolly P, Wheat LJ, et al. Histoplasmosis as a cause for a positive Fungitell (1→3)-β-D-glucan test. Med Mycol 2008;46:93–5.
48. Wingard JR. Have novel serum markers supplanted tissue diagnosis for invasive fungal infections in acute leukemia and transplantation? Best Pract Res Clin Haematol 2012;25:487–91.
49. Ostrosky-Zeichner L. Invasive mycoses: diagnostic challenges. Am J Med 2012;125:S14–24.
50. Mikulska M, Calandra T, Sanguinetti M, et al. The use of mannan antigen and anti-mannan antibodies in the diagnosis of invasive candidiasis: recommendations from the Third European Conference on Infections in Leukemia. Crit Care 2010;14:R222.
51. Pappas PG, Kauffman CA, Andes D, et al. Clinical practice guidelines for the management of candidiasis: 2009 update by the Infectious Diseases Society of America. Clin Infect Dis 2009;48:503–35.
52. Lain A, Elguezabal N, Moragues MD, et al. Contribution of serum biomarkers to the diagnosis of invasive candidiasis. Expert Rev Mol Diagn 2008;8:315–25.
53. Lehtonen L, Anttila VJ, Ruutu T, et al. Diagnosis of disseminated candidiasis by measurement of urine D-arabinitol/L-arabinitol ratio. J Clin Microbiol 1996;34:2175–9.
54. Khot PD, Fredricks DN. PCR-based diagnosis of human fungal infections. Expert Rev Anti Infect Ther 2009;7:1201–21.
55. Hall L, Le Febre KM, Deml SM, et al. Evaluation of the Yeast Traffic Light PNA FISH probes for identification of *Candida* species from positive blood cultures. J Clin Microbiol 2012;50:1446–8.
56. Farina C, Perin S, Andreoni S, et al. Evaluation of the peptide nucleic acid fluorescence in situ hybridization technology for yeast identification directly from positive blood cultures: an Italian experience. Mycoses 2012;55:388–92.
57. Morrell M, Fraser VJ, Kollef MH. Delaying the empiric treatment of *Candida* bloodstream infection until positive blood culture results are obtained: a potential risk factor for hospital mortality. Antimicrob Agents Chemother 2005;49:3640–5.
58. Balada-Llasat J, LaRue H, Kamboj K, et al. Detection of yeasts in blood cultures by the Luminex xTAG fungal assay. J Clin Microbiol 2012;50:492–4.
59. Babady NE, Miranda E, Gilhuley KA. Evaluation of Luminex xTAG fungal analyte-specific reagents for rapid identification of clinically relevant fungi. J Clin Microbiol 2011;49:3777–82.

60. Buelow DR, Gu Z, Walsh TJ, et al. Evaluation of multiplexed PCR and liquid-phase array for identification of respiratory fungal pathogens. Med Mycol 2012;50: 775–80.
61. Luong ML, Clancy CJ, Vadnerkar A, et al. Comparison of an *Aspergillus* real-time polymerase chain reaction assay with galactomannan testing of bronchoalveolar lavage fluid for the diagnosis of invasive pulmonary aspergillosis in lung transplant recipients. Clin Infect Dis 2011;52:1218–26.
62. Nguyen MH, Wissel MC, Shields RK, et al. Performance of *Candida* real-time polymerase chain reaction, β-D-glucan assay, and blood cultures in the diagnosis of invasive candidiasis. Clin Infect Dis 2012;54:1240–8.
63. Gu Z, Hall TA, Frinder M, et al. Evaluation of repetitive sequence PCR and PCR-mass spectrometry for the identification of clinically relevant *Candida* species. Med Mycol 2012;50:259–65.
64. White PL, Perry MD, Moody A, et al. Evaluation of analytical and preliminary clinical performance of Myconostica MycAssay *Aspergillus* when testing serum specimens for diagnosis of invasive aspergillosis. J Clin Microbiol 2011;49:2169–74.
65. Torelli R, Sanguinetti M, Moody A, et al. Diagnosis of invasive aspergillosis by a commercial real-time PCR assay for *Aspergillus* DNA in bronchoalveolar lavage fluid samples from high-risk patients compared to galactomannan enzyme immunoassay. J Clin Microbiol 2011;49:4273–8.
66. Lucignano B, Ranno S, Liesenfeld O, et al. Multiplex PCR allows rapid and accurate diagnosis of bloodstream infections in newborns and children with suspected sepsis. J Clin Microbiol 2011;49:2252–8.
67. Lau A, Halliday C, Chen SC, et al. Comparison of whole blood, serum, and plasma for early detection of candidemia by multiplex-tandem PCR. J Clin Microbiol 2010;48:811–6.
68. Great Basin Corporation. Available at: http://www.gbscience.com/. Accessed January 14, 2013.
69. RenDx Fungiplex panel. Available at: http://www.renishawdiagnostics.com/en/invasive-fungal-infection–17069. Accessed January 20, 2013.
70. T2 Biosystems. Available at: http://www.t2biosystems.com/Site/AboutUs/tabid/57/Default.aspx. Accessed January 20, 2013.
71. Zhao Y, Park S, Kreiswirth BN, et al. Rapid real-time nucleic acid sequence-based amplification-molecular beacon platform to detect fungal and bacterial bloodstream infections. J Clin Microbiol 2009;47:2067–78.
72. Dhiman N, Hall L, Wohlfiel SL, et al. Performance and cost analysis of matrix-assisted laser desorption ionization-time of flight mass spectrometry for routine identification of yeast. J Clin Microbiol 2011;49:1614–6.
73. Yan Y, He Y, Maier T, et al. Improved identification of yeast species directly from positive blood culture media by combining Sepsityper specimen processing and Microflex analysis with the matrix-assisted laser desorption ionization Biotyper system. J Clin Microbiol 2011;49:2528–32.
74. Alshawa K, Beretti J, Lacroix C, et al. Successful identification of clinical dermatophyte and *Neoscytalidium* species by matrix-assisted laser desorption ionization -time of flight mass spectrometry. J Clin Microbiol 2012;50:2277–81.
75. Schrodl W, Heydel T, Schwartze VU, et al. Direct analysis and identification of pathogenic *Lichtheimia* species by matrix-assisted laser desorption ionization time of flight analyzer-mediated mass spectrometry. J Clin Microbiol 2012;50:419–27.
76. Sampsonas F, Kontoyiannis DP, Dickey BF, et al. Performance of a standardized bronchoalveolar lavage protocol in a comprehensive cancer center: a prospective 2-year study. Cancer 2011;117:3424–33.

77. Reinwald M, Hummel M, Kovalevskaya E, et al. Therapy with antifungals decreases the diagnostic performance of PCR for diagnosing invasive aspergillosis in bronchoalveolar lavage samples of patients with haematological malignancies. J Antimicrob Chemother 2012;64:2260–7.
78. Avni T, Leibovici L, Paul M. PCR diagnosis of invasive candidiasis: systematic review and meta-analysis. J Clin Microbiol 2011;49:665–70.
79. White PL, Bretagne S, Klingspor L, et al. Aspergillus PCR: one step closer to standardization. J Clin Microbiol 2010;48:1231–40.
80. Forrest GN, Mankes K, Jabra-Rizk MA, et al. Peptide nucleic acid fluorescence in situ hybridization-based identification of Candida albicans and its impact on mortality and antifungal therapy costs. J Clin Microbiol 2006;44:3381–3.
81. Alexander BD, Ashley ED, Reller LB, et al. Cost savings with implementation of PNA FISH testing for identification of Candida albicans in blood cultures. Diagn Microbiol Infect Dis 2006;54:277–82.
82. Bergeron A, Porcher R, Menotti J, et al. Prospective evaluation of clinical and biological markers to predict the outcome of invasive pulmonary aspergillosis in hematological patients. J Clin Microbiol 2012;50:823–30.
83. Blennow O, Remberger M, Klingspor L, et al. Randomized PCR-based therapy and risk factors for invasive fungal infection following reduced-intensity conditioning and hematopoietic SCT. Bone Marrow Transplant 2010;45:17108.
84. Hardak E, Yigla M, Avivi I, et al. Impact of PCR-based diagnosis of invasive pulmonary aspergillosis on clinical outcome. Bone Marrow Transplant 2009;44: 595–9.
85. Hebart H, Klingspor L, Klingebiel T, et al. A prospective randomized controlled trial comparing PCR-based and empirical treatment with liposomal amphotericin B in patients after allo-SCT. Bone Marrow Transplant 2009;43:553–61.
86. Smith RM, Schaefer MK, Kainer MA, et al. Fungal infections associated with contaminated methylprednisolone injections—preliminary report. N Engl J Med 2012. [Epub ahead of print]. http://dx.doi.org/10.1056/NEJMoa1213978.
87. Balajee SA, Kano R, Baddley JW, et al. Molecular identification of Aspergillus species collected for the transplant-associated infection surveillance network. J Clin Microbiol 2009;47:3138–41.
88. Lyons JL, Roos KL, Marr KA, et al. Cerebrospinal fluid (1,3) β-D-glucan detection as an aid to diagnose iatrogenic fungal meningitis. J Clin Microbiol 2013. [Epub ahead of print]. http://dx.doi.org/10.1128/JCM.00061-13.
89. Chandler FW, Watts JC. Pathologic diagnosis of fungal infections. Chicago: ASCP Press; 1987.
90. Shinozaki M, Okubo Y, Sasai D, et al. Development and evaluation of nucleic acid-based techniques for an auxiliary diagnosis of invasive fungal infections in formalin-fixed and paraffin-embedded (FFPE) tissues. Med Mycol J 2012; 53:241–5.
91. Rickerts V, Khot PD, Myerson D, et al. Comparison of quantitative real time PCR with sequencing and ribosomal RNA-FISH for the identification of fungi in formalin fixed, paraffin-embedded tissue specimens. BMC Infect Dis 2011;11:202.
92. Munoz-Cadavid C, Rudd S, Zaki SR, et al. Improving molecular detection of fungal DNA in formalin-fixed paraffin-embedded tissues: comparison of five tissue DNA extraction methods using panfungal PCR. J Clin Microbiol 2010;48: 2147–53.

Advanced Techniques for Detection and Identification of Microbial Agents of Gastroenteritis

Sherry A. Dunbar, PhD[a], Hongwei Zhang, MD, PhD[a],
Yi-Wei Tang, MD, PhD[b],*

KEYWORDS

- Gastroenteritis • *Clostridium difficile* • Multiplex polymerase chain reaction
- Suspension array • Next-generation sequencing

KEY POINTS

- Current laboratory methods for diagnosis of gastroenteritis are laborious, have long turnaround times, and can be insensitive.
- Advancements in genomic and proteomic technologies have provided a variety of tools that are being adopted for clinical diagnostics.
- Several nucleic acid amplification–based assays have already been adopted for in vitro diagnostic use while next-generation sequencing is being explored for clinical microbiology applications, with cutting-edge proteomic technologies not far behind.
- These technologies are predicted to provide rapid and accurate diagnosis of infectious gastroenteritis, resulting in improved patient care.

INTRODUCTION

The role of diagnostic microbiology in gastroenterology is to determine whether suspected pathogenic microorganisms are present in test specimens collected from stool, blood, tissue, and other secretions of patients, and, if present, to identify them.[1,2] The gastrointestinal system, in health or disease, is a microbial milieu of unsurpassed variety and complexity. It varies in degree of colonization from the "buggiest" parties

Funding: The study was supported in part by a clinical trial contract between the Vanderbilt University Medical Center and the Luminex Corporation awarded to Yi-Wei Tang (VUMC 38228).

Disclosure: Sherry A. Dunbar and Hongwei Zhang are employees of Luminex Corporation, the commercial manufacturer of the xTAG Gastrointestinal Pathogen Panel.

[a] Luminex Corporation, 12212 Technology Boulevard, Austin, TX 78727, USA; [b] Clinical Microbiology Service, Department of Laboratory Medicine, Memorial Sloan-Kettering Cancer Center, 1275 York Avenue, S428, New York, NY 10065, USA
* Corresponding author.
E-mail address: tangy@mskcc.org

Clin Lab Med 33 (2013) 527–552
http://dx.doi.org/10.1016/j.cll.2013.03.003
0272-2712/13/$ – see front matter © 2013 Elsevier Inc. All rights reserved.

of the body, at both ends, to the nearly sterile environment of the small intestine and accessory glands. A community of at least 400 distinct species of bacteria, fungi, and protozoa has been identified in the resident flora of the normal gastrointestinal tract, and many more continue to be discovered by molecular approaches, especially next-generation sequencing (NGS) techniques.[3,4] The detection and differentiation of pathogenic among this milieu of commensal flora represents a major challenge to the clinical laboratory.[5]

Infectious diarrhea continues to be a worldwide problem and accounts for more than 2 million deaths annually.[6–8] For example, in the United States it is estimated that there are between 211 and 375 million episodes of acute diarrhea each year, and such episodes are responsible for more than 900,000 hospitalizations and 6000 deaths annually.[9,10] In addition to *Salmonella*, *Shigella*, and enterohemorrhagic *Escherichia coli* (EHEC), the list of potential enteric bacterial pathogens has been expanded to include microorganisms such as *Campylobacter jejuni*, *Aeromonas hydrophila*, *Yersinia enterocolitica*, and *Vibrio* species. *Clostridium difficile* is one of the leading causes of infectious antibiotic-associated diarrhea and pseudomembranous colitis worldwide. This fact is illustrated by the increased incidence and severity of *C difficile* infection, suggesting the emergence of a new hypervirulent strain.[11] Acute viral gastroenteritis is the second most common infectious disease worldwide.[8,12] Known enteric viral pathogens include rotavirus, norovirus, astrovirus, and adenovirus serotypes 40 and 41.[13–15] In recent years the number of reported gastroenteritis outbreaks of suspected viral etiology has increased, hence the need for rapid, sensitive, and reliable diagnostic assays.[14,15] Other parasites (*Giardia*, *Entamoeba histolytica*, and *Cryptosporidium*) have been reported to be pathogens causing gastroenteritis.[16,17]

Timely and accurate identification of suspected pathogens that are present in the stool specimens from patients with signs and symptoms of gastroenteritis is still a challenge in the clinical laboratory. Microscopic examination is conventionally required for parasite identification. An ova and parasite (O&P) examination for identification of the parasite form requires a trained technologist. However, in some cases microscopic examination is limited in distinguishing species. For example, one could not distinguish *E histolytica* (pathogenic species) from other nonpathogenic species, such as *Entamoeba dispar*.

Examination by electron microscopy (EM) can be used for a range of viruses, including adenovirus, norovirus, and rotavirus, but the method is cumbersome and requires significant expertise. EM was initially the only method for norovirus diagnosis, but its use has been limited owing to its low sensitivity and specificity. Various stool antigen tests have been available for the detection of different gastroenteritis pathogens. Although most antigen tests are simple and rapid, they usually lack sensitivity and specificity. Several comparison studies have shown that nonmolecular tests, such as the glutamate dehydrogenase (GDH) antigen test and enzyme immunoassay (EIA) for toxins A and B, are either less sensitive or less specific than molecular testing for *C difficile* infection detection.[18–20]

Bacterial stool cultures remain the mainstay of the laboratory evaluation of diarrheal illnesses. Selective agars are used to facilitate the isolation of suspicious enteric bacterial pathogens. Pure cultures obtained subsequently permit characterization and identification by morphologic and biochemical characteristics. These conventional methods, however, are time consuming, labor intensive, and require experienced clinical microbiologists. Identification and confirmation of suspicious colonies is highly nonspecific, and places a heavy burden on the laboratory in terms of biochemical and serologic testing.[21–23] Stool culture–based enteric bacterial pathogen detection and identification is a time-consuming process, with an estimated cost of $952 to $1200 per positive culture.[21-25] Current stool-culture procedures for the detection and identification of enteric bacterial pathogens require 3 to 5 days.

Recent advancements in genomic and proteomic techniques, as well as sample processing and extraction techniques, have enabled increased adoption of molecular tests for gastrointestinal pathogens by clinical laboratories.[2,26] **Table 1** provides an overview and comparison of conventional and molecular methods being used in the detection and identification of microbial pathogens. The next sections introduce and emphasize the advanced techniques developed in the past 25 years or so for laboratory diagnosis and monitoring of gastrointestinal tract infections. For the convenience of the reader, these techniques are divided into genomic and proteomic categories.

Table 1
Comparison of laboratory methods for detection and identification of microbial pathogens causing gastroenteritis

Testing Method	Current Applicability[a]	Pathogen Coverage	Advantages	Disadvantages
Electron microscopy	D	Viruses, such as noroviruses	Rapid	Limited application; subjective; less specific
Culture	A	Bacteria, such as *Salmonella* and *Shigella*	Gold standard; isolates used for antimicrobial susceptibility testing	Long TAT and HOT; sensitivity varies
Rapid antigen	B	A range of viruses and certain bacteria and toxins	Simple; rapid	Sensitivity varies; one antigen per test
Genomic assay, monoplex	A	*C difficile*	High sensitivity; short TAT	Inhibitor-related false negative; not for test of cure
Genomic assay, multiplex	A–C	Range of pathogens of interest	High sensitivity and specificity; one test provides multiple answers	Sensitivity for each pathogen may vary; inhibitor-related false negative
Genomic assay, NGS	D	Range of pathogens and commensals	Quantitative detection and identification of all existing microbials	Sensitivity may be low; undetermined clinical relevance
Proteomic assays	C–D	Range of pathogens of interest	Rapid; function correlation	Sensitivity may vary

Abbreviations: HOT, hands-on time; NGS, next-generation sequencing; TAT, test turnaround time.
[a] A, assays routinely used in clinical diagnosis; B, assays routinely used in clinical diagnosis with limited performance; C, assays with potential to be used in clinical diagnosis; D, assays available in research use only and not available in clinical diagnosis.

GENOMIC ASSAYS
Monoplex Molecular Assays

Numerous laboratory-developed tests (LDT) using molecular technologies have been at the forefront of an effort to implement more rapid and sensitive detection methods. The first real-time polymerase chain reaction (PCR) assay for the detection of *C difficile* was published in 2003 by Bélanger and colleagues,[27] stating that it is rapid (approximately 1 hour), sensitive, and specific, and allows detection of *C difficile* directly from feces samples. Several molecular diagnostic tests, including conventional and real-time PCR, have been developed for the detection and differentiation of *E histolytica*, *E dispar*, and *Entamoeba moshkovskii* in clinical samples.[28] In a recent review on norovirus diagnostics, it was noted that molecular testing provides high sensitivity and overall accuracy for norovirus detection.[29] Highly sensitive reverse transcription (RT)-PCR assays for norovirus have been under development by laboratories since 2003.[30,31]

In the past few years, commercially available molecular tests cleared by the Food and Drug Administration (FDA) for toxigenic *C difficile* detection have been implemented in routine diagnostic use. As of December 2012, 8 molecular assays for the detection of *C difficile* have received FDA clearance for in vitro diagnostic (IVD) use: (1) BD GeneOhm Cdiff Assay (cleared in January 2009); (2) Hologic Prodesse ProGastro Cd assay (cleared in April 2009); (3) Cepheid Xpert *C difficile* assay (cleared in June 2009) and Xpert*C difficile*/Epi (cleared in April 2011); (4) Meridian Bioscience Illumigene *C difficile* assay (cleared in July 2010); (5) Great Basin Corporation Portrait Toxigenic *C difficile* Assay (cleared in February 2012); (6) Quest Diagnostics Simplexa *C difficile* Universal Direct Test (cleared in April, 2012); (7) Nanosphere Verigene *C difficile* Test (cleared in December 2012); and (8) Quidel AmpliVue *C difficile* Test (cleared in December 2012). The reader is referred to a recent review on the applications and key features of the first 4 assays.[32] **Table 2** summarizes the key features of the tests. Here an overview is provided of the testing principles and overall performance of these 8 molecular tests.

The BD GeneOhm Cdiff Assay is a real-time PCR-based in vitro diagnostic test for the detection of the *C difficile* toxin B gene (*tcdB*) in human liquid or soft stool specimens from patients suspected of having *C difficile*–associated disease (CDAD). The assay uses molecular beacon technology whereby the amplified DNA target is detected with a molecular beacon, a hairpin-forming single-stranded oligonucleotide labeled at one end with a quencher and at the other end with a fluorescent reporter dye (fluorophore). In the absence of the target nucleic acid sequence, the fluorescence is quenched. The presence of the targeted nucleic acid sequence results in beacon/target hybridization and, consequently, emission of fluorescence. The assay is run on a Smart-Cycler thermocycler, and the SmartCycler DX software (Cepheid, Sunnyvale, CA) provides the diagnostic result. The established sensitivity, specificity, and positive and negative predictive values compared with the Wampole *C difficile* Toxin B test from TechLab (Blacksburg, VA) are 90.9% (40/44), 95.2% (340/357), 70.2% (40/57), and 98.8% (340/344), respectively. When compared with toxigenic culture, the sensitivity, specificity, and positive and negative predictive values are 83.6%, 98.2%, 89.5%, and 97.1%, respectively.[33]

The Prodesse ProGastro Cd assay (Hologic, Inc, Bedford, MA) is a real-time TaqMan assay targeting *tcdB* only. This assay requires a sample processing and extraction step. The stool sample is diluted in Stool Transport and Recovery buffer. On centrifugation, the internal control is added, and nucleic acids from the sample are extracted and purified using the NucliSENS easyMAG automated extractor

Table 2
Overview of the 8 FDA-cleared C difficile molecular assays

Assay	GeneOhm Cdiff Assay	ProGastro Cd Assay	Xpert C difficile and C difficile/Epi	Illumigene C difficile	Portrait Toxigenic C difficile Assay	Simplexa C difficile Universal Direct Test	Verigene C difficile Test	AmpliVue C difficile
Company	BD	GenProbe/Prodesse	Cepheid	Meridian	Great Basin	Quest	Nanosphere	Quidel/BioHelix
Target gene	tcdB	tcdB	tcdB, cdtA and cdtB tcdC gene single-base deletion	tcdA	tcdB	tcdB	tcdA, tcdB, tcdC mutation and cdtA	tcdA
Sample processing	Heat lysis	With S.T.A.R. buffer	Closed system (cartridge based)	Heat lysis	Close-in system	Heat lysis	Close-in system (cartridge based)	Heat lysis
Nucleic acid extraction	No	easyMAG	Close-in system (cartridge based)	No	Close-in system	No	Close-in system (cartridge based)	No
Internal control	Yes	Yes	Yes	Yes	Yes	Yes	Yes	Yes
Test principle	Real-time PCR (Molecular Beacons)	Real-time PCR (TaqMan)	Real-time PCR (TaqMan)	LAMP	Isothermal amplification	Real-time PCR (Scorpion)	Gold nanoparticles for nucleic acid detection	Isothermal amplification
Amplification	SmartCycler	SmartCycler	GeneXpert	Heating block	Portrait Analyzer	3M Integrated Cycler	No	Heating block
Detection	SmartCycler DX software	SmartCycler DX software	GeneXpert	Illumipro-10 Incubator/Reader	Portrait Analyzer Chip-based	3M Integrated Cycler	Verigene Processor SP and Reader	Detection cassette
Turnaround time	2 h	3 h	45 min to 1 h	~1 h	~1.5 h	~1 h	~2 h	~1.5 h
Batch/random access	Batch	Batch	Random access	Random access	Random access	Batch	Limited random access (4/test)	Batched amplification

Abbreviations: LAMP, loop-mediated isothermal amplification; S.T.A.R., stool transport and recovery buffer.

(bioMerieux, Marcy l'Etoile, France). The nucleic acids are added to *C diff* Mix for PCR amplification and detection using specific oligonucleotide primers and probes targeting the *tcdB* gene of toxigenic strains of *C difficile*. The probes are dual-labeled with a reporter dye attached to the 5′-end and a quencher dye attached to the 3′-end. If the target nucleic acid sequence is present, the primers and probes anneal to the template followed by primer extension and template amplification. The 5′-3′ exonuclease activity of *Taq* polymerase cleaves the probe, separating the reporter dye from the quencher and generating an increase in fluorescent signal. The amount of fluorescence at any given cycle depends on the amount of amplification product present. When compared with the Wampole *C difficile* Toxin B TOX-B test, the Prodesse ProGastro Cd had sensitivity, specificity, and positive and negative predictive values of 83.3%, 95.6%, 69.4%, and 98%, respectively.[34]

The Cepheid Xpert *C difficile* assay is a real-time PCR assay cleared for detection of the *tcdB* gene, and is run on the Cepheid GeneXpert Dx System. The subsequent clearance of Xpert *C difficile*/Epi includes the qualitative detection of toxin B and presumptive identification of 027/NAP1/BI strains of toxigenic *C difficile*. Both Xpert assays are run on an automated, single-use cartridge-based system. A swab is used to collect stool sample and is subsequently inserted into a vial containing the "Sample Reagent" provided with the IVD. After brief vortexing of the vial with a swab intended for use with the Xpert *C difficile*/Epi assay, the eluted material and 2 single-use reagents (Reagent 1 and Reagent 2, provided with the assay) are transferred to 2 uniquely labeled chambers in the disposable fluidic cartridge, 1 for the Xpert *C difficile* target and 1 for the NAP1 target. The user then selects a test from the system-user interface and places the cartridge into the GeneXpert Dx System. The instrument is fully automated and completely integrated for additional sample preparation, amplification, and real-time detection. This closed system requires minimum hands-on time and provides a result in less than 1 hour. Cepheid also manufactures a multiplex assay using TaqMan-based primers and probes (Life Technologies, Carlsbad, CA) specific for the *tcdB* gene, binary toxin genes (*cdtA* and *cdtB*), and *tcdC* gene single-base deletion at nucleotide 117, to detect toxigenic *C difficile* and presumptively detect ribotype 027. When compared with the cytotoxicity neutralization assay, Xpert *C difficile* showed a sensitivity of 97% and a specificity of 93% for *C difficile* toxin detection. The assay showed 100% sensitivity and 98% specificity for ribotyping when compared with PCR ribotyping.[35] Similar findings for Xpert *C difficile*/Epi performance was reported by Babady and colleagues.[36]

Meridian's Illumigene *C difficile* assay (Meridian Bioscience, Inc, Cincinnati, OH) was FDA cleared in July 2010. Instead of using the most commonly applied nucleic acid amplification technology (PCR), Illumigene *C difficile* uses a technology called loop-mediated isothermal DNA amplification (LAMP).[37] Moreover, the assay target region is different from the aforementioned assays in that it is designed to detect the pathogenicity locus (PaLoc) of toxigenic *C difficile*. The *C difficile* PaLoc is a gene segment present in all known toxigenic *C difficile* strains, and codes for both *tcdA* and *tcdB*. The Illumigene *C difficile* assay detects the PaLoc by targeting a partial DNA fragment on *tcdA*. This region is an intact region occurring in all known A+B+ and A−B+ toxinotypes. The assay uses specifically designed primers targeting the PaLoc for specific and continuous isothermal DNA amplification. A by-product of this amplification, magnesium pyrophosphate, forms a white precipitate leading to a turbid reaction solution. The presence of turbidity signifies a positive reaction, whereas the absence of turbidity represents a negative reaction. The results of the assay are determined using the Meridian Illumipro-10 Incubator/Reader. The assay kit includes a Sample Preparation Apparatus and a Test Device. The Sample

Preparation Apparatus is filled with phosphate-buffered saline containing formalin-treated *Staphylococcus aureus*, and is used for specimen dilution and preparation. No extraction is required because the sample is heated for inactivation. The overall turnaround time is less than an hour. A study by Norén and colleagues[38] has shown that the Illumigene *C difficile* assay had a sensitivity and specificity of 98% when compared with a composite reference method using the cytotoxin B assay and toxigenic culture. Furthermore, the Illumigene *C difficile* assay performance was compared with the real-time PCR-based BD GeneOhm Cdiff assay, and 2 antigen assays (Wampole QUIK CHEK COMPLETE and TechLab TOX A/B QUIK CHEK) for the detection of toxigenic *C difficile*.[39] After discrepant analysis by toxigenic culture, the Illumigene *C difficile* assay performed comparably with the BD GeneOhm Cdiff assay, with a similar sensitivity of 95.2% but a slightly lower specificity of 96.6%. The 2 antigen tests in the study showed much poorer sensitivity (47.6% for QUIK CHEK and 52.4% for TOX A/B II) than the 2 molecular tests.

The Portrait Toxigenic *C difficile* assay (Great Basin Corp, Salt Lake City, UT) is an automated closed system that performs sample extraction, isothermal helicase-dependent amplification, and chip-based detection. Great Basin's assay uses a novel Hot Start approach: ribonuclease-mediated amplification (RMA). In the RMA approach, DNA primers contain a single RNA base linkage near a blocked 3′-end. By blocking the 3′-end, no amplification may occur unless temperature is elevated to greater than 50°C, when a thermostable version of the enzyme RNase H2 is activated. If the blocked primer is hybridized to a target DNA sequence, RNase H2 will cut the primer at the RNA base, removing the block and permitting DNA amplification. This approach prevents the primer artifacts during amplification. In a multicenter clinical study, the Portrait assay showed 98.2% sensitivity and 92.8% specificity when compared with a toxigenic bacterial culture/cell cytotoxin neutralization assay (TBC/CCNA) for the detection of toxigenic *C difficile* in 549 stool specimens.[40]

Quest Diagnostics Simplexa *C difficile* Universal Direct Test (Quest Diagnostics, Madison, NJ) is a real-time PCR assay targeting *tcdB* for the detection of toxigenic *C difficile* from liquid or unformed stool specimens. The assay requires heat treatment of the stool specimen (no extraction required) followed by an amplification step using bifunctional fluorescent probe-primers together with reverse primers (Scorpion Technology) targeting a well-conserved region of the *tcdB* gene. The assay is intended to be used on the 3M Integrated Cycler instrument (3M, St Paul, MN). The Simplexa *C difficile* Universal Direct Test had a sensitivity of 90% and a specificity of 93% when using direct toxigenic culture as a reference method (Ferreira S, personal communication, 2012).

The Nanosphere Verigene *C difficile* Test (Nanosphere, Inc, Northbrook, IL) uses the Verigene system based on gold nanoparticle technology for the direct detection of nucleic acid through a microarray-based capture platform. The system consists of a sample processer (Processor *SP*), an automated system that handles both sample preparation and test processing, and a reader that performs the detection step and generates the final result. All steps are performed on a single-use consumable (the test cartridge). The nucleic acid from a patient sample is sheared during the sample processing/extraction step, then hybridized to single-stranded DNA-capture oligonucleotides arrayed in replicate on a solid support and sequence-specific mediator oligonucleotides. This step is followed by further hybridization to the gold nanoparticle probes containing mediator oligonucleotide complementary sequence. Thus, the target nucleic acid is sandwiched between the sequence-specific capture and gold nanoparticle probes. A catalytic reaction deposits elemental silver onto the gold particle, which amplifies the signal from the gold nanoparticles. The amplified signal is then detected by the Verigene Reader. The Verigene C difficile Test targets tcd A, tcdB, tcdC (mutation), and cdtA genes, which allows the detection of toxigenic strains and 027/NAP1/BI strains. The Verigene processor can process up to 4 cartridges with a total turnaround time less than 2 hours. The assay had a sensitivity of 90% and specificity of 93.8% when compared with toxigenic culture (Buchan BW, personal communication, 2012). In the same study, the Verigene and Cepheid Xpert C difficile/Epi assays showed 100% agreement on the detection of tcdC and binary toxin (cdtA/cdtB) genes.

Quidel's AmpliVue C difficile test (Quidel Corp, San Diego, CA) is a disposable cassette-based assay that combines isothermal helicase-dependent amplification (BioHelix, Beverly, MA) with the company's lateral flow technology. AmpliVue requires no nucleic acid extraction step, with less than 80 minutes from sample to result. Although the assay does not involve nucleic acid extraction, it requires several steps to complete the heat lysis of the sample. A total of 50 μL of lysate is then transferred to a reaction tube preloaded with lyophilized reagents. After rehydration of the reaction by pipetting, the reaction tube is subjected to amplification at 64°C for 60 minutes. Detection is performed by placing the reaction tube into the Amplicon Cartridge, followed by inserting the Amplicon Cartridge into the Detection Cassette. The result can be read in about 10 minutes based on the color of the T line, with any pink to red visible line considered positive for toxigenic C difficile.[41]

Multiplex PCR-Based Detection and Identification of Gastrointestinal Pathogens

Further advancement in molecular technologies has enabled clinical laboratories to test for a panel of pathogens through a single reaction performed on a patient sample. Multiplex RT-PCR–based detection of multiple respiratory viral pathogens has become part of the routine diagnostic algorithm in clinical laboratories over the last 5 years.[42,43] With the success of multiplexing molecular detection in the respiratory arena, one would expect and anticipate such highly multiplexed molecular assays will become a reality for detection of gastroenteritis pathogens.[44–52] Indeed, effort and progress has been made in the past few years on this front, and there are a few multiplex RT-PCR–based LDTs as well as commercial assays available for multi-target detection and identification for gastroenteritis.

Several LDTs are generally focused on either a panel of viruses or a panel of bacteria suspected in gastroenteritis. Khamrin and colleagues[53] developed a novel multiplex RT-PCR assay that is able to identify 10 viruses in a single tube. The assay was designed to detect group A and C rotaviruses, adenovirus, norovirus GI, norovirus GII, sapovirus, astrovirus, Aichi virus, human parechoviruses, and human enteroviruses. This assay was shown to be useful as a rapid and cost-effective diagnostic tool for the detection of pathogenic viruses associated with diarrhea. Smaller panels have been developed using real-time PCR detection methods. One example is a viral panel targeting group C rotavirus, astrovirus, and subgenus F adenovirus in stool specimens.[54] A molecular screening approach developed by de Boer and colleagues[55] involved 2 internally controlled real-time multiplex PCRs (mPCRs) and was used for the simultaneous detection of 5 pathogens: Salmonella enterica, C jejuni, Giardia lamblia, Shiga toxin–producing E coli (STEC), and Shigella spp/enteroinvasive E coli (EIEC). The test was shown to yield a remarkable increase in pathogen positivity rate (19.2%) compared with conventional methods (6.4%), and was implemented in routine diagnostic use in December 2006.

Similarly, Liu and colleagues[56] developed a 1-step multiplex RT-PCR assay with microsphere-based fluorescence detection for norovirus GI and GII, rotavirus, astrovirus, sapovirus, and adenovirus. The assay was shown to be quantitative and nearly as sensitive as the corresponding singleplex quantitative real-time RT-PCR assay on analytical samples. In addition to being rapid, sensitive, and specific for the detection of the major viral causes of gastroenteritis, the quantitation provided by the assay is informative for clinical research, especially in the context of mixed infections. The same group developed a 7-plex PCR assay using Luminex bead–based detection to simultaneously screen for several of the major diarrhea-causing bacteria directly from fecal specimens (Aeromonas, C jejuni, Campylobacter coli, Salmonella, Shigella, EIEC, Vibrio, and Yersinia) so as to overcome laborious conventional diagnostic methods, such as culture, biochemical tests, and enzyme-linked immunosorbent assay (ELISA). The study found that the fluorescent signals obtained with this approach had statistically significant correlation with the cycle threshold (Ct) values from the real-time PCR assays ($P<.05$). This multiplex PCR assay enabled sensitive, specific, and quantitative detection of the major bacterial causes of gastroenteritis.[57] Recently the same group reported that 19 enteropathogens can be detected and identified simultaneously by multiplex PCR.[58] In another study using Luminex xMAP technology,[59] a multiplexed assay for the simultaneous identification of enteric viral pathogens, including rotavirus A (RVA), noroviruses (NoVs) (including genogroups GI and GII), sapoviruses (SaV), human astrovirus (HAstV), enteric adenoviruses (EAds), and human bocavirus 2 (HBoV2) was developed. The analytical sensitivity of the assay allowed detection of 10^3 (EAds, HBoV2, and RVA) and 10^4 (NoV GI and GII, SaV, and HAstV) copies per reaction mixture. Compared with conventional PCR, the Luminex-based assay yielded greater than 75% sensitivity and 97% specificity for each virus.

Several commercially available tests for detection of gastrointestinal pathogens are now available. Seegene's (Rockville, MD) Seeplex Diarrhea ACE Detection detects diarrhea-causing viruses and/or bacteria directly from stool and rectal swab. It is a multiplex RT-PCR system based on the company's DPO (Dual Priming Oligonucleotide) technology. This proprietary target-specific primer provides highly specific amplification of the nucleic acid sequence of interest. The system consists of 3 distinct multiplex panels, 1 for viruses and 2 for bacteria. The virus panel (Panel V) is designed to simultaneously detect rotavirus, norovirus GI, norovirus GII, enteric adenovirus, and astrovirus. The first bacterial panel (Panel B1) probes for Salmonella spp (S. bongori, and S enterica), Shigella spp (S flexneri, S boydii, S sonnei, and S dysenteriae), Vibrio spp (V cholerae, V parahaemolyticus, and V vulnificus), Campylobacter spp (C jejuni and C coli), and C difficile toxin B. The second bacterial panel 2 (Panel B2) targets Clostridium perfringens, Y enterocolitica, Aeromonas spp (A salmonicida, A. sobria A. bivalvium, and A. hydrophila), E coli O157:H7, and Verocytotoxin-producing E coli (VTEC). The overall workflow involves the following steps: (1) a multiplex RT-PCR amplification reaction, (2) auto-capillary electrophoresis to separate and analyze the PCR amplicons using an autocapillary electrophoresis device (MultiNA), and (3) data analysis using the ScreenTape System (Agilent Technologies, Inc, Santa Clara, CA).

A retrospective study by Higgins and colleagues[60] comparing the Seeplex Diarrhea Virus Panel with EM and/or real-time RT-PCR showed estimated diagnostic sensitivities of 100% for adenovirus, rotavirus, and norovirus GI, and 97% for norovirus GII. Diagnostic specificities after discordant analysis were 100% for adenovirus, rotavirus, and norovirus GI, and 99.4% for norovirus GII. By virtue of its multiplexing ability, the assay identified viral coinfections in 6.8% of stool specimens examined in this study. The overall turnaround time observed for a 96 sample run was 9 to 10 hours. The Seeplex Diarrhea-B1 ACE Detection Panel was also evaluated for its ability to detect Campylobacter species in stool specimens in comparison with culture and immunoassays. The study by Bessède and colleagues[61] demonstrated the poor sensitivity of culture methods for Campylobacter species and the advantage of the multiplex assay of detecting the presence of other bacterial pathogens.

The first molecular diagnostic test that detects a broad panel of viruses, bacteria, and parasites through a single, multiplex RT-PCR reaction is the xTAG Gastrointestinal Pathogen Panel (xTAG GPP). xTAG GPP has been available as an IVD since 2011, in Europe and then Canada, and now most recently the United States. The assay uses the Luminex xTAG Technology and the xMAP Technology platform to detect multiple targets in a single sample. The xTAG GPP can detect 15 major gastrointestinal pathogens. It detects 3 viruses (adenovirus 40/41, rotavirus A, norovirus GI/GII), 3 parasites (*Giardia, E histolytica*, and *Cryptosporidium*), and 9 bacterial pathogens (*Salmonella, Shigella, Campylobacter, C difficile* toxin A/B, Enterotoxigenic *E coli* (ETEC) LT/ST, *E coli* O157, STEC stx 1/stx 2, *V cholerae*, and *Y. enterocolitica*). The assay workflow begins with a sample pretreatment step involving bead beating followed by nucleic acid extraction and a single, multiplex, RT-PCR amplification step. Pretreatment breaks down parasitic cysts and preserves viral RNA for subsequent extraction and detection (**Fig. 1**). The assay includes an internal control, which monitors (1) the extraction process, (2) potential RT-PCR inhibition, and (3) RT and PCR steps. The overall assay turnaround time is approximately 5 hours (depending on the number of samples run on a 96-well plate) with bead-based detection on either the Luminex 100/200 or MAGPIX instruments. The data-acquisition protocol for individual bead populations is region-specific to accommodate local regulatory requirements. Qualitative calls are made via a desktop software module that enables user-defined data masking, thereby providing the option of reporting either the full pathogen panel or a defined subpanel.

The xTAG GPP assay provides overall high sensitivity and specificity for the probed target pathogens. The multicenter clinical study conducted for CE marking and Health Canada approval showed that the assay had 100% sensitivity and specificity for adenovirus 40/41, 94.7% sensitivity and 99.8% specificity for rotavirus A, and 93.5% sensitivity and 96.4% specificity for norovirus. Similarly, the assay showed 100% sensitivity for *Giardia* and *E histolytica*, and 91.7% for *Cryptosporidium*, with specificity of greater than 97% for all 3 parasites. For bacterial targets, overall performance is greater than 94% sensitivity and specificity, except for *Salmonella* with 84.6% sensitivity and 98.4% specificity. The sensitivity for *Y enterocolitica*, *V cholerae*, and STEC stx1/stx2 was not evaluated owing to the lack of clinical samples (**Table 3**). Clinical studies required for FDA approval included a large prospective cohort of pediatric and adult patients with a large enough representation of negative results to establish a high (>99%) negative predictive value for all analytes evaluated. The benefit of high negative predictive value from a multiplex test was also demonstrated with an LDT using a similar methodology (ie, xTAG Technology) for the detection of 15 pathogens, which was applied to screening for potential gastrointestinal microbial pathogens in pathogenesis of necrotizing enterocolitis.[62]

During the 2011 outbreak of a new aggressive EHEC strain in Germany, xTAG GPP was used by Kliniken der Stadt Köln GmbH, Cologne, to prescreen the exponentially increasing number of suspected cases. The assay was able to discriminate STEC from a broad panel of pathogens that are implicated in infectious diarrhea, providing the dual benefit of rapid time to result and high throughput.[63] The potential to significantly reduce the cost to the health care system is also noteworthy. More appropriate use of isolation rooms in hospitals for suspected hospital-acquired infectious gastroenteritis, reductions in hospital admissions for suspected community-acquired infectious gastroenteritis, and more rapid identification of potential local outbreaks from gastrointestinal pathogens are a few examples of health economic benefits that can be afforded through the implementation of a multiplexed molecular diagnostic approach.

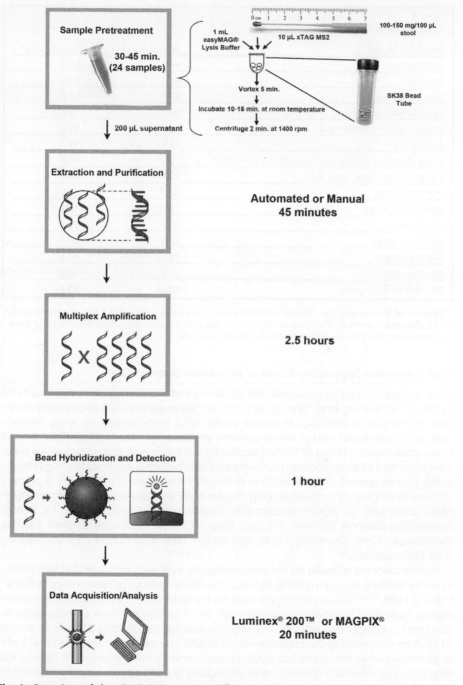

Fig. 1. Overview of the xTAG GPP assay workflow.

Table 3
xTAG GPP sensitivity and specificity

Target (Analyte)	Sensitivity (%)	Specificity (%)
Salmonella	84.6	98.4
Shigella	97.7	97.8
Campylobacter	97.5	97.8
Yersinia enterocolitica	N/A[a]	100.0
Enterotoxigenic *Escherichia coli* (ETEC) LT/ST	N/A[a]	97.0
E coli O157	94.1	98.8
Shiga-like toxin producing *E coli* (STEC) stx 1/stx 2	100.0	98.6
Clostridium difficile Toxin A/B	97.7	94.9
Vibrio cholerae	N/A[a]	100.0
Adenovirus 40/41	100.0	100.0
Rotavirus A	94.7	99.8
Norovirus GI/GII	93.5	96.4
Giardia lamblia	100.0	97.5
Cryptosporidium	91.7	99.9
Entamoeba histolytica	100.0	98.8

[a] Because of low sample size, clinical sensitivity was not assessed (N/A) for ETEC, *Y enterocolitica*, and *V cholerae*. However, analytical accuracy for these analytes was demonstrated in limit of detection and reactivity studies with culture isolates or plasmids.

Next-Generation Sequencing–Based GI Microbiota Determination

NGS applies to those technologies and platforms that allow cheaper, faster, and more in-depth sequencing than "first-generation" or "early-generation" sequencing methods, or Sanger sequencing. In recent years, NGS technologies have significantly reduced the time and cost of whole-genome sequencing; nevertheless, there are still many challenges in terms of clinical application of these new technologies. An overview of current NGS technology platforms and their potential applications to gastroenteritis microorganism determination is provided here. There are basically 5 primary NGS technologies: (1) pyrosequencing (Roche 454 Pyrosequencing and Qiagen PyroMark platforms); (2) SOLiD system (Life Technologies, Carlsbad, CA); (3) Solexa sequencing platform (Illumina, Inc, San Diego, CA); (4) HeliScope System (Helicos BioSciences Corp, Cambridge, MA); and (5) Ion Torrent semiconductor sequencing (Life Technologies).[64]

Pyrosequencing is based on the sequencing-by-synthesis principle that was developed by Mostafa Ronaghi and Pål Nyrén at the Royal Institute of Technology in Stockholm in 1996.[65,66] This technology is built on the detection of pyrophosphate release during nucleotide incorporation, rather than chain termination with dideoxynucleotides used in Sanger sequencing. The method enables sequencing of a single strand of DNA by synthesizing the complementary strand one base pair (bp) at a time. Light is generated when the nucleotide solution complements the first unpaired base of the template. The detection of which base was added at each step is based on detecting the activity of DNA polymerase with a chemiluminescent enzyme. The sequence of solutions that produce chemiluminescent signals is used to determine the sequence of the template. The template DNA can be immobilized by either solid-phase template preparation (streptavidin-coated magnetic beads) or liquid phase, such as enzymatic template preparation (apyrase + exonuclease). A limitation of pyrosequencing is that the lengths of individual reads are only about 300 to 500 nucleotides, shorter than the 800 to 1000 obtainable with chain termination methods (eg, Sanger sequencing). With the heavy commercial drive for the technology, this limitation is being challenged. Roche Diagnostics' 454 GS FLX+ system (454 Life Sciences, a Roche company, Branford, CT) claims to have read lengths of approximately 500 bp, and up to 1000 bp.

Pyrosequencing technology has been mainly used as a research tool in gastroenteritis for novel microorganism identification, genetic drift, and species identification of a specific pathogen. High-throughput pyrosequencing using the GS FLX Titanium platform (Roche 454 Life Sciences), which gave an average of 12,730 reads per sample, was used to identify a novel astrovirus (astrovirus VA1) associated with the 2008 outbreak of acute gastroenteritis in the Eastern Shore Health District of Virginia.[67] Using the Roche 454 NGS technology, novel pathogenic viruses including picornaviruses and circoviruses have been identified from patients with acute diarrhea and flaccid paralysis.[68–70]

Qiagen's PyroMark ID platform was used in a study to understand the diversity of Sites A and B for 1062 GII-4 NoV strains from clinical specimens associated with an outbreak of gastroenteritis (2000–2011) in England.[71] Persson and colleagues[72] recently developed a 2-step process for the species identification of *Campylobacter* from stool specimens. In this process, a real-time TaqMan assay was used for genus level identification of *C jejuni*, *Campylobacter coli*, *Campylobacter upsaliensis*, *Campylobacter lari*, and *Campylobacter fetus* followed by pyrosequencing for species identification. Pyrosequencing is probably the most widely used NGS technology in medical microbiology.[73]

The Applied Biosystems SOLiD system is based on Sequencing by Oligonucleotide Ligation and Detection (SOLiD). In this approach, sequencing is obtained by measuring sequential serial rounds of ligation of an oligonucleotide to the sequencing primer by a DNA ligase enzyme. Each ligation step is accompanied by fluorescence detection, after which a regeneration step prepares the extended primer for the next round of ligation.[64,74] The sequences generated using this technology could read up to 50 to 75 bp in length.

The Illumina Solexa sequencing platform is based on the sequencing-by-synthesis principle (similar to pyrosequencing), and is also like the Sanger method in that it relies on dye terminator nucleotides incorporated into the sequence by a DNA polymerase. Illumina Solexa terminators are reversible, permitting polymerization to proceed even after fluorophore detection. In this method, DNA fragments are immobilized on a flow cell surface, and bridge PCR is used for amplification. DNA sequencing is initiated with addition of the sequencing primer, DNA polymerase, and 4 reversible dye terminators. Fluorescence is recorded after incorporation by a 4-channel fluorescent scanner. The sequence read is about 100 bp in length using this technology.[64,75] The Illumina Genome Analyzer was used in the genome-wide association studies (GWAS) for rare variants associated with inflammatory bowel disease.[76] Similarly, this sequencing platform was used to understand the variation of a *Campylobacter concisus* genome from a biopsy of a child with Crohn disease.[77]

The HeliScope System by Helicos Biosciences allows sequencing directly from single DNA molecules. Although the technology is built on the sequencing-by-synthesis principle, it is an amplification-free method that can determine the nucleotide sequence of more than 280,000 individual DNA molecules simultaneously.[78] In brief, after DNA fragmentation, the template DNA sample is polyadenylated at the 3′ end with the final adenine labeled with Cy3. The poly-A template molecules are captured by hybridization to poly-T oligonucleotides immobilized on a flow cell surface. Because templates are fluorescently labeled, imaging can identify the array coordinates where a sequencing read is expected. The label is then cleaved, and sequencing proceeds by adding DNA polymerase and each of 4 Cy5-labeled nucleotides to the flow cell.[64] This technology only allows a read length of 25 bp.

Pacific Biosciences has developed a single-molecule real-time (SMRT) third-generation sequencing platform (PacBioRS system).[79] This technology can produce reads with average lengths of 3000 to 5000 bp, with longest reads of more than 20,000 bp. One advantage of single-molecule sequencing technology is that there is no need to generate a library (or amplification of the template), and it allows acquisition of sequence data from a small amount of input DNA. This technology has been used for sequencing ssDNA and dsDNA viruses, plasmid vector models for methylation studies, antibiotic resistance gene-carrying plasmids, and the entire genome of a clinically relevant microbial pathogen.[80] All were performed without the need for library preparation, and it was possible to generate sequence data within 8 hours from less than 1 ng of DNA without a PCR amplification step. The simplicity and speed of this platform illustrates its potential application in scenarios of acute disease and infectious outbreak.

The benchtop sequencing platform, Ion Proton System, developed by Ion Torrent (Life Technologies) is perhaps the most exciting sequencing platform described in 2012.[75,81] Instead of using light as an intermediary to sequence DNA, Ion Torrent uses semiconductor technology and simple chemistry, which allows low cost and scalability. Ion Torrent translates chemical signals into digital information. Ion Proton Chips use complementary metal-oxide semiconductor (CMOS) technology similar to that found in digital cameras, but instead of capturing light, the chip "sees" chemistry and translates it directly into digital data. The Ion PI Chip has 165 million wells, about 100-fold more than the Ion 314 Chip. The Ion PII Chip scales further to 660 million wells. Ion Proton Chips could deliver a human-scale genome, exome, or whole transcriptome in just a few hours, which is more rapid than any other sequencing technology.[81]

The performance of these recent sequencing platforms is yet to be evaluated and validated for clinical utility. A comparison study of Ion Torrent, Pacific Biosciences, and Illumina MiSeq sequencers was conducted by Quail and colleagues.[82] In this study, 4 microbial genomes, *Bordetella pertussis* (67.7% guanine-cytosine [GC] content, with some regions in excess of 90% GC content); *Salmonella pullorum* (52% GC), *Staphylococcus aureus* (33% GC), and *Plasmodium falciparum* (19.3% GC, with some regions close to 0% GC content) were used to test new sequencing technologies. The data from this study showed a higher raw error rate with the Ion Torrent PGM platform (~1.8%) than the Illumina platform (<0.4%). However, because of the sufficient coverage of Ion Torrent, the ability to call single-nucleotide polymorphisms (SNPs) is fairly comparable. On the other hand, the PacBio system was not as accurate in detecting SNPs. The use of single-molecule sequencing to detect low-level variants is yet to be proved. The Ion Torrent PGM sequencer coupled with Optical Mapping was successfully used to prospectively characterize the German EHEC O104:H4 outbreak.[83] Overall these exciting technologies are still to be further developed and tested for their unique applications.[82]

Limitations such as the cost, need for large amounts of DNA, the need of massive computing power, and the requirement of the appropriate software for the complex data analysis will continue to drive further development and maturation of NGS technologies.[75,84] NGS technologies in gastroenteritis clinical diagnostics may not be a reality in the near future, but they will certainly continue to play an important role in microbiology. There is still much effort being made in further advancing the technologies and decreasing costs. One may envision the possibility of NGS technologies being established as the main diagnostic means for microbial infections in clinical laboratories.

PROTEOMIC ASSAYS

Recently developed sensing strategies based on microscaled and nanoscaled biosensors, microfluidic lab-on-a-chip, and array technologies for detection of pathogenic bacteria are promising candidates for immunodetection of gastroenteritis agents in the clinical laboratory. Conventional bacterial identification methods, involving phenotypic tests or test of characteristic metabolites, can be time consuming and traditional immunoassay methods, such as radioimmunoassay and ELISA, have limitations including lengthy analysis times and expensive instrumentation. Biosensor technologies have several advantages over traditional methods, including (1) high sensitivity, (2) low detection limit, (3) high specificity, (4) reduced sample preparation time, (5) rapid analysis time, (6) portability, and (7) ease of use. This section reviews some of the newly developed proteomic assay technologies, and their application to the study of gastroenteritis and detection of enteric pathogens. Their capability for rapid and sensitive microbial detection, as shown in these early studies, illustrates their exciting potential as clinical diagnostic platforms in the future.

Biosensors

Biosensors function to convert receptor-binding recognition of the target into a detectable signal. Immunosensors are based on the interaction of antigens on the target cells, and immobilized antibodies and the bound complexes can be detected by various label and label-free detection systems, including fluorescence, electrical/electrochemical impedance, cantilever, quartz crystalline microbalance, surface plasmon resonance, and magnetoresistivity.[85]

Luo and colleagues[86] used electrospinning to fabricate a nitrocellulose nanofibrous membrane, which was functionalized to detect E coli O157:H7 and bovine viral diarrhea virus (BVDV) in a biosensor that integrated magnetic separation, capillary immunoassay, and direct-charge electrical measurement. Pathogen detection was achieved by incubating the sample with antibody-functionalized conductive magnetic nanoparticles to bind any pathogens present in the test sample. The captured pathogens are removed from the test sample by magnetic separation and are applied to the application pad on the sensor. By capillary action, the target pathogen enters the capture pad and is bound by the immobilized secondary antibody, forming a sandwich complex. The accumulated complexes produce electron transport across the silver electrodes where the direct charge transfer between electrodes is proportional to the pathogen concentration. Equilibrium was achieved within 8 minutes and the sensing response for E coli O157:H7 was linear from 0 to 10^4 CFU/mL, with a limit of detection of 61 CFU/mL. The limit of detection for BVDV was 10^3 cell culture infective dose (CCID)/mL.

A novel electrochemical impedimetric immunosensor was described based on Fe_3O_4 nanoparticles for the detection of C jejuni in stool.[87] This label-free immunosensor was developed by immobilizing monoclonal antibodies to the C jejuni FlaA protein on Fe_3O_4 nanoparticles surface-modified with O-carboxymethylchitosan. Antibody-antigen interactions were characterized using atomic force microscopy and electrochemical impedance spectroscopy. Binding of C jejuni could be detected at 10 minutes by relative change in electron-transfer resistance, but 40 minutes was required to achieve saturated equilibrium. Detection limit for C jejuni was 10^3 CFU/mL and the sensor demonstrated a linear dose response to 10^7 CFU/mL. Intra-assay coefficient of variation (CV) was 4.8%, and precision of fabrication reproducibility between sensors was within 6.3% for a concentration of 10^5 CFU/mL. Specificity was verified using Salmonella spp and E coli at concentrations up to 10^4 CFU/mL, and only a slight change in impedance could be observed with increasing concentration (relative standard deviation of <5%).

Ho and colleagues[88] applied ganglioside-sensitized liposomes in a flow-injection immunoanalysis system for the detection of cholera toxin. This immunodetection system used a microcapillary with anticholera toxin antibody immobilized on its inner surface and ganglioside (GM_1) liposomes containing sulforhodamine B (SRB) dye. GM_1, which has specific affinity toward cholera toxin, was inserted into the phospholipid bilayer during liposome synthesis. Samples are introduced into the system by injection and the cholera toxin is captured by the antibodies on the microcapillary column. The toxin is subsequently bound by GM_1 present on the liposomes. Bound liposomes are ruptured and the fluorescent intensity of the released SRB is used to determine the concentration of cholera toxin in the test sample. A calibration curve using cholera toxin standard demonstrated a dynamic range of 3 orders of magnitude from 10 ag/mL to 10 fg/mL. Intra-assay reproducibility was very good, with CV at 5.8%, and the limit of detection was approximately 1.1 zmol, or 66 ag/mL, which was 7-fold more sensitive than a comparable liposome-based assay using lateral flow.

Berkenpas and colleagues[89] developed a shear horizontal surface acoustic wave device fabricated on langasite for the detection of E coli O157:H7 in liquid samples. Surface acoustic wave (SAW) devices directly measure a physical property change caused by the presence of an analyte, and provide a less complicated, label-free detection system. SAW devices can be miniaturized, which makes it possible to integrate them into array systems, and they can be fabricated in large quantities inexpensively by photolithographic processes widely used in the semiconductor industry. Langasite was selected as the substrate because of its characteristic properties that make this family of crystals suitable for operation in liquids.[90] Biotinylated anti-E coli or anti-O157:H7 antibody was applied to gold thin film slides preconjugated with NeutrAvidin (Thermo Fisher Scientific, Inc, Rockford, IL). The experimental setup for flow-through testing incorporated a syringe pump, temperature controller, and software to measure the magnitude and phase of the transmission coefficient sensor response at a fixed frequency. Sensors were also evaluated by a "dip-and-dry" method whereby bacteria were applied and bound to the antibody-conjugated surface for 2 hours, rinsed 5 times, and allowed to dry before measurement. Sensors were subsequently imaged by fluorescence microscopy to quantify bacterial binding. The flow-through method produced reduced variation in sensor response, similar to that of negative controls, and was thought to be due to a relatively large distance of the E coli from the sensor surface. The dip-and-dry method produced a significant and measurable response, which confirmed the viability of this method for potential development into an inexpensive portable detector for E coli O157:H7.

BVDV was detected using a conductometric biosensor that incorporated polyaniline in the biosensor architecture.[91] In this study a lateral-flow biosensor was developed, which used BVDV-specific antibodies as the sensing element and 5 polyaniline compounds as transducer and signal amplifier. The biosensor that used polyaniline synthesized with perchloric acid was found to be most sensitive, with a detection limit of 10^3 CCID/mL. Sensitivity using other polyaniline compounds ranged from 10^4 to 10^5 CCID/mL.

Ditcham and colleagues[92] developed an optoelectric immunosensor for detection of BVDV antigens in crude cell lysates. Binding of viral antigens prepared from crude cell lysates was determined using the laser-induced surface second harmonic generation (SSHG) technique. SSHG is a 1-step label-free optical process that coverts 2 incident photons into a single emission photon when high-intensity light is incident upon the surface or interface between media. The signal originates from the field and structural discontinuity of the interface. In this study, binding by 2 monoclonal antibodies in both ELISA plates and glass coverslips was evaluated. The light collected from antigen-antibody binding reactions was passed through a 532-nm filter and detected with a photomultiplier tube. The sensors were further processed by incubation with labeled secondary antibody and peroxidase-conjugated antispecies detection antibody to obtain results by ELISA for comparison. The highest antigen concentration produced a higher surface second harmonic (SSH) signal than that from negative control samples, but the signal decreased rapidly with 2-fold dilution of the antigen preparation. SSH results from the assay on plates correlated well with ELISA results on plates ($R^2 = 0.86$) and on coverslips ($R^2 = 0.96$), but the signals were lower than those obtained from biosensors on coverslips. Regression analysis showed that correlation of SSH results from coverslips to ELISA was $R^2 = 0.75$ and 0.67 in experiments using either both monoclonal antibodies or a single monoclonal antibody for antigen binding.

Multiplex Protein/Antigen Liquid Array

The clinical spectrum of gastroenteritis is wide, and the severity of symptoms reflects the degree of intestinal inflammation resulting from the host-pathogen interaction. Host protein profiles may have the potential to indicate infectious disease status, and arrays comprising specific protein biomarkers that can be used in various combinations may provide a sensitive and specific minimally invasive diagnostic method for a variety of infections.[93,94]

Chronic inflammatory bowel diseases (Crohn disease and ulcerative colitis) affect more than 1 million individuals and, although the etiology is unknown, studies have suggested that the cause is multifactorial and the result of inflammatory responses to commensal microorganisms in susceptible hosts who are exposed to environmental triggers.[95] Blood-based and stool-based protein biomarkers, including cytokines and antibodies, can be helpful in the diagnosis and management of these patients. Levels of C-reactive protein and the fecal biomarkers calprotectin and lactoferrin can help differentiate inflammatory bowel disease (IBD) from noninflammatory diarrheal illnesses, whereas antineutrophil cytoplasmic antibodies and anti–*Saccharomyces cerevisiae* antibodies can be used to differentiate Crohn disease from ulcerative colitis. Advances in multiplex proteomic array profiling technology have sparked interest in using the technique for assessment of IBD at cellular and subcellular levels, and with future development could be used in the identification of active disease by differentiating types of IBD and predicting or monitoring response to therapy.

Multiplex arrays for the quantitation of cytokines have also proved to be useful for monitoring the course of infectious gastroenteritis. Enocksson and colleagues[96] determined rectal nitrous oxide (NO) levels and used multiplex liquid array (Fluorokine MAP; R&D Systems, Minneapolis, MN) to measure levels of proinflammatory cytokines in stools of patients with infectious gastroenteritis. In general, high NO levels were found in the acute phase of infection, which gradually dropped in the subacute phase, and during the convalescent phase reached the levels found in normal controls. Stool interleukin (IL)-1β levels were elevated in 82% of patients and decreased with clinical improvement. IL-1β levels were higher among patients with bacterial enteritis than in patients with CDAD or negative stool cultures, but the difference was not statistically significant. Interferon (IFN)-γ, IL-4, and tumor necrosis factor (TNF)-α were detected in stool samples from 18%, 33%, and 11% of patients, respectively. The investigators were unable to establish a significant correlation between stool IL-1β levels and the rectal NO levels during the acute phase of the disease in this study, and furthermore noted that because high NO levels have been shown in patients with noninfectious

IBD, these conditions would need to be considered in the differential diagnosis when using these tools in diagnostic procedures.

DePaolo and colleagues[97] used a multiplex cytokine array (Beadlyte; EMD Millipore, Billerica, MA) to measure mucosal and serum cytokine levels, in combination with the chemokine CCL2, to study the role of CCL2 in murine gastric S enterica infection. On infection with Salmonellae, mucosal expression of CCL2 is rapidly upregulated and then systemically expressed in the spleen. Mucosal and serum IL-6 and TNF-α levels were significantly elevated in homozygous CCL2-negative (CCL2$-$/$-$) mice. CCL2$-$/$-$ mice also had a more rapid decline, greater mortality, and significantly higher levels of bacteria in the liver in comparison with wild-type mice. Macrophages in CCL2$-$/$-$ mice infected with Salmonellae or treated with Salmonella lipopolysaccharide also showed increased proinflammatory cytokine production, suggesting an important regulatory function for CCL2 during innate immune response to Salmonella infection.

A bead-based 4-member multiplex antigen array was developed to detect circulating antibodies to viruses in cattle, and compared the performance to that of individual ELISA assays used in veterinary diagnostics and surveillance.[98] Crude lysates of cultured viruses were used as capture antigens coupled to the fluorescent beads, and tested with a panel of field serum samples. The results for 2 of the assays (bovine herpes virus 1 and parainfluenza 3 virus) showed sensitivities and specificities similar to those of the separate ELISAs. The performance of the assays for BVDV and bovine respiratory syncytial virus was not as good as that of the corresponding ELISAs, owing to low signal strength that led to higher assay variability and reduced ability to distinguish positive from negative samples. Use of recombinant antigen for BVDV led to increased signal and improved performance in the array. The results demonstrated that viral lysate antigens used in ELISA may or may not perform as well when used as capture moiety in a bead-based array system, and suggest that differences in performance may be associated with the differences in available surface area in microtiter plate wells and microspheres. The study did demonstrate the potential for the multiplex antigen liquid array method for routine serologic testing if appropriate antigens can be identified, and that it may be possible to combine the use of viral lysates and recombinant antigens into workable array systems.

In a proof-of-concept study by Griffin and colleagues,[99] a 7-plex antigen bead array was developed for detection of salivary immunoglobulin (Ig)G and IgA responses to waterborne pathogens. Saliva is an attractive specimen for use in epidemiologic testing in the community because sampling is noninvasive, and is ideal for multiplex arrays where only a small sample size is needed for simultaneous testing of all assay members. Antigen-specific antibody or control serum was used to confirm coupling of the antigens to beads and control proteins, and a separate duplex assay for total IgG and total IgA were used to control for antibody cross-reactivity and to assess saliva variability. The method was tested using 200 prospectively collected saliva specimens from 20 subjects and 10 paired sera from a subset of the test cases. The strongest salivary antibody responses were found in chronic infections (Helicobacter pylori and Toxoplasma gondii), and correlated with positive IgG responses determined by commercial ELISA. A strong increase in antinorovirus salivary antibody was observed after an episode of acute diarrhea and vomiting in 1 subject. The array was also capable of detecting seroconversion to Cryptosporidium using control sera from infected children. The study demonstrated the application of antigen array technology for assessment of proteins present in salivary samples, and the potential of salivary antibody detection as a useful indicator of specific infections.

Real-Time Cell Analysis System

Cell-based screening technologies have emerged as a method of choice for high-content screening in research and drug discovery to identify compounds that produce desired changes in cell phenotypes.[100] Classic detection methods use fluorescence, radioisotope, luminescence, or light absorption; however, these methods can be costly and complex, and labeled compounds may interfere with physiologic conditions. Label-free detection allows the monitoring of cellular events (eg, cell number, viability, morphology) in real time without the incorporation of labels.[101] There are several advantages to using label-free detection methods, including (1) homogeneous assay format, (2) noninvasive measurement closer to physiologic conditions, (3) kinetic and real-time measurement, (4) reduced time and cost, and (5) less interference in detection by exogenous compounds.

ACEA Biosciences (San Diego, CA) has developed a label-free electrical impedance detection method and used it for real-time electronic sensing of cell-based assays. Solly and colleagues[102] found that the real-time cell electronic sensing (RT-CES) system, when compared with classic analysis methods, provided comparable results for cell number, cell proliferation, cytotoxicity, cytoprotection, cell growth inhibition, and apoptosis analyses, and concluded that the label-free system was a useful tool for measurement of certain cellular parameters. Virus neutralization assays were applied to the real-time cell analysis (RTCA) system to measure neutralizing antibody concentrations following a single vaccination with a monovalent, unadjuvanted, inactivated 2009 H1N1 influenza vaccine.[103]

Yu and colleagues[104] applied the RT-CES system to assess the functional activation of G-protein–coupled receptors (GPCRs) in different signaling pathways, and compared the results with those of standard assays, including fluorescence microscopy and Western blot. The RT-CES system provided rapid, precise, and specific measurements for GPCR activation. The investigators concluded that the system offered a convenient, sensitive, and quantitative method for assessing GPCR activity, independent of the particular pathway. Furthermore, because multiple treatments could be applied to the same reaction well over time and monitored in real time, they could also study desensitization and receptor cross-talk on the same platform.

A novel cell-based immunocytotoxicity assay was developed for detecting C difficile toxins in porcine clinical samples. He and colleagues[105] used a monoclonal antibody to C difficile toxin A (TcdA), which enhanced the activity of TcdA on cells expressing Fc γ receptor I, and used RT-CES to detect the biological activity of TcdA as a function of cell index (CI). C difficile toxins disrupt cell attachment and cause cell rounding, leading to a decrease in CI and cell spreading. A rapid decrease in CI was recorded within hours after the addition of toxins to the cells at doses of 1 to 1000 ng/mL. At 20 hours' incubation, doses as low as 0.1 pg/mL rendered complete loss of CI when the anti-TcdA antibody was present. The RT-CES assay was found to be considerably more sensitive than the standard cytotoxin B assay with a reduced turnaround time (2–4 hours) and a rapid and easy-to-perform workflow, and provided results that could be collected in real time in an automatic manner. The investigators concluded that the cell-based immunocytotoxicity assay had good potential as a diagnostic method for C difficile infection.

Ryder and colleagues[106] described an RTCA system for assessment of C difficile toxin in human stool by monitoring the dynamic response of HS27 cells to C difficile toxin B (TcdB) as a function of CI. Purified C difficile toxin inoculated into negative stool samples was used to determine the analytical sensitivity of the assay, which showed a limit of detection of 0.2 ng/mL at 15 to 18 hours. Concentrations of 3.2 ng/mL could be detected in 30 minutes. No cross-reactivity with cholera or diphtheria toxins was observed at concentrations of 1 to 100 ng/mL, and nontoxigenic *C difficile*, *C fallax*, or *C perfringens* could not be detected. Sensitivity and specificity were assessed by parallel testing using real-time PCR and a glutamate dehydrogenase/toxin A/B EIA. RTCA had an overall sensitivity of 87.5% and overall specificity of 99.6%, which was higher than with EIA but lower than with real-time PCR. A significant correlation between toxin concentration and clinical severity before antibiotic treatment was observed, and toxin concentrations were significantly lower after treatment, demonstrating the RTCA system as a functional tool for assessment of *C difficile* infections. A similar system has been used to quantitatively detect *V cholerae* toxin directly from stool specimens (Jin D, personal communication, 2012).

CONCLUDING REMARKS

There is much need for rapid and accurate detection and identification of microbial pathogens that cause gastroenteritis so as to facilitate appropriate treatment and patient management. Technological innovations in microbiology, immunology, and molecular biology have significantly expanded and improved the capabilities of diagnostic microbiology in the detection and identification of pathogens causing gastroenteric infections. Some technologies are commercially available and are gradually being implemented for routine clinical diagnostic services.

Screening of populations at risk for a group of possible microbial pathogens is an exciting area of development in molecular microbiology.[7,24,107,108] This concept is very important for the quick detection and identification of various microbial pathogens that cause diarrhea. There are numerous etiologic agents that can cause debilitating gastroenteritis in immunosuppressed patient populations, including parasites (eg, *Giardia*, *Cryptosporidium*), viruses (eg, rotaviruses and noroviruses), and typical bacterial pathogens (*E coli* variants, *Salmonella*, *Shigella*, and *Campylobacter*). Traditionally, different methods of detection are used for each group of pathogens, which require special media and equipment, expensive facilities for the culture of mycobacteria, expertise in the identification of parasites in O&P stool preparations, virology facilities, the specific media for bacterial enteric pathogens.

Advanced genomic and proteomic techniques can cover a clinical specimen for panels of probable pathogens. One example is to develop a GI Chip by coupling multiplex PCR amplification with a matrix probe hybridization. The multiplex PCR uses multiple primer sets within a single reaction tube to amplify microbial pathogen-specific nucleic acids extracted from the stools of patients with gastroenteritis. After amplification, an array containing a panel of specific oligonucleotide probes is used to identify the microorganism-specific PCR products. Several GI Chip devices using this combination are commercially available, and are predicted to be used in routine diagnostic microbiology.

REFERENCES

1. Tang YW, Persing DH. Diagnostic microbiology. In: Schaechter M, editor. Encyclopedia of microbiology. 3rd edition. Oxford (United Kingdom): Elsevier Press; 2009. p. 308–20.
2. Pawlowski SW, Warren CA, Guerrant R. Diagnosis and treatment of acute or persistent diarrhea. Gastroenterology 2009;136(6):1874–86.
3. Lozupone CA, Stombaugh JI, Gordon JI, et al. Diversity, stability and resilience of the human gut microbiota. Nature 2012;489(7415):220–30.

4. Wilson KH. Natural biota of the human gastrointestinal tract. In: Blaser MJ, Smith PD, Ravdin JI, et al, editors. Infections of the gastrointestinal tract. 2nd edition. Philadelphia: Lippincott Williams & Wilkins; 2002. p. 45–56.
5. Brugere JF, Mihajlovski A, Missaoui M, et al. Tools for stools: the challenge of assessing human intestinal microbiota using molecular diagnostics. Expert Rev Mol Diagn 2009;9(4):353–65.
6. Kosek M, Bern C, Guerrant RL. The global burden of diarrhoeal disease, as estimated from studies published between 1992 and 2000. Bull World Health Organ 2003;81(3):197–204.
7. Thielman NM, Guerrant RL. Clinical practice. Acute infectious diarrhea. N Engl J Med 2004;350(1):38–47.
8. Bresee JS, Marcus R, Venezia RA, et al. The etiology of severe acute gastroenteritis among adults visiting emergency departments in the United States. J Infect Dis 2012;205(9):1374–81.
9. Guerrant RL, Van Gilder T, Steiner TS, et al. Practice guidelines for the management of infectious diarrhea. Clin Infect Dis 2001;32(3):331–51.
10. Jones TF, McMillian MB, Scallan E, et al. A population-based estimate of the substantial burden of diarrhoeal disease in the United States; FoodNet, 1996-2003. Epidemiol Infect 2007;135(2):293–301.
11. McDonald LC, Killgore GE, Thompson A, et al. An epidemic, toxin gene-variant strain of Clostridium difficile. N Engl J Med 2005;353(23):2433–41.
12. Glass RI, Parashar UD, Estes MK. Norovirus gastroenteritis. N Engl J Med 2009; 361(18):1776–85.
13. Blanton LH, Adams SM, Beard RS, et al. Molecular and epidemiologic trends of caliciviruses associated with outbreaks of acute gastroenteritis in the United States, 2000-2004. J Infect Dis 2006;193(3):413–21.
14. de Wit MA, Koopmans MP, van Duynhoven YT. Risk factors for norovirus, Sapporo-like virus, and group A rotavirus gastroenteritis. Emerg Infect Dis 2003;9(12):1563–70.
15. Bok K, Green KY. Norovirus gastroenteritis in immunocompromised patients. N Engl J Med 2012;367(22):2126–32.
16. Katz DE, Taylor DN. Parasitic infections of the gastrointestinal tract. Gastroenterol Clin North Am 2001;30(3):797–815.
17. Mehta S, Fantry L. Gastrointestinal infections in the immunocompromised host. Curr Opin Gastroenterol 2005;21(1):39–43.
18. Chapin KC, Dickenson RA, Wu F, et al. Comparison of five assays for detection of Clostridium difficile toxin. J Mol Diagn 2011;13(4):395–400.
19. Quinn CD, Sefers SE, Babiker W, et al. C. Diff Quik Chek complete enzyme immunoassay provides a reliable first-line method for detection of Clostridium difficile in stool specimens. J Clin Microbiol 2010;48(2):603–5.
20. LaSala PR, Svensson AM, Mohammad AA, et al. Comparison of analytical and clinical performance of three methods for detection of Clostridium difficile. Arch Pathol Lab Med 2012;136(5):527–31.
21. Dusch H, Altwegg M. Evaluation of five new plating media for isolation of Salmonella species. J Clin Microbiol 1995;33(4):802–4.
22. Perez JM, Cavalli P, Roure C, et al. Comparison of four chromogenic media and Hektoen agar for detection and presumptive identification of Salmonella strains in human stools. J Clin Microbiol 2003;41(3):1130–4.
23. Perry JD, Ford M, Taylor J, et al. ABC medium, a new chromogenic agar for selective isolation of Salmonella spp. J Clin Microbiol 1999;37(3):766–8.

24. Bennett WE Jr, Tarr PI. Enteric infections and diagnostic testing. Curr Opin Gastroenterol 2009;25(1):1–7.

25. Gaillot O, di Camillo P, Berche P, et al. Comparison of CHROMagar *Salmonella* medium and hektoen enteric agar for isolation of Salmonellae from stool samples. J Clin Microbiol 1999;37(3):762–5.

26. Tang YW, Persing DH. Advances in the clinical microbiology of enteric infections. In: Blaser MJ, Smith PD, Ravdin JI, et al, editors. Infections of the gastrointestinal tract. 2nd edition. Philadelphia: Lippincott Williams & Wilkins; 2002. p. 1185–97.

27. Bélanger SD, Boissinot M, Clairoux N, et al. Rapid detection of *Clostridium difficile* in feces by real-time PCR. J Clin Microbiol 2003;41(2):730–4.

28. Fotedar R, Stark D, Beebe N, et al. Laboratory diagnostic techniques for *Entamoeba* species. Clin Microbiol Rev 2007;20(3):511–32 [table of contents].

29. Kirby A, Iturriza-Gomara M. Norovirus diagnostics: options, applications and interpretations. Expert Rev Anti Infect Ther 2012;10(4):423–33.

30. Gunson RN, Carman WF. Comparison of two real-time PCR methods for diagnosis of norovirus infection in outbreak and community settings. J Clin Microbiol 2005;43(4):2030–1.

31. Kageyama T, Kojima S, Shinohara M, et al. Broadly reactive and highly sensitive assay for Norwalk-like viruses based on real-time quantitative reverse transcription-PCR. J Clin Microbiol 2003;41(4):1548–57.

32. Svensson AM, LaSala PR. Pathology consultation on detection of *Clostridium difficile*. Am J Clin Pathol 2012;137(1):10–5.

33. Stamper PD, Alcabasa R, Aird D, et al. Comparison of a commercial real-time PCR assay for tcdB detection to a cell culture cytotoxicity assay and toxigenic culture for direct detection of toxin-producing *Clostridium difficile* in clinical samples. J Clin Microbiol 2009;47(2):373–8.

34. Stamper PD, Babiker W, Alcabasa R, et al. Evaluation of a new commercial TaqMan PCR assay for direct detection of the *Clostridium difficile* toxin B gene in clinical stool specimens. J Clin Microbiol 2009;47(12):3846–50.

35. Huang H, Weintraub A, Fang H, et al. Comparison of a commercial multiplex real-time PCR to the cell cytotoxicity neutralization assay for diagnosis of *Clostridium difficile* infections. J Clin Microbiol 2009;47(11):3729–31.

36. Babady NE, Stiles J, Ruggiero P, et al. Evaluation of the Cepheid Xpert *Clostridium difficile* Epi assay for diagnosis of *Clostridium difficile* infection and typing of the NAP1 strain at a cancer hospital. J Clin Microbiol 2010;48(12):4519–24.

37. Lalande V, Barrault L, Wadel S, et al. Evaluation of a loop-mediated isothermal amplification assay for diagnosis of *Clostridium difficile* infections. J Clin Microbiol 2011;49(7):2714–6.

38. Norén T, Alriksson I, Andersson J, et al. Rapid and sensitive loop-mediated isothermal amplification test for *Clostridium difficile* detection challenges cytotoxin B cell test and culture as gold standard. J Clin Microbiol 2011;49(2):710–1.

39. Boyanton BL Jr, Sural P, Loomis CR, et al. Loop-mediated isothermal amplification compared to real-time PCR and enzyme immunoassay for toxigenic *Clostridium difficile* detection. J Clin Microbiol 2012;50(3):640–5.

40. Buchan BW, Mackey TL, Daly JA, et al. Multicenter clinical evaluation of the Portrait toxigenic *C. difficile* assay for detection of toxigenic *Clostridium difficile* strains in clinical stool specimens. J Clin Microbiol 2012;50(12):3932–6.

41. Chow WH, McCloskey C, Tong Y, et al. Application of isothermal helicase-dependent amplification with a disposable detection device in a simple sensitive stool test for toxigenic *Clostridium difficile*. J Mol Diagn 2008;10(5):452–8.

42. Wu W, Tang YW. Emerging molecular assays for detection and characterization of respiratory viruses. Clin Lab Med 2009;29(4):673–93.
43. Yan Y, Zhang S, Tang YW. Molecular assays for the detection and characterization of respiratory viruses. Semin Respir Crit Care Med 2011;32(4): 512–26.
44. Ginocchio CC, Zhang F, Manji R, et al. Evaluation of multiple test methods for the detection of the novel 2009 influenza A (H1N1) during the New York City outbreak. J Clin Virol 2009;45(3):191–5.
45. Kim SR, Ki CS, Lee NY. Rapid detection and identification of 12 respiratory viruses using a dual priming oligonucleotide system-based multiplex PCR assay. J Virol Methods 2009;156(1–2):111–6.
46. Li H, McCormac MA, Estes RW, et al. Simultaneous detection and high-throughput identification of a panel of RNA viruses causing respiratory tract infections. J Clin Microbiol 2007;45(7):2105–9.
47. Mahony J, Chong S, Merante F, et al. Development of a respiratory virus panel test for detection of twenty human respiratory viruses by use of multiplex PCR and a fluid microbead-based assay. J Clin Microbiol 2007;45(9):2965–70.
48. Merante F, Yaghoubian S, Janeczko R. Principles of the xTAG respiratory viral panel assay (RVP Assay). J Clin Virol 2007;40(Suppl 1):S31–5.
49. Pierce VM, Hodinka RL. Comparison of the GenMark Diagnostics eSensor respiratory viral panel to real-time PCR for detection of respiratory viruses in children. J Clin Microbiol 2012;50(11):3458–65.
50. Rand KH, Rampersaud H, Houck HJ. Comparison of two multiplex methods for detection of respiratory viruses: FilmArray RP and xTAG RVP. J Clin Microbiol 2011;49(7):2449–53.
51. Raymond F, Carbonneau J, Boucher N, et al. Comparison of automated microarray detection with real-time PCR assays for detection of respiratory viruses in specimens obtained from children. J Clin Microbiol 2009;47(3):743–50.
52. Babady NE, Mead P, Stiles J, et al. Comparison of the Luminex xTAG RVP Fast assay and the Idaho Technology FilmArray RP assay for detection of respiratory viruses in pediatric patients at a cancer hospital. J Clin Microbiol 2012;50(7): 2282–8.
53. Khamrin P, Okame M, Thongprachum A, et al. A single-tube multiplex PCR for rapid detection in feces of 10 viruses causing diarrhea. J Virol Methods 2011; 173(2):390–3.
54. Mori K, Hayashi Y, Akiba T, et al. Multiplex real-time PCR assays for the detection of group C rotavirus, astrovirus, and Subgenus F adenovirus in stool specimens. J Virol Methods 2012. [Epub ahead of print]. http://dx.doi.org/10.1016/j.jviromet.2012.10.019.
55. de Boer RF, Ott A, Kesztyus B, et al. Improved detection of five major gastrointestinal pathogens by use of a molecular screening approach. J Clin Microbiol 2010;48(11):4140–6.
56. Liu J, Kibiki G, Maro V, et al. Multiplex reverse transcription PCR Luminex assay for detection and quantitation of viral agents of gastroenteritis. J Clin Virol 2011; 50(4):308–13.
57. Liu J, Gratz J, Maro A, et al. Simultaneous detection of six diarrhea-causing bacterial pathogens with an in-house PCR-Luminex assay. J Clin Microbiol 2012; 50(1):98–103.
58. Liu J, Gratz J, Amour C, et al. A laboratory developed Taqman array card for simultaneous detection of nineteen enteropathogens. J Clin Microbiol 2012; 51(2):472–80.

59. Liu Y, Xu ZQ, Zhang Q, et al. Simultaneous detection of seven enteric viruses associated with acute gastroenteritis by a multiplexed Luminex-based assay. J Clin Microbiol 2012;50(7):2384–9.

60. Higgins RR, Beniprashad M, Cardona M, et al. Evaluation and verification of the Seeplex Diarrhea-V ACE assay for simultaneous detection of adenovirus, rotavirus, and norovirus genogroups I and II in clinical stool specimens. J Clin Microbiol 2011;49(9):3154–62.

61. Bessède E, Delcamp A, Sifre E, et al. New methods for detection of campylobacters in stool samples in comparison to culture. J Clin Microbiol 2011;49(3):941–4.

62. Ullrich T, Tang YW, Correa H, et al. Absence of gastrointestinal pathogens in ileum tissue resected for necrotizing enterocolitis. Pediatr Infect Dis J 2012; 31(4):413–4.

63. Malecki M, Schildgen V, Kamm M, et al. Rapid screening method for multiple gastroenteric pathogens also detects novel enterohemorrhagic Escherichia coli O104:H4. Am J Infect Control 2012;40(1):82–3.

64. Metzker ML. Sequencing technologies—the next generation. Nat Rev Genet 2010;11(1):31–46.

65. Ronaghi M, Karamohamed S, Pettersson B, et al. Real-time DNA sequencing using detection of pyrophosphate release. Anal Biochem 1996;242(1):84–9.

66. Ronaghi M, Uhlen M, Nyren P. A sequencing method based on real-time pyrophosphate. Science 1998;281(5375):363–5.

67. Finkbeiner SR, Li Y, Ruone S, et al. Identification of a novel astrovirus (astrovirus VA1) associated with an outbreak of acute gastroenteritis. J Virol 2009;83(20): 10836–9.

68. Li L, Kapoor A, Slikas B, et al. Multiple diverse circoviruses infect farm animals and are commonly found in human and chimpanzee feces. J Virol 2010;84(4): 1674–82.

69. Li L, Victoria J, Kapoor A, et al. A novel picornavirus associated with gastroenteritis. J Virol 2009;83(22):12002–6.

70. Victoria JG, Kapoor A, Li L, et al. Metagenomic analyses of viruses in stool samples from children with acute flaccid paralysis. J Virol 2009;83(9):4642–51.

71. Zakikhany K, Allen DJ, Brown D, et al. Molecular evolution of GII-4 norovirus strains. PLoS One 2012;7(7):e41625.

72. Persson S, Petersen HM, Jespersgaard C, et al. Real-time TaqMan polymerase chain reaction-based genus-identification and pyrosequencing-based species identification of Campylobacter jejuni, C. coli, C. lari, C. upsaliensis, and C. fetus directly on stool samples. Diagn Microbiol Infect Dis 2012;74(1):6–10.

73. Siqueira JF Jr, Fouad AF, Rocas IN. Pyrosequencing as a tool for better understanding of human microbiomes. J Oral Microbiol 2012;4. [Epub ahead of print].

74. Ranade SS, Chung CB, Zon G, et al. Preparation of genome-wide DNA fragment libraries using bisulfite in polyacrylamide gel electrophoresis slices with formamide denaturation and quality control for massively parallel sequencing by oligonucleotide ligation and detection. Anal Biochem 2009;390(2):126–35.

75. Loman NJ, Misra RV, Dallman TJ, et al. Performance comparison of benchtop high-throughput sequencing platforms. Nat Biotechnol 2012;30(5):434–9.

76. Rivas MA, Beaudoin M, Gardet A, et al. Deep resequencing of GWAS loci identifies independent rare variants associated with inflammatory bowel disease. Nat Genet 2011;43(11):1066–73.

77. Deshpande NP, Kaakoush NO, Mitchell H, et al. Sequencing and validation of the genome of a Campylobacter concisus reveals intra-species diversity. PLoS One 2011;6(7):e22170.

78. Harris TD, Buzby PR, Babcock H, et al. Single-molecule DNA sequencing of a viral genome. Science 2008;320(5872):106–9.
79. Eid J, Fehr A, Gray J, et al. Real-time DNA sequencing from single polymerase molecules. Science 2009;323(5910):133–8.
80. Coupland P, Chandra T, Quail M, et al. Direct sequencing of small genomes on the Pacific Biosciences RS without library preparation. Biotechniques 2012; 53(6):365–72.
81. Rothberg JM, Hinz W, Rearick TM, et al. An integrated semiconductor device enabling non-optical genome sequencing. Nature 2011;475(7356):348–52.
82. Quail MA, Smith M, Coupland P, et al. A tale of three next generation sequencing platforms: comparison of Ion Torrent, Pacific Biosciences and Illumina MiSeq sequencers. BMC Genomics 2012;13:341.
83. Mellmann A, Harmsen D, Cummings CA, et al. Prospective genomic characterization of the German enterohemorrhagic *Escherichia coli* O104:H4 outbreak by rapid next generation sequencing technology. PLoS One 2011;6(7):e22751.
84. Nossa C, Tang YW, Pei Z. Pearls and pitfalls of genomics based microbiome analysis. Emerg Microb Infect 2012;1:e45.
85. Heo J, Hua SZ. An overview of recent strategies in pathogen sensing. Sensors (Basel) 2009;9(6):4483–502.
86. Luo Y, Nartker S, Miller H, et al. Surface functionalization of electrospun nanofibers for detecting *E. coli* O157:H7 and BVDV cells in a direct-charge transfer biosensor. Biosens Bioelectron 2010;26(4):1612–7.
87. Huang J, Yang G, Meng W, et al. An electrochemical impedimetric immunosensor for label-free detection of *Campylobacter jejuni* in diarrhea patients' stool based on O-carboxymethylchitosan surface modified Fe3O4 nanoparticles. Biosens Bioelectron 2010;25(5):1204–11.
88. Ho JA, Wu LC, Huang MR, et al. Application of ganglioside-sensitized liposomes in a flow injection immunoanalytical system for the determination of cholera toxin. Anal Chem 2007;79(1):246–50.
89. Berkenpas E, Millard P, Pereira da Cunha M. Detection of *Escherichia coli* O157:H7 with langasite pure shear horizontal surface acoustic wave sensors. Biosens Bioelectron 2006;21(12):2255–62.
90. Berkenpas E, Bitla S, Millard P, et al. Pure shear horizontal SAW biosensor on langasite. IEEE Trans Ultrason Ferroelectr Freq Control 2004;51(11):1404–11.
91. Tahir ZM, Alocilja EC, Grooms DL. Polyaniline synthesis and its biosensor application. Biosens Bioelectron 2005;20(8):1690–5.
92. Ditcham WG, Al-Obaidi AH, McStay D, et al. An immunosensor with potential for the detection of viral antigens in body fluids, based on surface second harmonic generation. Biosens Bioelectron 2001;16(3):221–4.
93. Natesan M, Ulrich RG. Protein microarrays and biomarkers of infectious disease. Int J Mol Sci 2010;11(12):5165–83.
94. Koene MG, Mulder HA, Stockhofe-Zurwieden N, et al. Serum protein profiles as potential biomarkers for infectious disease status in pigs. BMC Vet Res 2012;8:32.
95. Iskandar HN, Ciorba MA. Biomarkers in inflammatory bowel disease: current practices and recent advances. Transl Res 2012;159(4):313–25.
96. Enocksson A, Lundberg J, Weitzberg E, et al. Rectal nitric oxide gas and stool cytokine levels during the course of infectious gastroenteritis. Clin Diagn Lab Immunol 2004;11(2):250–4.
97. DePaolo RW, Lathan R, Rollins BJ, et al. The chemokine CCL2 is required for control of murine gastric *Salmonella enterica* infection. Infect Immun 2005; 73(10):6514–22.

98. Anderson S, Wakeley P, Wibberley G, et al. Development and evaluation of a Luminex multiplex serology assay to detect antibodies to bovine herpes virus 1, parainfluenza 3 virus, bovine viral diarrhoea virus, and bovine respiratory syncytial virus, with comparison to existing ELISA detection methods. J Immunol Methods 2011;366(1–2):79–88.

99. Griffin SM, Chen IM, Fout GS, et al. Development of a multiplex microsphere immunoassay for the quantitation of salivary antibody responses to selected waterborne pathogens. J Immunol Methods 2011;364(1–2):83–93.

100. Gasparri F. An overview of cell phenotypes in HCS: limitations and advantages. Expert Opin Drug Discov 2009;4(6):643–57.

101. Proll G, Steinle L, Proll F, et al. Potential of label-free detection in high-content-screening applications. J Chromatogr A 2007;1161(1–2):2–8.

102. Solly K, Wang X, Xu X, et al. Application of real-time cell electronic sensing (RT-CES) technology to cell-based assays. Assay Drug Dev Technol 2004;2(4):363–72.

103. Sun F, Zhang Y, Tian D, et al. Responses after one dose of a monovalent influenza A (H1N1) 2009 inactivated vaccine in Chinese population—a practical observation. Vaccine 2011;29(38):6527–31.

104. Yu N, Atienza JM, Bernard J, et al. Real-time monitoring of morphological changes in living cells by electronic cell sensor arrays: an approach to study G protein-coupled receptors. Anal Chem 2006;78(1):35–43.

105. He X, Wang J, Steele J, et al. An ultrasensitive rapid immunocytotoxicity assay for detecting *Clostridium difficile* toxins. J Microbiol Methods 2009;78(1):97–100.

106. Ryder AB, Huang Y, Li H, et al. Assessment of *Clostridium difficile* infections by quantitative detection of tcdB toxin by use of a real-time cell analysis system. J Clin Microbiol 2010;48(11):4129–34.

107. Wistrom J, Jertborn M, Ekwall E, et al. Empiric treatment of acute diarrheal disease with norfloxacin. A randomized, placebo-controlled study. Swedish Study Group. Ann Intern Med 1992;117(3):202–8.

108. Wong CS, Jelacic S, Habeeb RL, et al. The risk of the hemolytic-uremic syndrome after antibiotic treatment of *Escherichia coli* O157:H7 infections. N Engl J Med 2000;342(26):1930–6.

Molecular Approaches and Biomarkers for Detection of *Mycobacterium tuberculosis*

Robert F. Luo, MD, MPH[a,b,*], Niaz Banaei, MD[a,b,c]

KEYWORDS

- *Mycobacterium tuberculosis* • Molecular diagnostics
- Nucleic acid amplification tests • Biomarkers

KEY POINTS

- Tuberculosis continues to be a public health emergency worldwide.
- There is a significant and pressing need for improved diagnostic tests for tuberculosis.
- Molecular tests can accurately and rapidly diagnose tuberculosis and drug resistance compared with conventional smear microscopy and culture.
- Biomarker-based tests may allow for simple and noninvasive methods of diagnosing TB.

INTRODUCTION

Tuberculosis (TB) continues to be a major public health problem worldwide. In 2011, there were nearly 9 million new cases of tuberculosis and 1.4 million deaths.[1] After the human immunodeficiency virus (HIV), TB ranks as the second leading cause of death due to infection; however, unlike HIV, no rapid point-of-care test exists to diagnose TB. Sputum smear microscopy, developed more than a century ago, remains the most common laboratory test for diagnosing TB around the world, despite having a sensitivity of as low as 30% to 60%.[2,3] Microbiological culture is considered the diagnostic gold standard, but results can take weeks to obtain and laboratories with culture capacity are often not available in resource-limited settings.[4]

In recent years, there has been renewed interest in culture-free diagnostics for TB. Advances in molecular diagnostics and biomarker identification for TB have been

[a] Department of Pathology, Stanford University School of Medicine, 300 Pasteur Drive, L235, Stanford, CA 94305, USA; [b] Clinical Microbiology Laboratory, Stanford University Medical Center, 3375 Hillview Avenue, Palo Alto, CA 94304, USA; [c] Department of Medicine, Stanford University School of Medicine, 300 Pasteur Drive, L134, Stanford, CA 94305, USA
* Corresponding author. Department of Pathology, Stanford University School of Medicine, 300 Pasteur Drive, L235, Stanford, CA 94305.
E-mail address: rluo2@stanford.edu

Clin Lab Med 33 (2013) 553–566
http://dx.doi.org/10.1016/j.cll.2013.03.012   labmed.theclinics.com
0272-2712/13/$ – see front matter © 2013 Elsevier Inc. All rights reserved.

coupled with the understanding that new tests should be accurate, rapid, and inexpensive to be most useful, particularly in the regions of the world with the highest prevalence of TB where resources are the most limited.[5] Correct and timely diagnosis of TB facilitates prompt initiation of tailored treatment, thereby helping to reduce the transmission of TB and development of drug resistance.[6] Although much work has been done regarding the diagnosis of latent TB, this review focuses on molecular diagnostics and biomarkers for active TB and emphasizes the diagnosis of pulmonary TB, the most common form of TB worldwide.

MOLECULAR DIAGNOSTICS FOR TUBERCULOSIS
Commercial Nucleic Acid Amplification Tests for Mycobacterium tuberculosis Detection

Commercial nucleic acid amplification tests (NAATs) are the most commonly used molecular diagnostic tests for TB.[7] In 1995, the first commercial test, Gen-Probe's Amplified *Mycobacterium tuberculosis* Direct Test (San Diego, CA), was approved by the US Food and Drug Administration (FDA) for use directly on smear-positive sputum samples.[8] Based on transcription-mediated amplification, the test targets a ribosomal RNA gene sequence specific for *M tuberculosis* complex using isothermal RNA transcription followed by DNA synthesis. The following year, a second test, the Amplicor *M tuberculosis* test (Roche Molecular Systems, Branchburg, NJ), based on polymerase chain reaction (PCR) amplification of a target sequence in the ribosomal RNA gene, was also approved in the United States for smear-positive samples.[9] Both tests demonstrated greater than 95% sensitivity and 100% specificity in detecting *M tuberculosis* complex in smear-positive sputum samples compared with culture. These tests also were shown to have 50% to 80% sensitivity for smear-negative sputum samples, although only the Gen-Probe test was eventually approved by the FDA for this purpose and for use on extrapulmonary samples.[10,11] A major limitation of these tests is that they include separate nucleic acid extraction and amplification steps.

Based on the improved performance of NAATs over smear microscopy and rapid turnaround time compared with culture, the US Centers for Disease Control and Prevention recommended that a NAAT should be done on at least 1 respiratory specimen from any patient with suspected TB, in addition to conventional smear and culture.[12] Although not FDA approved, several other commercial tests using different molecular amplification approaches have been developed for use outside the United States, including the Abbott LCx *M tuberculosis* test (Abbott Park, IL), which relies on ligase chain reaction amplification, the BD ProbeTec Direct test (Sparks, MD), which uses strand-displacement amplification, and the Hain GenoType Mycobacteria Direct test (Nehren, Germany), based on transcription-mediated amplification.[13–15] Although availability of these assays varies by country, numerous meta-analyses examining the performance of commercial NAATs have confirmed the high specificity of the tests, with variable estimates of sensitivity, depending on specimen type and smear status, although sensitivity was typically high (85%–100%) for smear-positive sputum specimens.[7,15,16] Sensitivity estimates were typically low for extrapulmonary specimens and smear-negative samples (33%–93%).[15,17,18]

Laboratory-Developed Tests for M tuberculosis Detection

In parallel to the increase in commercial NAAT assays for the detection of *M tuberculosis*, several laboratories have developed their own tests for diagnosing TB. In the United States, laboratory-developed or in-house tests can be used for patient care as long as they have been validated following methods appropriate for each laboratory. Guidance can be provided by the College of American Pathology, New York State, Clinical Laboratory Improvement Amendment, and Clinical and Laboratory Standards Institute standards.[12,19] In-house tests are also commonly used in developing countries because they can be less expensive than commercial kits and avoid import and shipping fees. Most laboratory-developed tests are based on PCR amplification of DNA sequences specific to *M tuberculosis*.[20] Because each test uses different conditions, it can be difficult to make generalizations about their performance as design and assay characteristics reported in the literature vary significantly compared with commercial assays. Reported sensitivities and specificities have ranged from 9% to 100% and 6% to 100%, respectively, depending on assay type, population tested, and specimen type.[16,20,21] However, tests that targeted IS6110, a genomic sequence often present in multiple copies, tended to have higher sensitivity.[20,22] Because in-house tests have variable performances, it is up to the laboratory director to ensure sufficient assay sensitivity and specificity for the patient population served and to document assay performance for test users and applicable regulatory and accreditation agencies. Laboratories that rarely see TB cases may defer NAAT testing to public health or private reference laboratories.

Commercial NAATs for Simultaneous Molecular Detection of M tuberculosis and Drug Resistance

With the spread of drug-resistant strains of *M tuberculosis*, NAATs have also been recognized as important tools for identifying patients who need individualized treatment regimens. In 2011, there were an estimated 630,000 cases of multidrug-resistant TB, defined as a *M tuberculosis* isolate with resistance to 2 of the best first-line treatment drugs, isoniazid and rifampicin.[1] However, it is believed that only a small fraction of patients with multidrug-resistant TB are actually diagnosed because of the lack of drug susceptibility testing in many resource-limited settings worldwide.[23] To address this problem, NAATs that can simultaneously diagnose TB and assess for drug resistance have been developed and implemented with increasing frequency.

In 2008, the World Health Organization endorsed 2 commercial line probe assays for the rapid diagnosis of multidrug-resistant TB in settings with a high TB burden: Innogenetics INNO-LiPA Rif.TB test (Ghent, Belgium) and the Hain Genotype MTBDR test (Nehren, Germany).[24] Line probe assays rely on PCR amplification of target gene sequences followed by hybridization with probes printed on strips, which detect either wild-type or mutated sequences (**Fig. 1**). Both assays have uncoupled extraction and amplification steps; DNA extraction must be performed as a separate procedure from PCR amplification. Both of these line probe assays allow for simultaneous diagnosis of *M tuberculosis* and identification of the most common mutations that confer drug resistance.

The INNO-LiPA test only detects resistance to rifampicin with probes to the *rpoB* gene and is only marketed for use on cultured *M tuberculosis* isolates. The MTBDR test checks for resistance to rifampicin and isoniazid with probes to the *rpoB* and *katG* genes and has been validated for use on either cultured isolates or directly on sputum specimens. An expanded version of the MTBDR test, the MTBDRplus, was later developed to replace the MTBDR test and includes additional probes for the gene *inhA* for isoniazid resistance; a third version, the MTBDRsl, tests for resistance to ethambutol as well as second-line drug classes of quinolones and aminoglycosides.[24,25] The INNO-LiPA test has shown a sensitivity and specificity of more than 95% for the detection of *M tuberculosis* and rifampicin resistance from cultured isolates and a sensitivity of more than 80% on direct pulmonary specimens, although it is indicated for research use only on direct specimens by the manufacurer.[24,26] The

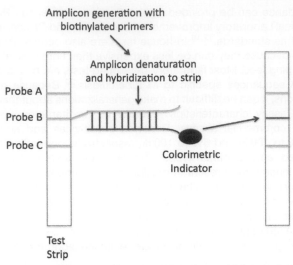

Fig. 1. Line probe assays. After DNA extraction, PCR is done with biotinylation of amplicons. Amplicons are denatured and biotinylated single-stranded fragments hybridize to a complementary target probe, if present, on the test strip. Enzymatic detection of biotin allows for colorimetric visualization of a positive test strip line.

MTBDRplus test demonstrates sensitivities and specificities for detection of *M tuberculosis* and rifampicin resistance of greater than 95% in multiple studies, on both cultured isolates and smear-positive sputum samples. The sensitivity of isoniazid resistance detection is slightly lower at approximately 80% to 90% on culture and sputum samples, although specificity remains greater than 95%.[26–28]

Simplified Molecular Diagnostics

Following the endorsement of line probe assays, in 2010, the World Health Organization also endorsed Cepheid's GeneXpert Xpert MTB/RIF test (Sunnyvale, CA) for simultaneous rapid detection of *M tuberculosis* complex and rifampicin resistance.[29] The Xpert system is currently the only commercial TB test that is performed on demand with complete automation of sample processing, extraction, amplification, and result interpretation. The Xpert MTB/RIF test uses real-time PCR and molecular beacons to provide results in less than 2 hours, and detection of rifamipicin resistance is intended as a proxy for multidrug-resistant TB. A large multicenter study demonstrated that the Xpert MTB/RIF test has sensitivity of more than 98% on smear-positive sputum specimens and 72.5% on smear-negative sputum, with a specificity of more than 99%.[30] In the same study, the sensitivity for detection of rifampicin resistance was 99%. Multiple studies have confirmed its ability to provide accurate rapid results in a variety of settings.[31,32] The Xpert MTB/RIF test is currently undergoing FDA clearance in the United States and development of an assay for second-line drug resistance testing is underway.

The Xpert MTB/RIF test has heralded a new era of automated molecular diagnostics. With little sample handling required and automation of nearly the entire process, the assay can be run by a health worker after minimal training. In addition, other than the GeneXpert instrument itself, no other specialized laboratory equipment or additional biosafety precautions are required in TB clinics and hospitals, as the assay has the same infectious risk as routine smear microscopy.[33] With the price of the test dropping for resource-limited countries, several studies have shown that implementation of this test will be cost-effective as well as efficacious in improving TB case finding.[34,35]

Also recognizing the need for automated and low-tech molecular diagnostics for use in resource-limited settings, the loop-mediated isothermal amplification (LAMP) test was developed to provide a rapid and simpler alternative to other NAATs. LAMP relies on multiple primer sets to produce a large amount of DNA amplicon under isothermal conditions (**Fig. 2**).[36] Visualization of results can be done by direct fluorescent detection or turbidity measurement, obviating the need for a more complicated instrument and electricity to detect labeled DNA amplicons or probes. In addition, the number of steps needed for preanalytical processing has been reduced compared with many conventional NAATs. Studies have demonstrated more than 90% sensitivity in smear-positive sputum specimens and greater than 99% specificity.[37,38]

Future of Molecular Diagnostics

A summary of the test characteristics of the various NAATs for TB is summarized in **Table 1**. NAATs for TB have not only improved and accelerated the diagnosis of TB; they have also shown potential to be used successfully in developing countries with the highest burden of disease.[31] Many groups continue to work on making NAATs even faster, simpler, and cheaper, while still preserving high standards of accuracy and safety.[39] New exciting platforms are also being explored, such as microchips that can be used for immediate point-of-care diagnosis, although extensive feasibility testing is still required.[40] In addition, more complex molecular techniques, including sequencing entire genes for resistance mutations and even whole genome

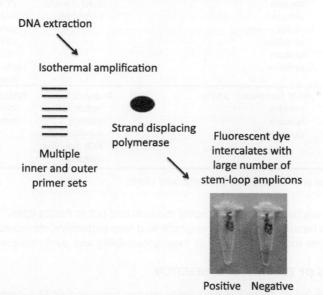

Fig. 2. LAMP. After DNA extraction, isothermal amplification is done with multiple nesting inner and outer primer sets. A polymerase with high strand-displacement activity creates stem-loop amplicon structures, which continue to lengthen and quickly produce a large amount of DNA. Visualization can be done with a fluorescent dye that intercalates with DNA. (*Adapted from* Aryan E, Makvandi M, Farajzadeh A, et al. A novel and more sensitive loop-mediated isothermal amplification assay targeting IS6110 for detection of *Mycobacterium tuberculosis* complex. Microbiol Res 2010;165(3):211–20; with permission.)

Table 1
Test characteristics of NAATs for TB

Method	Sensitivity	Specificity	Speed	Economy	Convenience
Commercial NAATs[a]	>95% smear-positive sputum samples 50%–80% smear-negative sputum samples	>95%	Half day	Requires PCR machine and molecular biology supplies	Requires nucleic acid extraction
Laboratory developed	Widely variable (9%–100%) depending on assay and specimen type	Widely variable (6%–100%) depending on assay and specimen type	Half day	Less expensive than commercial NAATs	Requires assay design Requires nucleic acid extraction
Line probe assays	>95% for cultured isolates 80%–95% for smear-positive sputum samples	>95%	Half day	Requires PCR machine and molecular biology supplies	Simultaneous detection of drug resistance Requires nucleic acid extraction
Xpert MTB/RIF	>98% for smear-positive sputum samples 73% for smear-negative sputum samples	>99%	2 h	Requires GeneXpert machine and cartridges	Automates extraction and PCR Simultaneous detection of rifampicin resistance Undergoing FDA clearance
LAMP	>90% for smear-positive sputum samples	>99%	Half day	Requires molecular biology supplies but no PCR machine needed	Requires nucleic acid extraction

[a] Excluding line probe assays, Xpert MTB/RIF, and LAMP.

sequencing, are being explored in novel medical and public health uses.[41,42] As these technologies become more commonplace and less expensive, molecular testing for TB will become more widespread as their accessibility and performance improves.

BIOMARKERS OF TUBERCULOSIS INFECTION

In contrast to NAAT testing, which relies on the presence of *M tuberculosis* DNA, biomarker detection may provide a useful alternative, especially when specimens may be paucibacillary or difficult to obtain.[5] Biomarkers can either be from the bacterium itself, or from responses within the human body to TB infection.[43] The use of biomarkers for the diagnosis of active TB is less advanced than NAAT testing and much research remains to be done on biomarkers from blood, urine, breath, sputum, and extrapulmonary sites of TB disease.

Blood Biomarkers

Interferon γ release assays (IGRAs), including Qiagen's QuantiFERON-TB Gold In-Tube assay (Hilden, Germany) and Oxford Immunotec's T-SPOT.TB test (Abingdon, UK), measure the in vitro release of interferon γ in blood by effector T cells as they are stimulated with antigens specific to *M tuberculosis*. Although IGRAs were developed as a replacement for the tuberculin skin test for diagnosing latent tuberculosis infection, they have limited usefulness in diagnosing active TB, as they cannot reliably distinguish between latent and active disease and may have poor sensitivities, especially in children and immunocompromised patients.[44] Pooled analyses of their sensitivity for active TB range from 35% to 92%.[45–47] IGRAs may be useful as an adjunct to other clinical and diagnostic criteria for TB, but should not be used as a standalone test.[48] Other blood-based biomarkers of TB infection, including neopterin, soluble intercellular adhesion molecule, and procalcitonin, have been proposed as possible targets for a diagnostic test, but not enough research exists yet on their sensitivity and specificity for active TB.[43]

Another type of blood biomarker test that has not proved useful is serology. Estimates of test accuracy for antibody detection for TB have varied by as much as 0% to 100%; the quality of evidence in most of the published literature has been low.[49] Because of the poor performance of these tests, the World Health Organization released a policy statement in 2011 that strongly recommended against the use of serology tests for diagnosing TB, the first time it has recommended against the use of a diagnostic test.[50] Some countries such as India have started to ban the import and sale of serologic tests. However, despite these findings, the use of serologic tests remains widespread worldwide because of their unregulated availability in private clinics; they are inexpensive and other, more effective, rapid point-of-care tests are lacking in these settings.[51]

Urine Biomarkers

Urine represents a noninvasive clinical sample that may be particularly useful in patients from whom sputum is difficult to collect (eg, children) or is low yield (eg, patients infected with HIV). Urine has been shown to contain several pathogen-derived biomarkers. Transrenal mycobacterial DNA are small DNA fragments of bacterial genome released during cell lysis that have been detected in the urine of patients with active TB, although only small-scale studies have looked at the diagnostic efficacy of DNA fragment detection.[52] Another *M tuberculosis*–derived molecule that has been extensively studied is lipoarabinomannan (LAM), a cell wall glycolipid that can represent up to 1.5% of the total dry weight of *M tuberculosis*.[53] The sensitivity of detection of urinary LAM enzyme Immunoassay for the diagnosis of TB has ranged from 13% to 93%, with specificity between 87% and 99%.[54] Although the performance of the urinary LAM assay is low in immunocompetent patients (pooled sensitivity of 18%), it does show improved performance in patients infected with HIV; most other tests show reduced sensitivity in the setting of severe immune deficiency.[55] The Alere Determine TB-LAM Ag lateral flow test (Walnut Creek, CA) is a simple, low-cost, urinary LAM test that may be helpful for the diagnosis of TB in patients with very low CD4 counts, with a sensitivity of 67% in this population (**Fig. 3**).[56]

Breath Biomarkers

TB infection is believed to result in the release of volatile organic compound metabolites that may be detected in the breath of patients.[57] Breath, like urine, has advantages over sputum in terms of ease of noninvasive specimen collection and

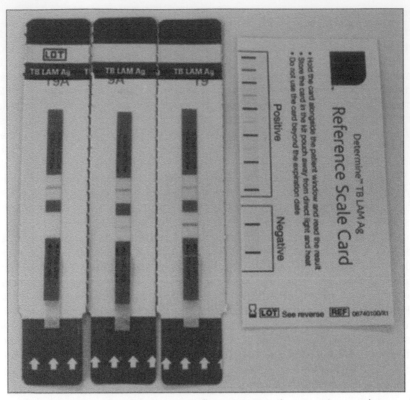

Fig. 3. Alere Determine TB-LAM Ag lateral flow test. Sample test strips are shown, along with a reference card for interpreting the results. All the strips show the upper control band. The strip on the left has a negative test band, whereas the other 2 strips have positive test bands of different intensities. (*From* Lawn SD, Kerkhoff AD, Vogt M, et al. Diagnostic accuracy of a low-cost, urine antigen, point-of-care screening assay for HIV-associated pulmonary tuberculosis before antiretroviral therapy: a descriptive study. Lancet Infect Dis 2012;12(3):201–9; with permission.)

potential usefulness in populations from whom it may be difficult to obtain quality sputum samples. Several companies have developed and assessed point-of-care technologies for direct detection of volatile compounds from breath in patients with TB.[58,59] A gas chromatography–based device developed by Menssana Research (Newark, NJ) to identify a pattern of volatile organic compounds that distinguished patients with active TB from healthy controls was shown to have a sensitivity and specificity of approximately 70% in a multicenter international study. Another device, the DiagNose, developed by eNose (Zutphen, Netherlands), uses a series of metal oxide sensors to detect volatile compounds in breath. Sensitivity of 77% and specificity of 87% have been reported in an initial validation study in Bangladesh.[60] Further optimization of biomarker detection from breath may help improve test sensitivity, especially with portable devices for simple point-of-care screening of suspected patients.[60,61]

Sputum Biomarkers

Several *M tuberculosis* proteins have been proposed as potential diagnostic biomarkers in sputum, although none has been developed into an actual diagnostic test yet. Aptamers, or oligonucleotides that bind to specific target peptides, have been designed for tuberculosis antigens, such as CFP10, ESAT-6, and MPT64, and can be detected through enzyme-linked immunoassays.[62–64] Similarly, proteins specific to TB such as Antigen85 have also been proposed as diagnostic markers.[64,65] One recent study demonstrated detection of down to 10 colonies of mycobacteria in a spiked sputum sample using a fluorescent probe specific to an *M tuberculosis* β-lactamase, BlaC.[65] Such biomarkers may prove useful if present in concentrations much higher than the number of individual bacteria, and if each enzymatic target can catalyze multiple reactions to amplify the amount of detectable signal produced in an assay.

Other biomarkers in sputum include enzymes and markers produced by the host in response to infection. For example, interferon γ has shown mixed usefulness in assisting with the diagnosis of TB in respiratory samples.[66,67] Although it is not useful in the blood, interferon γ has shown more promise for diagnosing TB in extrapulmonary samples, such as cerebrospinal fluid and pleural fluid.[68–70] Similarly, adenosine deaminase and alkaline phosphatase levels have been examined in sputum and extrapulmonary samples, but have not been shown to be diagnostic of TB as a standalone marker.[71–73] A test combining multiple biomarkers into a simple diagnostic array may ultimately prove useful as an initial screening test for TB.

The Future of Biomarkers

A summary of biomarkers for TB is presented in **Table 2**. Development of biomarker-based diagnostics for TB will only continue to accelerate as new biomarkers are discovered and novel assays are developed to detect them. Advances will likely be made along 3 major avenues: transcriptomics, or RNA markers of gene expression by the host; proteomics, or protein molecules indicating TB infection; and metabolomics, or metabolites produced by the host or the bacterium.[74] Transcriptome research has already demonstrated a differential RNA signature in the blood of patients with active TB compared with healthy controls and individuals with latent TB infection, although more studies need to be done to profile patients infected with other pulmonary diseases.[75] Similarly, proteomic and metabolomics research is already underway

Table 2
Summary of candidate biomarkers for TB

Specimen Type	Example Biomarkers	Advantages	Current Status
Blood	Interferon γ Neopterin Procalcitonin TB antibodies	Commercial tests approved for latent TB	Variable sensitivity (35%–92%) for active TB for interferon γ, other biomarkers still under research, antibody serologies not effective
Urine	Lipoarabinomannan (LAM) Transrenal DNA	Specimen easily obtained	LAM assays show variable sensitivities (13%–93%); other biomarkers still under research
Breath	Volatile organic compounds	Specimen easily obtained	Few prototypes tested, sensitivities 70%–77%, specificities 70%–87%
Sputum	TB-specific β-lactamase TB antigens (CFT10, MPT64) Adenosine deaminase	Specimen already routinely collected from patients with TB	Still under research

in blood, sputum, urine, and breath specimens as described earlier. As more bio-markers are identified and validated, some may even prove useful as a test of treatment response and cure in addition to diagnosis.[76,77] Candidate biomarkers have even been proposed for distinguishing drug-susceptible and drug-resistant *M tuberculosis*, although little research has been published on this topic.[78] Even though biomarker discovery is currently less developed than nucleic acid tests for TB, biomarkers may ultimately prove the most fruitful in producing low-cost, rapid, point-of-care tests in easily accessible samples such as breath and urine.

SUMMARY

The ability to diagnose TB in infected individuals worldwide continues to be unacceptably poor. It is estimated that only 50% to 60% of cases are diagnosed in resource-poor regions of Africa and Asia.[1] Traditional diagnostic methods either have low sensitivity, such as smear microscopy, or require advanced laboratories with specific biocontainment facilities and liquid and solid culture capabilities, and can take weeks to months to produce results. To provide patients with correct and timely treatment and reduce further transmission of *M tuberculosis*, improved diagnostics must be available in places with the highest burden of TB. This not only requires that the diagnostics have high accuracy but also that they be low cost, simple, and designed for use in settings that lack adequate laboratory resources for conventional mycobacteriology, including trained technologists and reliable electricity.

The recent development of novel diagnostics and ongoing efforts to develop new biomarker assays can fulfill all of these criteria. Existing NAATs with high performance characteristics, such as the Xpert MTB/RIF test, can be used by workers safely and effectively after minimal training for the rapid diagnosis of TB. The future development of biomarker tests on breath or urine may prove even more useful if their accuracy can be optimized, especially in pediatric and HIV-infected populations for whom nucleic acid testing has not been as successful. As new tests are developed, clinical and operational studies will be needed to show if and how these tests affect patient and public health outcomes. Continued investment and interest in improving existing diagnostics and the development of new diagnostics will be required to advance molecular and biomarker-based technologies and to expand access to these technologies to resource-poor countries around the world.

REFERENCES

1. World Health Organization. Global tuberculosis report. Geneva (Switzerland): World Health Organization; 2012.
2. Steingart KR, Henry M, Ng V, et al. Fluorescence versus conventional sputum smear microscopy for tuberculosis: a systematic review. Lancet Infect Dis 2006;6(9):570–81.
3. Hepple P, Ford N, McNerney R. Microscopy compared to culture for the diagnosis of tuberculosis in induced sputum samples: a systematic review. Int J Tuberc Lung Dis 2012;16(5):579–88.
4. Storla DG, Yimer S, Bjune GA. A systematic review of delay in the diagnosis and treatment of tuberculosis. BMC Public Health 2008;8:15.
5. McNerney R, Maeurer M, Abubakar I, et al. Tuberculosis diagnostics and biomarkers: needs, challenges, recent advances, and opportunities. J Infect Dis 2012;205(Suppl 2):S147–58.
6. Weyer K, Carai S, Nunn P. Viewpoint TB diagnostics: what does the world really need? J Infect Dis 2011;204(Suppl 4):S1196–202.

7. Greco S, Girardi E, Navarra A, et al. Current evidence on diagnostic accuracy of commercially based nucleic acid amplification tests for the diagnosis of pulmonary tuberculosis. Thorax 2006;61(9):783–90.
8. Centers for Disease Control and Prevention. Nucleic acid amplification tests for tuberculosis. MMWR Morb Mortal Wkly Rep 1996;45(43):950–2.
9. Piersimoni C, Callegaro A, Nista D, et al. Comparative evaluation of two commercial amplification assays for direct detection of *Mycobacterium tuberculosis* complex in respiratory specimens. J Clin Microbiol 1997;35(1):193–6.
10. Guerra RL, Hooper NM, Baker JF, et al. Use of the amplified mycobacterium tuberculosis direct test in a public health laboratory: test performance and impact on clinical care. Chest 2007;132(3):946–51.
11. Rapid diagnostic tests for tuberculosis: what is the appropriate use? American Thoracic Society Workshop. Am J Respir Crit Care Med 1997;155(5):1804–14.
12. Centers for Disease Control and Prevention. Updated guidelines for the use of nucleic acid amplification tests in the diagnosis of tuberculosis. MMWR Morb Mortal Wkly Rep 2009;58(1):7–10.
13. McHugh TD, Pope CF, Ling CL, et al. Prospective evaluation of BDProbeTec strand displacement amplification (SDA) system for diagnosis of tuberculosis in non-respiratory and respiratory samples. J Med Microbiol 2004;53(Pt 12): 1215–9.
14. Jouveshomme S, Cambau E, Trystram D, et al. Clinical utility of an amplification test based on ligase chain reaction in pulmonary tuberculosis. Am J Respir Crit Care Med 1998;158(4):1096–101.
15. Parsons LM, Somoskövi A, Gutierrez C, et al. Laboratory diagnosis of tuberculosis in resource-poor countries: challenges and opportunities. Clin Microbiol Rev 2011;24(2):314–50.
16. Ling DI, Flores LL, Riley LW, et al. Commercial nucleic-acid amplification tests for diagnosis of pulmonary tuberculosis in respiratory specimens: meta-analysis and meta-regression. PLoS One 2008;3(2):e1536.
17. Pai M, Flores LL, Pai N, et al. Diagnostic accuracy of nucleic acid amplification tests for tuberculous meningitis: a systematic review and meta-analysis. Lancet Infect Dis 2003;3(10):633–43.
18. Pai M, Flores LL, Hubbard A, et al. Nucleic acid amplification tests in the diagnosis of tuberculous pleuritis: a systematic review and meta-analysis. BMC Infect Dis 2004;4:6.
19. Clinical and Laboratory Standards Institute. Document EP12–A2. User protocol for evaluation of qualitative test performance. Wayne (PA): CLSI; 2008.
20. Flores LL, Pai M, Colford JM, et al. In-house nucleic acid amplification tests for the detection of *Mycobacterium tuberculosis* in sputum specimens: meta-analysis and meta-regression. BMC Microbiol 2005;5:55.
21. Greco S, Rulli M, Girardi E, et al. Diagnostic accuracy of in-house PCR for pulmonary tuberculosis in smear-positive patients: meta-analysis and metaregression. J Clin Microbiol 2009;47(3):569–76.
22. Luo RF, Scahill MD, Banaei N. Comparison of single-copy and multicopy real-time PCR targets for detection of *Mycobacterium tuberculosis* in paraffin-embedded tissue. J Clin Microbiol 2010;48(7):2569–70.
23. Caminero JA. Multidrug-resistant tuberculosis: epidemiology, risk factors and case finding. Int J Tuberc Lung Dis 2010;14(4):382–90.
24. World Health Organization. Molecular line probe assays for rapid screening of patients at risk of multidrug-resistant tuberculosis. Geneva (Switzerland): World Health Organization; 2008.

25. Ignatyeva O, Kontsevaya I, Kovalyov A, et al. Detection of resistance to second-line antituberculosis drugs by use of the genotype MTBDRsl assay: a multi-center evaluation and feasibility study. J Clin Microbiol 2012;50(5):1593–7.

26. Morgan M, Kalantri S, Flores L, et al. A commercial line probe assay for the rapid detection of rifampicin resistance in *Mycobacterium tuberculosis*: a systematic review and meta-analysis. BMC Infect Dis 2005;5:62.

27. Bwanga F, Hoffner S, Haile M, et al. Direct susceptibility testing for multi drug resistant tuberculosis: a meta-analysis. BMC Infect Dis 2009;9:67.

28. Ling DI, Zwerling AA, Pai M. GenoType MTBDR assays for the diagnosis of multidrug-resistant tuberculosis: a meta-analysis. Eur Respir J 2008;32(5): 1165–74.

29. World Health Organization. Rapid implementation of the Xpert MTB/RIF diagnostic test. Geneva (Switzerland): World Health Organization; 2011.

30. Boehme CC, Nabeta P, Hillemann D, et al. Rapid molecular detection of tuberculosis and rifampin resistance. N Engl J Med 2010;363(11):1005–15.

31. Boehme CC, Nicol MP, Nabeta P, et al. Feasibility, diagnostic accuracy, and effectiveness of decentralised use of the Xpert MTB/RIF test for diagnosis of tuberculosis and multidrug resistance: a multicentre implementation study. Lancet 2011;377(9776):1495–505.

32. Scott LE, McCarthy K, Gous N, et al. Comparison of Xpert MTB/RIF with other nucleic acid technologies for diagnosing pulmonary tuberculosis in a high HIV prevalence setting: a prospective study. PLoS Med 2011;8(7):e1001061.

33. Banada PP, Sivasubramani SK, Blakemore R, et al. Containment of bioaerosol infection risk by the Xpert MTB/RIF assay and its applicability to point-of-care settings. J Clin Microbiol 2010;48(10):3551–7.

34. Andrews JR, Lawn SD, Rusu C, et al. The cost-effectiveness of routine tuberculosis screening with Xpert MTB/RIF prior to initiation of antiretroviral therapy: a model-based analysis. AIDS 2012;26(8):987–95.

35. Vassall A, van Kampen S, Sohn H, et al. Rapid diagnosis of tuberculosis with the Xpert MTB/RIF assay in high burden countries: a cost-effectiveness analysis. PLoS Med 2011;8(11):e1001120.

36. Boehme CC, Nabeta P, Henostroza G, et al. Operational feasibility of using loop-mediated isothermal amplification for diagnosis of pulmonary tuberculosis in microscopy centers of developing countries. J Clin Microbiol 2007;45(6): 1936–40.

37. Geojith G, Dhanasekaran S, Chandran SP, et al. Efficacy of loop mediated isothermal amplification (LAMP) assay for the laboratory identification of *Mycobacterium tuberculosis* isolates in a resource limited setting. J Microbiol Methods 2011;84(1):71–3.

38. Mitarai S, Okumura M, Toyota E, et al. Evaluation of a simple loop-mediated isothermal amplification test kit for the diagnosis of tuberculosis. Int J Tuberc Lung Dis 2011;15(9):1211–7, i.

39. Pai NP, Pai M. Point-of-care diagnostics for HIV and tuberculosis: landscape, pipeline, and unmet needs. Discov Med 2012;13(68):35–45.

40. Fang X, Chen H, Xu L, et al. A portable and integrated nucleic acid amplification microfluidic chip for identifying bacteria. Lab Chip 2012;12(8):1495–9.

41. Köser CU, Ellington MJ, Cartwright EJ, et al. Routine use of microbial whole genome sequencing in diagnostic and public health microbiology. PLoS Pathog 2012;8(8):e1002824.

42. Gardy JL, Johnston JC, Ho Sui SJ, et al. Whole-genome sequencing and social-network analysis of a tuberculosis outbreak. N Engl J Med 2011;364(8):730–9.

43. Wallis RS, Pai M, Menzies D, et al. Biomarkers and diagnostics for tuberculosis: progress, needs, and translation into practice. Lancet 2010;375(9729): 1920–37.
44. Vesenbeckh SM, Schönfeld N, Mauch H, et al. The use of interferon gamma release assays in the diagnosis of active tuberculosis. Tuberc Res Treat 2012; 2012:768723.
45. Metcalfe JZ, Everett CK, Steingart KR, et al. Interferon-γ release assays for active pulmonary tuberculosis diagnosis in adults in low- and middle-income countries: systematic review and meta-analysis. J Infect Dis 2011;204(Suppl 4):S1120–9.
46. Rangaka MX, Wilkinson KA, Glynn JR, et al. Predictive value of interferon-γ release assays for incident active tuberculosis: a systematic review and meta-analysis. Lancet Infect Dis 2012;12(1):45–55.
47. Sester M, Sotgiu G, Lange C, et al. Interferon-γ release assays for the diagnosis of active tuberculosis: a systematic review and meta-analysis. Eur Respir J 2011;37(1):100–11.
48. Turtle L, Kemp T, Davies GR, et al. In routine UK hospital practice T-SPOT.TB™ is useful in some patients with a modest pre-test probability of active tuberculosis. Eur J Intern Med 2012;23(4):363–7.
49. Steingart KR, Flores LL, Dendukuri N, et al. Commercial serological tests for the diagnosis of active pulmonary and extrapulmonary tuberculosis: an updated systematic review and meta-analysis. PLoS Med 2011;8(8):e1001062.
50. World Health Organization. Commercial serodiagnostic tests for the diagnosis of tuberculosis: policy statement. Geneva (Switzerland): World Health Organization; 2011.
51. Grenier J, Pinto L, Nair D, et al. Widespread use of serological tests for tuberculosis: data from 22 high-burden countries. Eur Respir J 2012;39(2):502–5.
52. Cannas A, Goletti D, Girardi E, et al. *Mycobacterium tuberculosis* DNA detection in soluble fraction of urine from pulmonary tuberculosis patients. Int J Tuberc Lung Dis 2008;12(2):146–51.
53. Chan J, Fan XD, Hunter SW, et al. Lipoarabinomannan, a possible virulence factor involved in persistence of *Mycobacterium tuberculosis* within macrophages. Infect Immun 1991;59(5):1755–61.
54. Minion J, Leung E, Talbot E, et al. Diagnosing tuberculosis with urine lipoarabinomannan: systematic review and meta-analysis. Eur Respir J 2011;38(6): 1398–405.
55. Lawn SD, Edwards DJ, Kranzer K, et al. Urine lipoarabinomannan assay for tuberculosis screening before antiretroviral therapy diagnostic yield and association with immune reconstitution disease. AIDS 2009;23(14):1875–80.
56. Lawn SD, Kerkhoff AD, Vogt M, et al. Diagnostic accuracy of a low-cost, urine antigen, point-of-care screening assay for HIV-associated pulmonary tuberculosis before antiretroviral therapy: a descriptive study. Lancet Infect Dis 2012; 12(3):201–9.
57. Phillips M, Basa-Dalay V, Bothamley G, et al. Breath biomarkers of active pulmonary tuberculosis. Tuberculosis (Edinb) 2010;90(2):145–51.
58. Kolk A, Hoelscher M, Maboko L, et al. Electronic-nose technology using sputum samples in diagnosis of patients with tuberculosis. J Clin Microbiol 2010;48(11): 4235–8.
59. Phillips M, Basa-Dalay V, Blais J, et al. Point-of-care breath test for biomarkers of active pulmonary tuberculosis. Tuberculosis (Edinb) 2012;92(4):314–20.
60. Bruins M, Rahim Z, Bos A, et al. Diagnosis of active tuberculosis by e-nose analysis of exhaled air. Tuberculosis (Edinb) 2012;93(2):232–8.

61. Kolk AH, van Berkel JJ, Claassens MM, et al. Breath analysis as a potential diagnostic tool for tuberculosis. Int J Tuberc Lung Dis 2012;16(6):777–82.
62. Qin L, Zheng R, Ma Z, et al. The selection and application of ssDNA aptamers against MPT64 protein in *Mycobacterium tuberculosis*. Clin Chem Lab Med 2009;47(4):405–11.
63. Rotherham LS, Maserumule C, Dheda K, et al. Selection and application of ssDNA aptamers to detect active TB from sputum samples. PLoS One 2012; 7(10):e46862.
64. Flores LL, Steingart KR, Dendukuri N, et al. Systematic review and meta-analysis of antigen detection tests for the diagnosis of tuberculosis. Clin Vaccine Immunol 2011;18(10):1616–27.
65. Xie H, Mire J, Kong Y, et al. Rapid point-of-care detection of the tuberculosis pathogen using a BlaC-specific fluorogenic probe. Nat Chem 2012;4(10):802–9.
66. Li H, Yang L, Zheng CY, et al. Use of bronchoalveolar lavage enzyme-linked immunospot for diagnosis of smear-negative pulmonary tuberculosis. Int J Tuberc Lung Dis 2012;16(12):1668–73.
67. Cattamanchi A, Ssewenyana I, Nabatanzi R, et al. Bronchoalveolar lavage enzyme-linked immunospot for diagnosis of smear-negative tuberculosis in HIV-infected patients. PLoS One 2012;7(6):e39838.
68. Greco S, Girardi E, Masciangelo R, et al. Adenosine deaminase and interferon gamma measurements for the diagnosis of tuberculous pleurisy: a meta-analysis. Int J Tuberc Lung Dis 2003;7(8):777–86.
69. Jiang J, Shi HZ, Liang QL, et al. Diagnostic value of interferon-gamma in tuberculous pleurisy: a metaanalysis. Chest 2007;131(4):1133–41.
70. Juan RS, Sánchez-Suárez C, Rebollo MJ, et al. Interferon gamma quantification in cerebrospinal fluid compared with PCR for the diagnosis of tuberculous meningitis. J Neurol 2006;253(10):1323–30.
71. Liang QL, Shi HZ, Wang K, et al. Diagnostic accuracy of adenosine deaminase in tuberculous pleurisy: a meta-analysis. Respir Med 2008;102(5):744–54.
72. Xu HB, Jiang RH, Li L, et al. Diagnostic value of adenosine deaminase in cerebrospinal fluid for tuberculous meningitis: a meta-analysis. Int J Tuberc Lung Dis 2010;14(11):1382–7.
73. Jadhav AA, Jain A. Sputum adenosine deaminase and alkaline phosphatase activity in pulmonary tuberculosis. Arch Physiol Biochem 2012;118(1):6–9.
74. Maertzdorf J, Weiner J, Kaufmann SH. Enabling biomarkers for tuberculosis control. Int J Tuberc Lung Dis 2012;16(9):1140–8.
75. Wang C, Yang S, Sun G, et al. Comparative miRNA expression profiles in individuals with latent and active tuberculosis. PLoS One 2011;6(10):e25832.
76. Kumar SG, Venugopal AK, Mahadevan A, et al. Quantitative proteomics for identifying biomarkers for tuberculous meningitis. Clin Proteomics 2012;9(1):12.
77. Fu YR, Yi ZJ, Guan SZ, et al. Proteomic analysis of sputum in patients with active pulmonary tuberculosis. Clin Microbiol Infect 2012;18(12):1241–7.
78. Zhang L, Wang Q, Wang W, et al. Identification of putative biomarkers for the serodiagnosis of drug-resistant *Mycobacterium tuberculosis*. Proteome Sci 2012;10:12.

Automation in the Clinical Microbiology Laboratory

Susan M. Novak, PhD*, Elizabeth M. Marlowe, PhD

KEYWORDS

- Clinical microbiology • Preanalytical automation • Total laboratory automation
- Efficiency • Quality

KEY POINTS

- Today there are more skilled technicians leaving the workforce than entering, which has resulted in a looming critical shortage of skilled laboratory workers. At the same time, laboratory testing is expected to increase with universal health care and an aging baby boomer population.
- Automation will play a key role in addressing workforce shortages while improving efficiency and maintaining quality in the clinical microbiology laboratory.
- Automation options range from preanalytical specimen processors to total laboratory automation (TLA) with digital imaging that allows for remote work-up of specimens and diagnostic telemedicine that will have an impact on patient care.
- The cost of laboratory automation will depend on the level of automation required. Future studies are needed to fully understand the financial and clinical impact of total automation on clinical laboratory workflow and patient outcomes.

THE CLINICAL MICROBIOLOGY LABORATORY TODAY

The role of the clinical microbiology laboratory is to assist in the diagnosis of infectious diseases. This role is critical to patient care, patient outcomes, and infection control. This is an era of newly emerging and re-emerging pathogens and increasing antimicrobial resistance. Couple this with a global society that has allowed for increased mobility of emerging pathogens and antibiotic-resistant superbugs across continents, and the role of the clinical microbiology laboratory cannot be understated. Additionally, if a bioterrorism event were to occur, the clinical microbiology laboratory would be a front line of protection to accurately identify the presence of a looming threat to the community.

The authors have nothing to disclose.
Southern California Permanente Medical Group, Regional Reference Laboratories, 11668 Sherman Way, North Hollywood, CA, USA
* Corresponding author.
E-mail address: susan.m.novak@kp.org

An illustrative example of this is the case of Andrew Speaker, who in 2007 created a tuberculosis scare after he traveled from Atlanta, Georgia, to Paris, Greece, Italy, Prague, and Canada and then back across the United States border, all while infected with multidrug-resistant tuberculosis.[1] This diagnosis was made with techniques that were developed over 40 years ago and require weeks to yields answers. Much in microbiology is still manual and requires highly skilled technologists to analyze and interpret cultures to provide organism identification and antimicrobial susceptibility profile. Improved techniques are on the horizon, the Xpert MTB/RIF assay (Cepheid, Sunnyvale, California) is a fully automated molecular assay that can detect *Mycobacterium tuberculosis* as well as rifampicin resistance from a direct specimen in 2 hours. Currently this assay is labeled for research use only, but is close to United States Food and Drug Administration approval and already in use outside the United States.

Most of the traditional methods in clinical microbiology are culture based, which requires the plating of specimens to growth media as they are received into a laboratory. The manual processing and plating of specimens is a way of life for bacteriology. Culture work-up today is manual and subjective and depends on a skilled technologist to read the plates and identify the pathogens. Over the past several decades, automation has made some inroads into clinical microbiology laboratories. Automation has had impacts on the area of bacterial identification and susceptibility testing with the introduction of the Vitek (bioMérieux, Marcy l'Etoile, France), MicroScan (Siemens, Malvern, Pennsylvania, and Newark, Delaware), and Phoenix (Becton Dickinson and Company, Franklin Lakes, NJ (BD)) systems. These systems allowed microbiology to move most of the testing from tubed biochemical identification and susceptibility testing methods to plates and cards with wells that can be incubated, monitored, and read automatically. Additionally, automated blood culture instruments that allow for the continuous monitoring of incubated blood culture bottles and flag cultures when positive was a leap ahead of the manual method of detecting positive blood cultures, both in terms of sensitivity and time to detection of positive cultures and workflow in laboratories. The manual method of working up blood cultures requires visual examination of bottles, subculturing of negatives, and 7 days of incubation. The streamlined use of staffing resources and improved methodologies has made adoption of these instruments commonplace.

With the advance of modern molecular techniques, the implementation of methods from translational research to the clinical laboratory has become easier. The use of polymerase chain reaction (PCR)-based tests have become more integrated in the routine microbiology laboratory. Historically molecular testing in the clinical laboratory has required the use of typically 3 unidirectional separate PCR rooms which make testing more complex. Currently in the United States, there are Food and Drug Administration–approved PCR assays that fully automate nucleic acid extraction, amplification, and detection in a closed single-use device. These advances have made this technology not only more accessible to smaller laboratories and nearer to patients. These systems have gone from a single pathogen target with an internal control to systems that now have the ability to detect 15 or more pathogens in a single specimen as a panel with a turnaround time of approximately 1 hour. Genome sequencing and gene arrays, although not widely used in clinical microbiology, could result in a further transformation of traditional diagnostic approaches.

CHALLENGES IN THE CLINICAL LABORATORY

Operational challenges to clinical microbiology laboratories have also grown. In the midst of changing technology, laboratories are challenged with budget cuts, a shrinking workforce, and legislation-mandated testing. At the same time, laboratories are expected to maintain quality for optimal patient care. Clinical laboratories and their role, however, are evolving. Laboratories are an active part of the way medicine is practiced. It has been estimated that as many as 70% of all medical decisions are based on laboratory results (Marc D. Silverstein, MD, unpublished data, 2003). Historically, microbiology laboratory results have relied on the growth of cultures that could delay patient results. New technology allows for rapid detection of pathogens directly from specimens. The tools now available are increasingly becoming more sophisticated and more accessible. These tools and the power behind them have the ability to substantially improve the quality and delivery of service, given that the necessary supporting teams (ie, infection prevention and antimicrobial stewardships) are in place. The pressure to become lean or eliminate waste along the entire stream of workflow, while maintaining quality, has left laboratories seeking ways to continually improve how patient care is delivered.

At the dawn of universal health care coverage in the United States, perhaps one of the most daunting challenges facing laboratories is who will perform the increasing volume of work and do so within budgetary constraints. The pipeline of laboratory workers is such that there are fewer skilled laboratory workers entering the workforce than leaving it, and the average medical technologist is approaching retirement age.[2–4] At the same time, there is a significant shortage of graduates from accredited laboratory science programs each year, so these programs simply cannot meet the demand to fill these positions.[2] There has also been a dramatic decline in the number of technologist training programs; 71% have closed from 1970 to 2007.[5] This decrease in technologist pool correlates with the projection that annually there is a greater than or equal to 70% shortfall of skilled laboratory workers.[3] These highly trained and skilled workers are college educated, certified, and/or licensed (depending in the state where they work) and a vanishing resource in this country. Similar to the nursing shortage this country faced more than a decade ago, the situation has hit the tipping point to becoming a crisis.

In part to mitigate this problem, in California, a medical laboratory technologist (MLT) licensure was implemented. MLTs are midlevel laboratory professionals. Under the supervision of a clinical laboratory scientist, an MLT can perform limited routine testing in a clinical laboratory and operate, maintain, and troubleshoot automated diagnostic instrumentation. MLTs can perform phlebotomy and moderately complex testing and supervise lower level laboratory workers. California currently has 6 approved MLT training programs in operation.[4]

Other solutions to improving the workforce crisis are to improve salary and increase public knowledge of laboratory science as a career choice. Change, however, will not happen quickly enough. Laboratories are increasingly asked to improve turnaround time and do more with less as budgets continue to shrink. TLA in clinical microbiology laboratories is one piece of the solution to addressing the workforce shortages that could improve efficiency and quality.

LIQUID MICROBIOLOGY—A PREREQUISITE TO PLATING AUTOMATION

Diagnosis of an infectious disease often requires the appropriate specimen collection from a clinically relevant site. Adequate specimen collection is extremely important to obtain quality results for patient care. Historically, collection swabs have been wound rayon-tipped swabs that are placed in a semisolid transport medium after collection. It is important to note about the rayon swab (**Fig. 1**) that, based on the tip structure, it is easy for a specimen to become trapped in the filaments that make up the tip of the

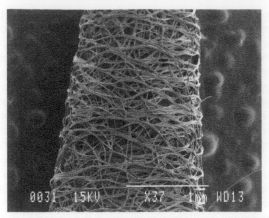

Fig. 1. Electron micrograph image of the tip of a rayon specimen collection swab. (*Courtesy of* Copan Diagnostics, Murrieta, CA; with permission.)

swab, thus reducing the amount of organism available for the plated media and pathogen recovery. Some culture types may require plating 5 or more different types of media, so little if any specimen may be remaining on the swab after being rolled across several plates.

To improve on the recovery of pathogens in a swab sample, Copan Diagnostics (Brescia, Italy) introduced the novel nylon flocked ESwab to microbiology in 2006. The ESwab is the only liquid based, multipurposed collection and transport system currently on the market. Perpendicular nylon fibers, as shown in **Fig. 2**, allow efficient collection and mitigate trapping of specimen due to the soft brush-like structure; hence, most of the available specimen attached to the flocked swab is eluted in the tube (approximately 90%) after it comes in contact with the liquid medium. Due to the homogenous nature of the specimen in the liquid Amies medium when plated, there is an equivalent distribution of the specimen on all plates, no matter how many plates are inoculated for a given specimen, contrary to conventional swabs. Because the transport medium is a liquid, the ESwab device is amenable for use on

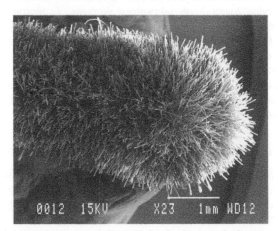

Fig. 2. Electron micrograph image of the tip of a flocked swab showing the increased surface area. (*Courtesy of* Copan Diagnostics, Murrieta, CA; with permission.)

automated plating instruments (**Fig. 3**). Studies show good viability of aerobic, anaerobic, and fastidious bacteria for up to 48 hours at room and refrigerated temperatures with the ESwab.[6–8] The performance of the ESwab compared with other swab systems for aerobic bacteria has been well documented.[7]

PREANALYTICAL AUTOMATION IN THE CLINICAL MICROBIOLOGY—HISTORICAL PERSPECTIVE

Historically, microbiology laboratories have been less automated than other clinical laboratories, such as chemistry. Laboratories in the United States and Europe have automated the preanalytical area of microbiology with the implementation of plating instruments. The reduction or elimination of repetitive tasks associated with manual plating can lead to efficiencies in labor savings and a reduction in ergonomic injuries.

The first semiautomated plating instrument, the Isoplater (Vista Technology, Edmonton, Alberta, Canada), was developed 23 years ago. Over the past several years, newer, more sophisticated plating instrumentation has been developed, such as the Innova (BD), InoquIA (part of TLA [discussed later] [BD Kiestra], Walk-Away Specimen Processor (WASP) (Copan Diagnostics), and PREVI Isola (bioMérieux). The newer instruments automate the plating of liquid specimens regardless of the specimen container type or size. All of these newer instruments can be interfaced with various laboratory information systems (LISs) that are currently available on the market. Interfaces with LISs are commonplace in laboratories for most instruments and can improve efficiency and patient safety in the laboratory setting. Reading of the primary specimen barcode and labeling of the plated media with patient identifiers allows for traceability and positive patient identification of all specimens. Some instruments are more versatile in that they have added features and functionality in addition to plating the primary specimen. These descriptions contained in this article are meant to highlight certain features on the various plating instruments and are not an exhaustive list of all the features available. **Fig. 4** summarizes and compares the fully automated preanalytical specimen processors currently on the market. For a more extensive list of instrument characteristics that should be taken into account when choosing a system, readers are referred to an article by Greub and Prod'hom.[9]

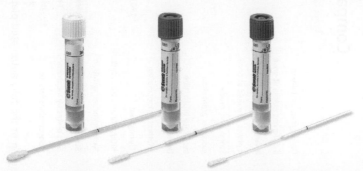

Fig. 3. Various ESwab collection and transport systems. White cap includes 1 regular-sized FLOQSwab (sampling sites: nose, throat, vaginal, and wounds). Green cap includes 1 minitip-sized FLOQSwab (sampling sites: eye, ear, nasal passages, and urogenital). Blue cap includes 1 flexible minitip-sized FLOQSwab (sampling sites: nasopharynx and pediatric sample collection). (*Courtesy of* Copan Diagnostics, Murrieta, CA; with permission.)

Comparison of Automated Specimen Processors

	PREVI Isola	Innova	WASP	InoqulA
De-cap/cap containers	No	Yes	Yes	Yes
# different media at once	5	6	9	12
# samples at once (max)	114	200	72	288
# plates streaked at once	1	1	1	Up to 5 at once
Streak only mode	No	Yes	Yes	Yes – MI module
Inoculate gram slide	No	No	Yes	Yes
Inoculate broth tube	No	No	Yes-Copan only	Yes
Detect ESwab presence	No	Yes	No	No
Method of Inoculation	Pipette	Re-useable loop	Re-useable loop	Pipette
Throughput	~180 inoculations/hr	~130 inoculations/hr	~130 inoculations/hr	250+ inoculations/hr
Integrate into track system	Future	No	Future	Yes - today
Sample vortex/agitation	No	Yes	Yes	Yes
Streaking Method	Spiral- plastic comb	Custom- loop	Custom- loop	Custom- rolling bead
Sort plates by incubator	Yes - standard	Yes - standard	Yes	Yes
Consumables/Waste	Streaking comb, pipette tip, extra cap	Re-useable loop	Re-useable loop	Re-useable bead, pipette tip

Fig. 4. Comparison of the fully automated plating instruments currently on the market.

ISOPLATER

The first semiautomated plating instrument developed was the Isoplater in 1989, and this device continues to be used in many laboratories. The instrument is semiautomated, meaning that the primary specimen must first be applied to the agar plate before placed on the instrument for streaking. Because specimens are planted onto the media before placed on the Isoplater, there is no requirement for a liquid sample. The streaking is performed with a wire loop and the pattern is a spiral streak (depicted in **Fig. 5**). This streaking pattern is unique and not the normal 4-quadrant streaking pattern that most technologists are familiar with in a clinical laboratory. There is a learning curve that technologists experience when moving from a 4-quadrant streak to a spiral streak pattern. With time and practice, technologists can easily make the transition to reading a spiral streak pattern. At Kaiser Permanente Regional Reference Laboratories, technologists adapted readily to the use of spiral streak pattern generated by the Isoplater. Other plating instruments in the authors' laboratory generate the 4-quadrant streak pattern but technologists have no problem reading plates that contain varied streak patterns. The Isoplater cannot be interfaced to an LIS, and barcodes or patient identifiers must be applied manually to the plates.

INOCULAB

In 2002, the InocuLAB (formerly Dynacon, now BD) was introduced to the market as an instrument that fully automated the plating process for liquid specimens (**Fig. 6**). The InocuLAB can decap the specimen container, inoculate the agar plate, and recap the container for future storage, adding to increased time savings and standardization within a laboratory. The InocuLAB can be programmed with several streaking patterns and a reusable wire loop is used for inoculating and streaking the specimen onto the plate. The InocuLAB can hold 40 specimens for primary plating. Becton Dickinson plans to phase out the InocuLAB and replace it in the market with Innova and InoquIA.

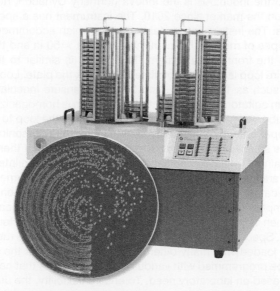

Fig. 5. Isoplater. The Isoplater is a first-generation semiautomated streak-only plating instrument. (*Courtesy of* Vista Technology Inc, Edmonton, Alberta Canada; with permission.)

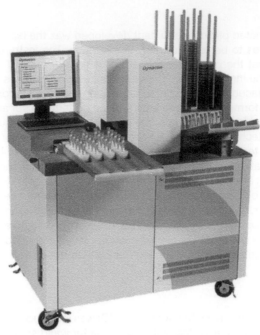

Fig. 6. InocuLAB. The InocuLAB is the first plating instrument that fully automated the decapping/capping and plating process for liquid specimens. (*Courtesy of* Becton Dickinson, Franklin Lakes, NJ; with permission.)

INNOVA

The successor to the InocuLAB is the Innova (formerly Dynacon, now BD) **(Fig. 7)**, which has been on the market since 2010. The instrument has a specimen capacity of 200 containers. The instrument contains 6 silos, which accommodate 270 plates and 6 different types of media. The instrument is 60 in × 50 in and the user only requires access to the front of the system. The Innova is similar to the InocuLAB in that a reusable wire loop is used to inoculate and streak the plate. Loops are available in various sizes, such as 1 μL, 10 μL, and 30 μL. To ensure inoculation quality, the Innova includes an agitator/shaker so that the specimen is homogenized before delivery to the plate/tube. An internal camera takes a picture of the loop to ensure the loop is straight for proper entry into the specimen container. An ultrasonic level senor ensures that there is sufficient volume in the specimen container. If there is not enough volume, the container is skipped and flagged so the operator can intervene when the other specimens are finished plating. The Innova was the first instrument to have a universal capper/decapper that can adjust to various-sized specimen transport containers. For example, the decapping/capping mechanism can uncap a urine boric acid tube and then adjust automatically to uncap a stool vial after the boric acid tube is recapped. Specimen containers are loaded in flexible metal racks, which allow the Innova to be loaded with many different-sized containers at the same time. The Innova can also be programmed with various plating protocols that can be configured by an end user based on laboratory need. To ensure flexibility, the user can program each drawer (a total of 5) with a unique plating protocol or the system can obtain the protocol information for each specimen container from the LIS. This is perhaps an

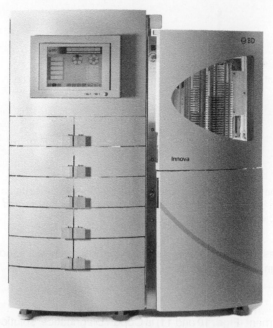

Fig. 7. Innova. The instrument has a specimen capacity of 200 containers and accommodates 270 plates and up to 6 different types of media. (*Courtesy of* Becton Dickinson, Franklin Lakes, NJ; with permission.)

important feature for smaller to medium-sized laboratories that might only have 1 plating instrument due to specimen volume and require added flexibility.

INOQULA

In 2012, BD acquired Kiestra, a Dutch company specializing in automation for the microbiology laboratory. Kiestra has been in the business of laboratory automation for 17 years, and installed its first system in a clinical microbiology laboratory in 2006. Kiestra has modular and full automation systems in operation with placements located in Europe, Australia, and the Middle East. The InoqulA (**Fig. 8**) has a dimension of 160 in × 36 in. The instrument has a capacity of 612 plates and can be loaded with 12 different media types. Compared with the other instruments discussed in this review, this system has the largest capacity. The system has customizable container racks and a flexible decapper so that different-sized containers can be processed by the system. A calibrated pipette is used to inoculate plates, broth tubes, and slides according to the sample protocol set by the end user. The instrument has a unique streaking technology that uses a magnetic rolling bead (shown in **Fig. 9**) to streak the plate using customizable patterns (spiral, 4 quadrant, biplate, and so forth). The beads can be reused after sterilization or disposed of. The instrument can streak up to 5 plates at one time with the rolling bead technology, enabling high throughput. So, for example, if a sample requires 7 plates to be inoculated, the InoqulA can streak 296 plates per hour.

The InoqulA also has a manual interactive mode that is designed for specimens that are not suitable for fully automated plating, such as tissues, catheter tips, and other

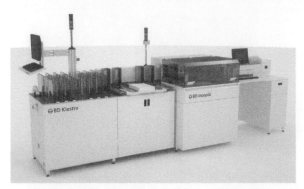

Fig. 8. InoculA. The InoculA is part of the Kiestra TLA line. The instrument has a capacity of 612 plates and can be loaded with 12 different media types. (*Courtesy of* Becton Dickinson, Franklin Lakes, NJ; with permission.)

nonliquid samples. In this mode, plates are automatically selected, barcoded, and streaked, while an operator manually inoculates the plates.

WASP

The WASP instrument (**Figs. 10** and **11**) is Copan Diagnostics' solution to preanalytical specimen processing automation, including plating and streaking, Gram slide preparation, and broth inoculation. The WASP has a footprint of 43.5 in × 81.5 in × 76 in and accommodates loading of up to 378 plates at once. There are 9 silos on the instrument that can accommodate up to 9 different types of media and can be loaded while the instrument is operating. The throughput of the instrument is approximately 180 bi-plates/hour. The instrument has a universal capping/decapping mechanism that allows for the plating of a wide variety of specimen types. The bidirectional interface allows for random loading of specimen types as the instrument queries the LIS to determine the specific plating protocol needed for that specimen type. The WASP includes a vortexer and a spinner so that the specimen is adequately homogenized for even specimen delivery and distribution during inoculation. Reusable metal loops are available in 3 sizes: 1 μL, 10 μL, and 30 μL. Each loop device comprises 2 individual loops, each of which (per the manufacturer) can process up to 15,000 plates. The

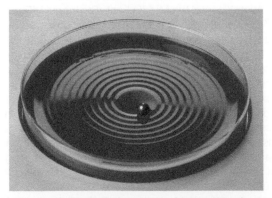

Fig. 9. Petri dish streaked with magnetic bead technology using the InoculA. (*Courtesy of* Becton Dickinson, Franklin Lakes, NJ; with permission.)

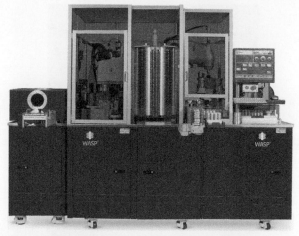

Fig. 10. WASP, front view. The instrument accommodates loading up to 378 plates at once. There are 9 silos on the instrument that can accommodate 9 different types of media. (*Courtesy of* Copan Diagnostics, Murrieta, CA; with permission.)

loops are incinerated between samples and inoculation is driven by specimen barcode. The WASP automatically selects the correct loop size based on the sample-type protocol. The WASP can use 2 loops on a single plate simultaneously, for example on a urine culture biplate, thus improving the throughput of the instrument. A variety of streak patterns can be programmed based on user need. For quality-control purposes, there is a camera that takes a picture of the loop each time an inoculation is made to assure a specimen is plated. The overall plating throughput varies depending on the streaking protocol.

In addition to plating functionality, the WASP includes a module that prepares a slide for Gram stain. The Gram SlidePrep Module (attached to the WASP, Copan) prepares not only the smear but will also ink jet the patient information directly onto the slide. The WASP contains another internal station called the warehouse carousel. This carousel can be loaded, for example, with Kirby-Bauer, optochin disks and bacitracin disks, to be planted on either primary or secondary plates for susceptibility testing or to aid in organism identification (**Fig. 12**). The WASP also includes a feature that allows inoculation of a mass spectrometer template. A study on the performance of the WASP was performed at Geisinger Health System,[10] which assessed cross-contamination, accuracy of the results, and quality of plating. Plated media results were comparable when WASP-inoculated plates were evaluated against routine plating methods.[10]

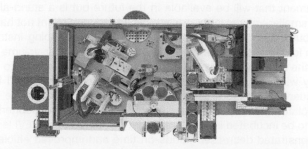

Fig. 11. WASP, top view. (*Courtesy of* Copan Diagnostics, Murrieta, CA; with permission.)

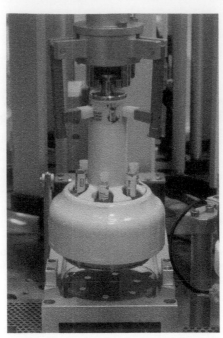

Fig. 12. WASP, warehouse carousel. (*Courtesy of* Copan Diagnostics, Murrieta, CA; with permission.)

PREVI ISOLA

The PREVI Isola (**Fig. 13**) is bioMérieux's product for preanalytical specimen plating. The instrument has a footprint of 66.5 in × 58.7 in × 35.7 in and accommodates 150 plates and 5 different types of media at once. The PREVI Isola has a unique streaking pattern, using a comb mimicking 16 loops streaking simultaneously, using a greater surface area of the agar that was shown to provide improved separation of organisms (**Fig. 14**). The spiral streaking pattern is similar to the Isoplater (described previously). Single-use, disposable specimen applicators (combs) are required for specimen inoculation of the primary specimen; the user also has the option to use 1 applicator per specimen. The throughput of the instrument is approximately 180 plates streaked per hour. The system also has the capability of streaking a biplate.

The PREVI Isola does not have the capability to decap and recap specimens, so these steps are manual. bioMérieux has in development an automated decapping/capping instrument that will be available in the future but is a stand-alone piece of equipment. In smaller-volume laboratories, this added step might not have an impact on efficiency but the necessary space needed for the decapping instrument might prove an issue for laboratories with limited floor space. In larger-volume laboratories, the impact of the lack of the capping/decapping functionality needs to be assessed but most likely will have an impact on efficiency savings. The PREVI Isola has the capability of querying the LIS similar to the other systems and can be programmed to segregate plates into separate canisters based on the atmospheric conditions the plates are to be incubated in. One study that compared the PREVI Isola to manual methods demonstrated decreased hands-on time and improved efficiency with the PREVI Isola.[11]

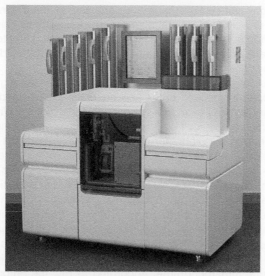

Fig. 13. PREVI Isola. The instrument accommodates 150 plates and 5 different types of media at once. (*Courtesy of* bioMérieux SA, Marcy l'Etoile, France.)

DIGITAL MICROBIOLOGY

Manufacturers have made progressive steps and have incorporated digital imaging into routine bacteriology incubators that have been in use for decades. The next generation of incubators will have a digital camera incorporated with an incubator for direct culture plate imaging. This digital imaging technology will allow clinical microbiology to develop and expand in ways that many would not have imagined. As part of the full automation package, the new incubators can be linked to the plating

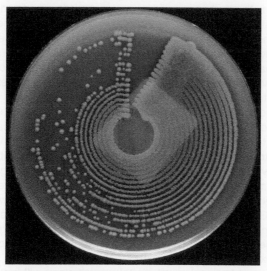

Fig. 14. Petri dish streaked using PREVI Isola. (*Courtesy of* bioMérieux SA, Marcy l'Etoile, France.)

instrument by a conveyor system that moves specimens into the incubators. Due to space constraints or workflow considerations, some laboratories may choose to forgo the conveyor belt/track systems and transfer plates into the incubators manually. The exact location where a plate is placed within the incubator will be determined by the software of the specific system.

The respective software systems can be programmed to take digital images of the media plates at operator-defined times and intervals. Digital images of the colony growth on the agar plate are taken and stored within the system. When technologists begin work on a culture, they call up images of a culture on a computer screen at a workbench and analyze the plates for growth/no growth from the screen (**Fig. 15**). The digital technology will allow technologists to observe the plates under different lighting conditions and magnify the colonies on the plate for better resolution during pathogen work-up. The optics of digital cameras allow better analysis of multiple morphotypes of bacteria that might be present in a specific sample The optics in digital cameras can observe colony growth on an agar plate that is invisible to the human eye. The WASPLab system, for example, has a camera that is capable of imaging a colony at 15 megapixels with a depth of 1 cm. For white colonies on a dark background, the limit of visualization is approximately 0.1 mm. Earlier recognition of growth could reduce turnaround time. According to BD, the European laboratories with Kiestra automation have adjusted their workflows based on the generation of results by digital imagers (BD Kiestra, personal communication, 2012). Laboratories have moved to working up the specimens when the cultures are available for workup and scheduling technologists accordingly. As with any new technology, there will be a period of training and a learning curve that technologists go through. Productivity will increase gradually over time and as technologists become more comfortable with reading cultures digitally, so gains expected when automation is introduced will take time.

Digital microbiology brings clinical laboratories into the twenty-first century. Many institutions are already practicing and reaping the benefits of telemedicine. Laboratories that are in offsite locations with less-experienced technologists could receive assistance from more-experienced technologists when working up cultures. Another future application is that software could be programmed to read and discard negative cultures and transfer the results to an LIS for reporting without the need for a technologist to observe the plate. If chromogenic agar is used to work up specimens in a more timely fashion (where certain organisms turn a specific color on the medium), perhaps in the future software could be programmed to read the color of a colony and report a positive or negative result on that plate without technologist intervention.

Other benefits to digital microbiology are quality assurance and the ability to use stored images and cases for training purposes. When quality-related issues arise in a laboratory regarding cultures, frequently the plates are already discarded. As a result, little can be done to answer questions that might have been raised. With digital image collection, laboratory staff has the ability to review cultures for quality-assurance purposes that were worked up historically. Another advantage of being able to store images is for laboratories to develop a repository of unique isolates or challenging cultures for teaching and training purposes. bioMérieux is currently working with a laboratory in Berlin, Germany, to determine exactly what set of images is most useful to medical technologists. Studies of vary lighting conditions and backgrounds are under way so it can be determined which set of images is most useful to technologists on the bench (bioMérieux, personal communication, 2013).

Software developed to supplement digital microbiology will have functionality so that multiple cultures on the same patient can be viewed on 1 computer screen.

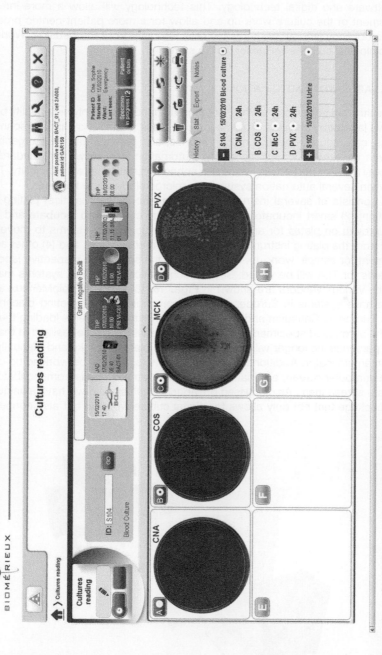

Fig. 15. Screen shot of MYLA courtesy of bioMérieux. Screen shots show an example of a computer screen with digital plate images. (Courtesy of bioMérieux SA, Marcy l'Etoile, France.)

This allows a broader-based assessment of all the cultures that are in a laboratory for a particular patient. For example, if both urine and blood cultures are growing a gram-negative rod, a technologist will be able to look at both cultures at the same time using the software and digital technology. This technology will allow a more integrated assessment of the culture work-up and allow for a more patient-centric process in the microbiology laboratory that is typically removed from the bedside. Work-up of microbiological cultures will never be the same.

TOTAL LABORATORY AUTOMATION

With health care reform comes the increased demand for not only high quality but cost effective laboratory services. Automation can result in efficiency and personnel cost savings, can reduce repetitive motion injuries, and perhaps can save organizations money in the area of workplace safety. Automation also allows for standardization in the way a task is performed, which can enhance quality and reproducibility. TLA occurs when several automation systems for microbiology come together.

TLA consists of several instrument components: (1) preanalytical plating instrumentation; (2) smart incubators containing digital cameras to incubate and photograph growth on plates for analysis; (3) track or conveyor systems to move plates to and from the plating instruments, incubators, and benches; and (4) other ancillary equipment for sample work-up. Depending on the size of the respective laboratory, the needs for TLA will be varied. Several schematics of the TLA systems manufactured by various vendors are shown in **Figs. 16–18**. Currently, bioMérieux and BD Kiestra have systems in Europe. All three companies are projecting placement of TLA in European, Canadian and US locations. With track systems loading the plates from the automated specimen processors, time savings will be realized in that laboratory personnel no longer will have to batch the plates in racks and manually place them in an incubator. Additionally, medical technologists will be working up cultures from a computer screen, eliminating the need to retrieve plates from incubators and manually screen them. As discussed previously, each system will have a unique software package that not only allows for digital culture work-up but also connects the

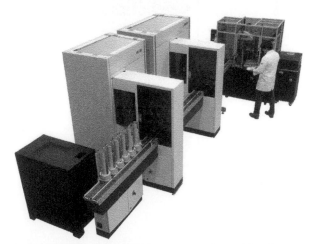

Fig. 16. WASPLab. Consists of WASP plating system, track, and incubator with digital camera. (*Courtesy of* Copan Diagnostics, Murrieta, CA; with permission.)

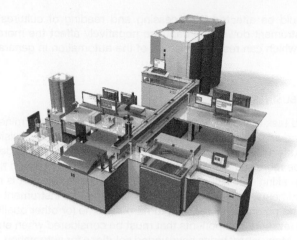

Fig. 17. BD Kiestra TLA. Consists of InoculA plating system, track system, and incubator with digital camera. (*Courtesy of* BD Kiestra B.V., 9207 JC Drachten, The Netherlands; with permission.)

various automation components that comprise a TLA solution for each vendor. bioMérieux is developing an ancillary instrument, called the Inoculum Preparation System, to inoculate the mass spectrometry template and tubes for susceptibility. Other vendors are developing similar instruments that can also inoculate a mass spectrometry template.

Mean time to failure data for track systems and digital incubators are not readily available because the instruments will be new to the market for bioMérieux and Copan, and BD Kiestra has been available solely in Europe. The Kiestra system tracks key performance indicators for their instruments, such as system availability, mean time between errors, and average time to repair. It is important with this instrumentation to ascertain reliability and mean time to failure before deployment in a laboratory setting for routine patient care. Poor reliability not only affects productivity in the workplace but also could have a significant negative impact on an operation that perhaps reduces personnel secondary to deployment of laboratory automation.

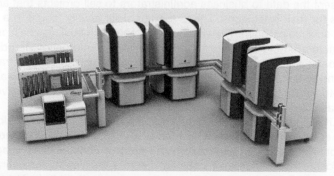

Fig. 18. bioMérieux. Full microbiology laboratory automation. Includes PREVI Isola, track system and smart incubator system with digital camera. (*Courtesy of* bioMérieux SA, Marcy l'Etoile, France.)

Patient care could be affected if processing and reading of cultures are delayed significantly. Instrument down time can also negatively affect the morale of laboratory personnel, which can result in mistrust of the automation in general and toward administration.

DEVELOPING A BUSINESS CASE

The complicated task of laboratories and manufacturers is to determine the automation necessity and provide a solid business case to support the acquisition of equipment. Automation manufacturers must realize that the relationship developed with customers will be more symbiotic than what exists today. Information that end users will need when making a decision about TLA solutions includes (but is not limited to) footprint of instruments, cost, mean time to failure of all the instrument components, labor savings, and potential decrease in turnaround time (or other quality indicators). These are just a few core components that must be considered when embarking on a solution for TLA. Many laboratories have varied solutions for automation. The question that remains is how the various TLA vendors will interface with automation, such as the Vitek, MicroScan, or Bactec (BD), already present in laboratories into a fully automated solution for each individual laboratory.

In 2010, health care expenditures in the United States approached $2.6 trillion. Compare this to 1980, when those costs were more than 10 times less, at $256 billion.[12] According to the Congressional Budget Office, laboratory spending is approximately 4% of health care expenditures, accounting for approximately $60 billion annually. Laboratory testing continues to grow every year because of newer, more specialized testing (that is often proprietary), consumer demand, and an aging population. It has been estimated that a majority, or approximately two-thirds, of health care decisions are based on laboratory results (Marc D. Silverstein, MD, unpublished data, 2003). Laboratories are unique, however, within the hospital setting. Conceivably, it is possible to run a hospital with most laboratory testing sent out. Consolidation of laboratory services and outreach programs has led to lower costs while generating revenue. Thus, hospital-based laboratories have competition. If there is a more cost-effective way to do something and address the lack of skilled laboratory workers, there is a threat that testing could be outsourced.

For laboratories to remain competitive, they must be able to make the case for new technology, namely automation, to administration. Part of the challenge is to know how to present a business case. In other words, technical directors have to learn how to present the data to business administrators to sell projects that are the best investments for their institutions. These are not skills readily taught in a laboratory or graduate science program. The first step to preparing a business case is to understand the factors driving the need for new technology/automation. In addition, it is important to understand who the stakeholders are (physicians, administration, technologists, and so forth) and educate them on the importance of laboratory automation. In the end, administrators will want to know what it will cost, what it will save, and how long it will take to get a return on investment (ROI).

Simply put, the key to selling the idea of automation in clinical microbiology laboratories is the cost difference between the manual and automated approaches. With the TLA components (described previously), the cost of consumables, reagents, and plates will, for the most part, remain constant. Factors, such as implementing ESwabs, to move to liquid microbiology could have an impact on cost analysis. The largest gain will be with the reduction in labor costs, with additional gains in quality, efficacy, reduced ergonomic injuries, and improved safety. The manual labor costs are

Table 1
Costs saved with automated microbiology specimen processor

Method	No. of FTEs/D	# D/Wk Plate	Annual Labor Costs[a]	Labor Savings/Y
Manual	2.5	7	$129,872.50	—
Automated	1.0	7	$51,949	$77,923.50

Abbreviation: FTE, Full Time Equivalent.
[a] Based on median laboratory assistant I cost with bonuses, benefits, and time off according to Salary.com, January 2013.

determined by calculating the total number of annual hours of staff time required to perform a procedure manually and multiplying those hours by the cost of labor (wages including benefits). The automated labor costs are determined by calculating the estimated annual hours of staff time required to perform a procedure in an automated fashion and multiplying those hours by the cost of labor (wages including benefits) (**Table 1**). Next, it is important to calculate the cost of acquisition; this includes the capital cost of the equipment, service contracts, cost of remodeling (if applicable), cost of interfacing equipment, and the cost of project planning/implementation/validation of the equipment (**Table 2**).

The ROI is calculated by determining the annual staff cost savings of the automated system (manual labor costs − automated labor costs) and dividing that by the cost of acquisition. This calculation determines how long it takes to recuperate the cost of converting to an automated process (**Table 3**). The ROI is meant to be a simplistic way to initially estimate if a project is worth the effort of a more-extensive cost analysis/pro forma.[13] This quantitative total has also been referred to as the economic justification index (EJI). An EJI of 0.5 equals 2 years, 1 is equal to 1 year, and 2 equals 6 months of a payback period for the reduction in costs.[14] Factors that are more difficult to quantify need to be monitored so gains to the organization due to reduced ergonomic injuries, quality, and turnaround time can be captured.

One approach to evaluating qualitative changes is to determine their strategic justification index (SJI). The SJI is determined by assigning a value of 0 to 2 (0 = not important, 1 = moderately important, and 2 = very important) to 6 change factors. These factors are quality, safety, procedure enhancement, audit trail, more timely decisions, and flexibility. The SJI is determined by dividing the sum of the 6 change factors by 12 (highest possible score). An SJI of 1 is equal to a very high value, indicating all 6 change factors are very important to the organization.[14]

To determine overall project justification, the EJI and SJI for the automation can be plotted on an X-Y graph, with a minimum of 0 and maximum of 1 (**Fig. 19**). This approach was originally proposed by the Zymar Corporation and later modified by Hamilton and colleagues[14,15] as a simple go/no-go tool for use before investing

Table 2
Cost of automated microbiology specimen processor

	Year 1	Year 2	Year 3	Year 4	Year 5	Total
Automation capital	$250,000					$250,000
LIS	$10,500					$10,500
Service Contract	—	$12,500	$12,500	$12,500	$12,500	$50,000
Total	$260,500	$12,500	$12,500	$12,500	$12,500	$310,500

Table 3	
ROI for an automated microbiology specimen processor	
Annual labor savings	$77,923.50
Five-year costs	$310,500.00
Payback period	3.98 y

time in a more detailed justification (Zynmark Corporation, unpublished data, 1988). An EJI of greater than 1 (meaning less than 1 year for ROI) most likely occurs in large-volume laboratories where the business case is more justifiable. The cost of TLA could potentially lend itself to more laboratory consolidation due to economies of scale. As a rule of thumb, companies like to see an ROI with a payback period of less than 4 years, but this may vary given what a company uses for expected lifetime of instrumentation.

For the most part, a stronger EJI is more compelling than a stronger SJI for the simple reason of being able to tangibly quantify a business case. If the EJI and SJI value of a project is low (ie, 0.25), this equates to only marginal justification, whereas an SJI and EJI value of 0.75–1 equates to a more compelling justification (see **Fig. 19**). In the end, these calculations provide a simple tool for determining if a project is worth the more detailed organization specific analysis while providing technical staff a means to communicate to nontechnical staff the justification of laboratory needs.

The total cost of ownership is another way to quantify the financial impact of deploying a new technology over the expected lifetime of the system. The gains quantified in annual payback can quickly disappear as equipment becomes degraded and less state of the art. There are costs to annually maintaining and upgrading equipment; although these costs are difficult to predict, they are beneficial to include in the planning process of automation.

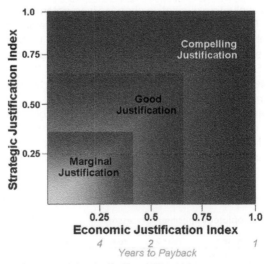

Fig. 19. Justification of automation. (*From* Hamilton SD. Justifying laboratory automation. SLA invited article. 2011. Available at: www.labautopedia.org/mw/index.php/justifying_laboratory_automation. This content is available under GNU free documentation License 1.2. Accessed January 2013.)

The cost of automation can vary greatly depending on the extent of automation. The most logical place to start with automation is the preanalytical instrumentation. Preanalytical automated microbiology processors costs range from $125,000 to $350,000, depending on manufacturer and instrument features. TLA costs are significantly higher and can run in the millions of dollars. Again, the cost of TLA will be laboratory dependent and vary by size of laboratory, specimen volume, and desired features of automation. Although the price tag seems high, the long-term the benefits are much larger. Laboratories in Europe have claimed increases in productivity by as much as 2.5-fold to 4-fold in a short time (Kiestra Lab Automation, unpublished data, 2012).[16]

Laboratories can use the tools discussed in this article to leverage the use of hospital resources to beat the odds and turn an expected administrative response from no to yes. The key to a successful business case is knowing how to present future value to an organization and quantify the gains. With any new technology, there are limitations to assessing costs beyond laboratory costs, particularly when there is a lack of published clinical impact studies. Automation will bring improvements in the quality of results and patient care. Those ROI studies will have to wait until the literature catches up and quality-improvement studies are in place. As Bob Dylan famously sang, "the times they are a-changing"; the face of clinical microbiology is in the midst of a metamorphis.

REFERENCES

1. 2007 Tuberculosis scare [Online Source]. 2013. 2-4-2013.
2. Best M. Strategic laboratory workforce planning—you can not afford not to do it [Magazine Article]. ASCP Laboratory Medicine 2004.
3. American Academy of Microbiology. Clinical micrbiology in the 21st century keeping the pace [Report]. American Academy of Microbiology. Washington, DC: ASM Press; 2008.
4. California Hospital Association. Critical roles: california allied healthcare workforce survey, report of key findings [Report]. Sacramento, CA: California Hospital Association; 2011.
5. The Lewin Group. Laboratory medicine: a National Status Report [Report]. Falls Church, VA: The Lewin Group; 2008.
6. Trotman-Grant A, Raney T, Dien BJ. Evaluation of optimal storage temperature, time, and transport medium for detection of group B Streptococcus in StrepB carrot broth. J Clin Microbiol 2012;50(7):2446–9.
7. Van Horn KG, Audette CD, Sebeck D, et al. Comparison of the Copan ESwab system with two Amies agar swab transport systems for maintenance of microorganism viability. J Clin Microbiol 2008;46(5):1655–8.
8. Van Horn KG, Audette CD, Tucker KA, et al. Comparison of 3 swab transport systems for direct release and recovery of aerobic and anaerobic bacteria. Diagn Microbiol Infect Dis 2008;62(4):471–3.
9. Greub G, Prod'hom G. Automation in clinical bacteriology: what system to choose? Clin Microbiol Infect 2011;17(5):655–60.
10. Bourbeau PP, Swartz BL. First evaluation of the WASP, a new automated microbiology plating instrument. J Clin Microbiol 2009;47(4):1101–6.
11. Mischnik A, Mieth M, Busch CJ, et al. First evaluation of automated specimen inoculation for wound swab samples by use of the Previ Isola system compared to manual inoculation in a routine laboratory: finding a cost-effective and accurate approach. J Clin Microbiol 2012;50(8):2732–6.

12. Centers for medicare and medicaid services OoANHSG [Report]. National Health Care Expeditures Data; 2012.
13. Young DS. Laboratory automation: smart strategies and practical applications. Clin Chem 2000;46(5):740–5.
14. Hamilton SD. Justifying laboratory automation. SLAS [Electronic Citation]. 11-30-2011.
15. Hamilton SD, Kramer GW, Russo MF. An Introduction to laboratory automation. 2011.
16. Matthews S, Deutekom J. The future of diagnostic bacteriology. Clin Microbiol Infect 2011;17(5):651–4.

MALDI-TOF Mass Spectrometry for Microorganism Identification

Tanis C. Dingle, PhD, Susan M. Butler-Wu, PhD*

KEYWORDS

- Mass spectrometry • Microbe identification • MALDI-TOF • Diagnosis

KEY POINTS

- MALDI-TOF MS is faster and more accurate than conventional identification methods for the identification of most bacterial and fungal clinical isolates.
- The identification of organisms by MALDI-TOF MS significantly decreases the turnaround time for the provision of definitive identification results to physicians.
- Some organisms currently cannot be reliably identified by this method, such as *Shigella* spp and *Streptococcus pneumoniae*.
- Direct-from-specimen organism identification, detection of antibiotic resistance, and epidemiology studies all are future possible applications for this method.

INTRODUCTION

The clinical microbiology laboratory plays a critical role in patient care by providing definitive knowledge of the cause of infection and antimicrobial susceptibility data to physicians. Rapid diagnostic methods are likely to improve patient outcomes (delayed initiation of effective antibiotic administration in patients with sepsis directly correlates with increased patient mortality).[1,2] Clinical microbiology has, however, traditionally been hampered by lengthy turnaround times for the provision of results to physicians. Conventional methods for identifying pathogens from a clinical specimen generally involve isolation of the organism in culture with subsequent examination of its phenotypic characteristics comprising a combination of microscopic and colony morphologies, along with an initial evaluation of growth on different culture media. Definitive identification typically requires additional overnight growth in vitro to ascertain reactivity of the organism with specific biochemical tests. Unfortunately, not all organisms can be readily identified using these methods and molecular diagnostic methods (eg, 16S rDNA sequencing) may be required. These methods are relatively rapid and can be used to identify uncommon or fastidious (ie, more difficult to grow) organisms.

Department of Laboratory Medicine, University of Washington Medical Center, Box 357110, 1959 Northeast Pacific Street, Seattle, WA 98195–7110, USA
* Corresponding author.
E-mail address: butlerwu@uw.edu

Clin Lab Med 33 (2013) 589–609
http://dx.doi.org/10.1016/j.cll.2013.03.001
0272-2712/13/$ – see front matter Published by Elsevier Inc.

labmed.theclinics.com

However, the cost and technical demands associated with these sequencing-based methods currently make them more suitable to the reference laboratory setting.

One of the newer and more powerful rapid methodologies being adopted in clinical microbiology laboratories worldwide is matrix-assisted laser desorption/ionization time-of-flight mass spectrometry (MALDI-TOF MS).[3–5] Long used in clinical chemistry, the first report of MS to characterize bacteria was described in 1975 by Anhalt and Fenselau.[6] Analyzing small molecules derived from lyophilized bacteria, the authors were able to differentiate taxonomically distinct organisms, although they were unable to differentiate between more closely related organisms (eg, *Escherichia* species and *Enterobacter* species). It was not until the 1980s when MALDI-TOF MS was developed, that the characterization of macromolecules by MS became possible.[7] Because of the ability of this technique to detect a large array of proteins rather than just small molecules, characterization of closely related species of organisms became possible.[8–10] In the late 1990s, application of the method to whole bacterial cells was found to produce characteristic and reproducible spectra that could be used to identify bacteria to the genus and species levels.[11–14] Barriers to clinical implementation at that time included the absence of commercially available systems, a dearth of standardized protocols, and poor reference database quality.

Only recently have commercially available and easy-to-use MALDI-TOF MS instruments come into more widespread use. This is readily evidenced by the ever-increasing number of publications describing the use of this method for identifying clinical isolates of microorganisms. This article reviews how MALDI-TOF MS and its superior efficacy in organism identification, in addition to its potential future applications, are likely to make it the new standard of practice in clinical microbiology.

PRINCIPLES OF MALDI-TOF MS FOR MICROBIAL IDENTIFICATION

The basic principle of intact cell MALDI-TOF MS is illustrated in **Fig. 1**. Briefly, microbial samples deposited on a target plate are overlaid with matrix solution, which cocrystalizes with the sample and lyses vegetative organisms.[15,16] More difficult to lyse microbes, such as certain Gram-positive bacteria, mycobacteria, yeast, and molds, often require an additional pretreatment with a strong organic acid or mechanical lysis (eg, bead-beating).[17–19] Once placed in the instrument, the samples are ionized by short laser pulses, forming gas phase ions with minimal fragmentation (ie, "soft ionization"), followed by acceleration of particles in a vacuum through an electric field. The amount of time each particle takes to reach the detector, or the so-called "time-of-flight," depends on its mass and charge. After all abundant proteins in the sample have been detected by the mass spectrometer, a spectral fingerprint is produced that is unique to the organism being analyzed. Studies have shown that the predominant proteins detected by MALDI-TOF MS are ribosomal proteins, although other highly abundant cytosolic proteins are also detected (eg, DNA-binding proteins and cold-shock proteins).[20–22] Identification of the organism being tested is then automatically determined using software that compares the spectral profile of the unknown organism with a reference database.

There are two commercially available MALDI-TOF MS systems for microbial identification (**Fig. 2**): the Bruker MALDI Biotyper (Bruker Daltonics, Billerica, MA) and the bioMérieux VITEK MS (bioMérieux, Durham, NC). Because the spectra obtained by MALDI-TOF MS are generally not completely identical to those already in the database, a "score value" (Bruker) or "confidence value" (bioMérieux) is assigned to each match based on the test organism's similarities to the reference spectra. For example, the MALDI Biotyper recommends that score values of greater than or equal

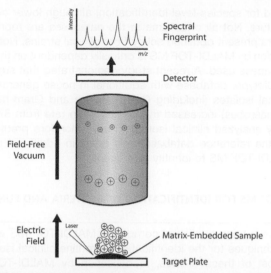

Fig. 1. Principle of MALDI-TOF MS for microbial identification. Microbial samples are deposited on a conductive metallic target plate and overlaid with a matrix solution composed of an organic acid. Once placed in the instrument, the samples are ionized by short laser followed by acceleration of variably charged particles through an electric field. The amount of time it takes for each particle to pass through a field-free tube, or time of flight (TOF), depends on its mass and charge and is measured by a detector. An organism-specific spectral fingerprint is generated and compared with thousands of spectral profiles in a database to obtain an identification of the organism. (*Courtesy of* Wigington K, Calgary, AB.)

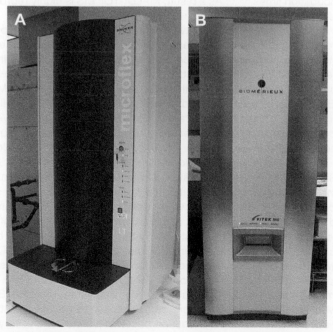

Fig. 2. (*A*) Bruker Daltonics MALDI Biotyper. (*B*) bioMérieux VITEK MS.

to 2.0 be obtained for species-level identification, although lower cutoffs have been used in the literature. Not all organisms in the databases are represented equally, nor are the spectra present obtained solely from clinical strains. Not surprisingly, organism identification by MALDI-TOF MS is critically dependent on the quality and accuracy of the database used. A recent study demonstrated that supplementation of the commercial Biotyper database with additional in-house generated spectra from 229 routine clinical isolates (including Gram-positive and Gram-negative bacteria, and yeast and anaerobes) increased the identification rate from 87.1% to 98% for 498 prospectively analyzed clinical isolates.[23] It is therefore predicted that further development of the reference databases will result in additional improvements in the ability of MALDI-TOF MS to identify pathogens.

USE OF MALDI-TOF MS FOR IDENTIFICATION OF BACTERIA AND FUNGI
Bacteria

Several studies have been published comparing MALDI-TOF MS with conventional microbiologic techniques for the identification of routine clinical isolates of bacteria (**Table 1**). In most of these studies, identification by MALDI-TOF MS has outperformed conventional methods. For example, in one study where 980 routine clinical isolates were prospectively analyzed by MALDI-TOF MS, 92% of isolates were correctly identified to the species-level compared with 83.1% of isolates identified using conventional identification methods.[19] Furthermore, conventional methods resulted in more incorrect genus-level identifications (1.6%) compared with MALDI-TOF MS (0.1%).[19] Because ribosomal proteins in the m/z 2- to 20-kDa range constitute the predominant peaks recorded by MALDI-TOF MS and expression of these proteins does not seem to vary under different cultivation conditions,[24,25] the performance of MALDI-TOF MS is not generally affected by culture media, cultivation conditions, or incubation times.[26–28] As a result, MALDI-TOF MS is highly reproducible for bacterial identification.

Although most published studies have used the Bruker MALDI Biotyper system, several have directly compared the performance of both available systems. In the first such study, the number of high-confidence identifications (as defined by the manufacturers of both instruments) obtained for 720 isolates was somewhat higher for the Bruker MS system (94.4%) than for the bioMérieux VITEK MS system (88.8%).[29] Both systems demonstrated more than 99% accuracy overall; however, lower accuracy was observed for Gram-negative anaerobes and several of the α-hemolytic Streptococcus species tested. In the latter case, only four of seven (57.1%) and five of seven (71.4%) of Streptococcus isolates yielding high-confidence identifications were correctly identified by the Bruker MS and bioMérieux MS, respectively. Misidentification would have been unlikely to alter patient management for the remainder of the incorrect results in the study (eg, an identification of Achromobacter xylosoxidans vs Achromobacter dentrificans). Importantly, 9 (69%) and 5 (38%) of 13 isolates that could not be identified by conventional identification methods were correctly identified by the Bruker MS and the bioMérieux MS, respectively.[29] Furthermore, where the results obtained by MALDI-TOF MS disagreed with those obtained using conventional methods, 16S rDNA sequencing resolved most disagreements in favor of the MALDI TOF MS result (75%–78.3%).[29] More recently, Carbonelle and colleagues[30] demonstrated that the Bruker and Shimadzu MALDI-TOF MS systems were comparable in terms of correct identifications to the species level for the 317 routine bacterial isolates analyzed with 94.9% and 93.4% correct identifications, respectively. Both systems had difficulty

Table 1
Performance of MALDI-TOF MS for routine bacterial identification[a]

Specimen Type	Study	N	System	Database	Database Supplemented?	Genus Level IDs (%)	Species Level IDs (%)	Organisms Misidentified or Unable to be Identified
Routine bacterial isolates	Seng et al,[5] 2009	1660	Bruker	Biotyper v2.0	No	95.4	84.1	Shigella species, Stenotrophomonas maltophilia, Streptococcus species and anaerobes
	Cherkaoui et al,[29] 2010	720	Bruker bioM	Biotyper SARAMIS	No / No	100 / 100	94.4 / 88.8	Gram-negative anaerobes and Streptococcus species
	van Veen et al,[19] 2010	980	Bruker	Biotyper v2.0	No	98.8	92	Streptococcus pneumoniae, viridans group Streptococci, Stenotrophomonas maltophilia
	Bizzini et al,[17] 2010	1371	Bruker	Biotyper v2.0	No	98.5	93.2	Shigella species, Streptococcus species and some Gram-negative rods
	Carbonelle et al,[30] 2012	317	Bruker bioM	Biotyper v2.0 SARAMIS v'08	No / No	97.4 / 97.2	94.9 / 93.4	Shigella sonnei, Streptococcus species, Enterobacter species
	Dubois et al,[31] 2012	767	bioM	VITEK	No	96.2	86.7	Aggregatibacter segnis, Shigella flexneri, Neisseria mucosa, Streptococcus species
Anaerobic bacteria	Veloo et al,[36] 2011	79	Bruker bioM	Biotyper v3.0 SARAMIS	No / No	60.8 / 70.9	50.6 / 60.8	Bacteroides species, Actinomyces species, Fusobacterium species
	Justesen et al,[87] 2011	290	Bruker bioM	Biotyper v3.1.1 SARAMIS v'10	No / No		67.2 / 49	Bacteroides species, Veillonella species, Fusobacterium species
	Fedorko et al,[37] 2012	152	Bruker	Biotyper v2.0.4	No	86	79	Fusobacterium species
	Fournier et al,[38] 2012	238	Bruker	Biotyper v3.0	No	Direct 87 Ext 91.6	Direct 66.4 Ext 77.7	Fusobacterium species, Propionibacterium species, Clostridium species
	Nagy et al,[39] 2012	283	Bruker	Biotyper v3.0	No	88	77	Bacteroides species

Abbreviations: bioM, bioMérieux; Direct, direct application; Ext, extraction.

a Because of the constantly evolving nature of MALDI-TOF MS databases, comparison between the results of older and newer studies is difficult. Conclusions should be drawn with caution.

identifying *Shigella sonnei* (misidentified as *Escherichia coli*) and *Streptococcus* species, consistent with other published studies.[5,17,31]

The performance of MALDI-TOF MS for the identification of genera that tend to be more recalcitrant to identification using routine methods has also been studied. For example, an analysis of 659 Gram-positive organisms (including *Nocardia, Listeria, Actinomyces,* and *Bacillus* species) by MALDI-TOF MS demonstrated that 98.5% of isolates were correctly identified to the species level (excluding *Listeria* species).[32] Furthermore, MALDI-TOF MS was capable of distinguishing between closely related species of *Corynebacterium* (*C diphtheriae, C pseudotuberculosis, C ulcerans*), which are generally more challenging to differentiate. MALDI-TOF MS also correctly identified Gram-positive organisms that typically require sequencing-based techniques for definitive identification to the species level (*Nocardia* and *Actinomyces* species). However, most *Listeria* isolates tested (93%) could only be identified to the genus level because of indistinguishable spectra produced by multiple species.[32]

The identification of nonfermenting Gram-negative bacilli (NFGNB) (which include *Pseudomonas aeruginosa* and members of the *Burkholderia cepacia* complex) from patients with cystic fibrosis (CF) is particularly challenging for laboratories. Because of chronic colonization of the CF airway by these organisms, many isolates fail to produce typical phenotypic characteristics, have become biochemically inert, and thus are not reliably identified using conventional biochemical-based methods.[33,34] Even though molecular methods perform excellently for the identification of NFGNB, these are laborious and expensive to perform. When 200 NFGNB isolates from patients with CF were analyzed, MALDI-TOF MS outperformed conventional methods with regards to speed and reliability.[34] The Bruker MALDI Biotyper outperformed the bioMerieux VITEK MS for these isolates (97% vs 89.5%), although the Bruker system more frequently required an additional extraction step.[34] MALDI-TOF MS identification for NFGNB is rapid and reliable, and is likely to facilitate more timely management of infection and colonization in patients with CF than the current standard of practice.[33,34]

Accurate and timely identification of *Mycobacterium* species is critical not only for initiating the most appropriate antimicrobial therapy, but also for infection prevention purposes (eg, discontinuing respiratory precautions for patients infected with nontuberculosis *Mycobacterium* species). Nevertheless, the identification of *Mycobacterium* species using conventional methods is particularly cumbersome and time consuming. These organisms were traditionally identified based on growth characteristics, biochemical testing, pigment production, and high-performance liquid chromatography, with testing often taking weeks to perform. Even though these methods have largely been replaced by nucleic acid probe assays and DNA sequencing of specific genes (eg, *hsp65* and *rpoB*), a more cost-effective testing option is highly desirable. Because of the mycolic acid-rich cell wall and infectious nature of *Mycobacterium tuberculosis*, MALDI-TOF MS for *Mycobacterium* identification is generally preceded by a heat-killing and protein extraction step. The manufacturers of both available instruments have recommended protocols that involve a combination of heat, ethanol treatment, and mechanical lysis. In addition, one recent study has described a procedure that reproducibly produces high-quality spectra for this group of organisms that involves a combination of heating at 95°C for 30 minutes, micropestle dispersion, and protein extraction using formic acid and glass beads. This strategy led to successful MALDI-TOF MS identification of 90 (87%) of 104 mycobacterial isolates to the species level using an in-house–developed database, with 13 of these isolates identified only to the genus level.[35] Although MALDI-TOF MS could identify members of the *M tuberculosis* complex, it could not separate them to the species level.

In contrast to the organisms described thus far, the identification of anaerobic bacteria by MALDI-TOF MS has been somewhat problematic (see **Table 1**). In one study from 2011, both commercially available MALDI-TOF MS systems were compared for the identification of 79 isolates representing 19 different genera of anaerobic Gram-positive and Gram-negative bacteria. The bioMérieux VITEK MS demonstrated superior performance to the Bruker system, identifying more anaerobes to the genus level (70.9% vs 60.8%, respectively).[36] These findings were critically dependent on the composition and quality of the database used; when organisms absent from the database were excluded from the analysis, correct genus identifications were obtained in 76.7% and 75% of cases for the bioMérieux VITEK MS and Bruker MS systems, respectively.[36] Several more recent studies evaluating the Bruker MS for identification of anaerobes have achieved improved rates of identification to the species level (77%–79%) most likely resulting from enhanced database quality and the inclusion of a prior extraction step (see **Table 1**).[37–39] Overall, the identification of anaerobes by MALDI-TOF MS seems to be less reliable than for aerobic bacteria. A variety of explanations are possible including culture age, composition of the media used for organism growth, the quantity of organism tested, and the database used. Further studies are required to determine whether additional optimization is possible for anaerobic bacteria.

Yeasts and Molds

Immunocompromised patients are at increased risk for the development of invasive fungal infections, yet can present with nonspecific signs and symptoms of infection. Delayed initiation of antifungal therapy has been shown to correlate with higher mortality and prompt identification of the cause of infection is essential in enabling physicians to select the most appropriate treatment. Because of important differences in the intrinsic resistance of closely related organisms to antifungal agents, timely identification of fungal isolates is imperative. Examples of this intrinsic resistance include fluconazole resistance in *Candida krusei* and amphotericin B resistance in *Candida lusitaniae*. The current standard of practice for the identification of fungi is slow. This is particularly so for filamentous fungi, where identification of mold isolates primarily relies on the microscopic examination of reproductive structures produced during in vitro growth. The formation of these structures can be a lengthy process and one that does not always occur, despite the best efforts of the laboratory. In the absence of additional molecular-based testing, the identification of such isolates can only be resulted to physicians as "mycelia sterilia." Unfortunately, this identification result provides no indication to the physician as to the true identity of the organism.

The efficacy of MALDI-TOF MS for the identification of yeast and mold isolates has been examined in several studies (**Table 2**). In contrast to bacteria, a prior lysis and extraction step (involving multiple washes in absolute ethanol and formic acid) seems to be required. This requirement is believed to result from the thick, chitin-containing cell wall present in fungi.[40] However, a dramatically abbreviated procedure consisting of a formic acid overlay before the application of matrix solution seems to be a suitable alternative for most yeast clinical isolates.[40] In one study consisting of 241 yeast isolates (including *Candida*, *Cryptococcus*, *Rhodotorula*, and *Saccharomyces* species), 92% were correctly identified to the species level by MALDI-TOF MS.[41] Importantly, MALDI-TOF MS outperformed conventional methods for the identification of *C krusei* and *Candida dubliniensis*. Although minor differences were noted, the overall performance of MALDI-TOF MS did not seem to be influenced by either the culture media used (BHI agar, IMA, SAB) or the culture incubation time.[41] No major differences in performance were observed between the Bruker MALDI Biotyper and the bioMérieux

Table 2
Performance of MALDI-TOF MS for yeast and mold identification

Specimen Type	Reference	N	System	Database	Database Supplemented?	Genus Level IDs (%)	Species Level IDs (%)	Organisms Misidentified or Unable to be Identified
Yeasts	Marklein et al,[88] 2009 (250 Candida species)	267	Bruker	Biotyper v2.0	No		96	Candida norvegensis, C rugosa, C dubliniensis, C ciferrii (not present in original database, but identified successfully when supplemented)
					Yes		100	
	Stevenson et al,[89] 2010	194	Bruker	Biotyper v2.0.4	Yes	99	87.1	C rugosa, Cryptococcus neoformans
	van Veen et al,[19] 2010	61	Bruker	Biotyper v2.0	No	96.7	85.2	C dubliniensis (not in database)
	Bader et al,[42] 2011	1192	Bruker	Biotyper v3.0	No		97.6	Pichia species, several Candida species not in the database
			bioM	SARAMIS 3.3.1	No		96.1	
	Dhiman et al,[41] 2011	241	Bruker	Biotyper v2.0	No	93.4	87.6	Candida guilliermondii, Aureobasidium/Hormonema, C neoformans
Molds	Alanio et al,[43] 2011 (Aspergillus species)	140	Bruker	Andromas	Yes		98.6	Aspergillus fumigatus (no misidentifications)
	De Carolis et al,[44] 2012 (Aspergillus, Fusarium, Mucorales species)	103	Bruker	Biotyper v2.0	Yes	100	96.8	None
	Alshawa et al,[45] 2012 (dermatophytes)	381	Andromas	Andromas	Yes		91.9	Trichophyton metagrophytes var. interdigitale; spectral acquisition failed for 27 isolates

Abbreviation: bioM, bioMérieux.

VITEK MS systems for the identification of 1192 yeast isolates representing 36 species.[42] Both systems successfully differentiated closely related species (eg, *Candida glabrata* and *Candida bracarensis*) where biochemical methods were unable to do so. As with bacterial isolates, misidentification or the inability of MALDI-TOF MS to identify particular yeast isolates most often resulted from the absence of a corresponding reference spectrum for that species in the database.

Only recently has the clinical use of MALDI-TOF MS for the identification of mold isolates been evaluated. Thus far, the reference databases for filamentous fungi have been somewhat limited with respect to the depth and breadth of organism coverage.[3] However, recent data suggest that MALDI-TOF MS can be successfully applied to the identification of molds with appropriate database development. In one such study, a database of clinically relevant *Aspergillus* species was created that included spectra from both young and mature colonies. This approach led to accurate species identification (138 of 140 isolates) regardless of maturity of the organism tested.[43] The relatively poor representation of molds in currently available reference databases therefore requires laboratories interested in using this method to supplement the commercial databases with clinically relevant and diverse strains. De Carolis and colleagues[44] prospectively analyzed 103 clinical isolates of *Aspergillus*, *Fusarium*, and *Mucorales* after creating a reference database using culture collection strains. MALDI-TOF MS identified 96.8% of isolates to the species level, after nine organisms that were absent from their database were excluded from the analysis. Similarly, Alshawa and colleagues[45] created a database of 50 reference strains belonging to 12 clinically relevant species of dermatophytes. Using this database, 91.9% of the dermatophytes were correctly identified. However, this protocol was only validated for 3-week-old cultures and younger cultures were not evaluated. Thus, although MALDI-TOF MS shows great promise for these organisms, routine identification of molds by MALDI-TOF MS in the clinical laboratory is still in its infancy.

ADVANTAGES AND LIMITATIONS OF MALDI-TOF MS FOR MICROBIAL IDENTIFICATION

The major advantages and limitations associated with MALDI-TOF MS for organism identification are summarized in **Table 3**. Not only does MALDI-TOF MS outperform conventional methods for organism identification in terms of accuracy, it dramatically outperforms these methods with regards to speed. Thus, the primary advantage associated with MALDI-TOF MS is arguably the dramatically reduced turnaround time for result reporting to physicians (**Fig. 3**). Multiple studies have demonstrated improved turnaround times for microbial identification using MALDI-TOF MS compared with conventional methods. In 2009, Seng and colleagues[5] initially reported that MALDI-TOF MS results could be obtained from a given isolate within 6 to 8.5 minutes, compared with 5 to 48 hours for conventional identification methods. This turnaround time could be further improved by batching samples, a practice already common in most laboratories. Cherkaoui and colleagues[29] reported the ability to identify 10 batched isolates in less than 15 minutes by MALDI-TOF MS. More recently, the time to identification by MALDI-TOF MS in a prospective analysis of 952 microbial isolates yielded a definitive identification on average 1.45 days earlier compared with standard methods.[46] The improvement in time to identification by MALDI-TOF MS is even greater for organisms that are either fastidious or slow-growing (eg, HACEK, anaerobes, and so forth).[46] It has widely been speculated that the earlier provision of definitive organism identification to physicians has the potential to positively impact patient care by enabling physicians to target antimicrobial therapy earlier in the clinical course. Although this has not been directly investigated for cultured isolates, it has

Table 3
Advantages and limitations of MALDI-TOF MS for microbial identification

Advantages	Limitations
Rapid turnaround time	Unable to differentiate between certain highly related organisms
Low cost per test	High initial instrument cost
High throughput	Requires pure culture or well-isolated colonies
Reliable and reproducible	Breadth of databases needs improvement
Minimal isolate required (as little as a single colony)	Certain organisms (eg, fungi) require protein extraction before analysis
Ability to identify a broad range of microorganisms on a single platform	Unable to perform quantitation
Easy to use with respect to sample preparation, running, and data analysis	Ability to detect antibiotic resistance is variable
Errors in the initial identification process, such as Gram stain, do not impact the outcome of MALDI-TOF MS	Absence of practice guidelines for validation, implementation, or reporting of results
Preselection of phenotypic assays required for identification is unnecessary	At the time of writing, neither commercially available platform has Food and Drug Administration clearance for in vitro diagnostic use
Potential to identify organisms typically difficult to identify by conventional methods or organisms that require molecular methods to identify	
Potential to identify new disease-organism associations because MALDI-TOF MS databases are more comprehensive than typical phenotypic systems	

been addressed for the identification of organisms directly from positive blood cultures (discussed later).

The up-front instrumentation cost for MALDI-TOF MS is high (approximately $200,000), which has thus far limited implementation of this method to larger laboratories. However, the time to return of investment can be relatively short because of the low operating and consumable costs compared with conventional methods.[25,26,47] The cost per isolate for identification by MALDI-TOF MS has been estimated at only $0.50.[29,41] One recent study from a clinical microbiology laboratory that processes approximately 175,000 specimens annually for bacterial and fungal cultures suggested that incorporation of MALDI-TOF MS into the routine work flow can reduce reagent and labor costs by $102,424 (56.9%) annually compared with the continued use of traditional methodologies.[46] Another study evaluating the costs of bacterial identification suggested that the savings associated with the use of MALDI-TOF MS could be 89.3% compared with conventional methods. Implementation of MALDI-TOF MS into the laboratory work flow reduces the amount of hands-on technologist time required to perform organism identification enabling laboratory staff to instead engage in additional value-added activities.[5] Thus, despite the initial outlay of investment required for implementation of MALDI-TOF MS, the long-term savings associated with use of this method are likely to increase the prevalence of its use in clinical microbiology laboratories.

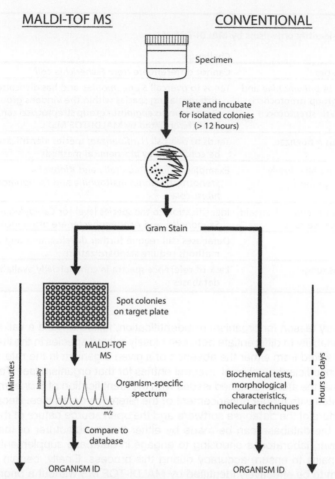

Fig. 3. Comparison of MALDI-TOF MS work flow versus conventional identification methods in the clinical microbiology laboratory. In comparison with the turnaround time for conventional methods (hours to days depending on the organism), MALDI-TOF MS provides organism identification within minutes. (*Courtesy of* Wigington K, Calgary, AB.)

MALDI-TOF MS is not without its limitations (see **Table 3**). Although MALDI-TOF MS is generally superior to conventional methods with respect to accuracy, this is not the case for all organisms. Specifically, the method is unable to differentiate between highly related organisms whose ribosomal proteins tend to be extremely well conserved, such as *E coli* and *Shigella* species (**Table 4** provides other examples). Thus, laboratories must perform additional testing using conventional methods on non–lactose fermenting isolates of *E coli* to rule out *Shigella* species. In addition, it has been repeatedly observed that MALDI-TOF MS systems tend to err on the side of caution with regards to the identification of certain pathogens that have less-pathogenic relatives. The major examples of this are *Streptococcus pneumoniae* and viridans group streptococci, and *Haemophilus influenzae* and certain noninfluenzae *Haemophilus* species (eg, *H haemolyticus*). Organisms yielding an identification of *S pneumoniae* or *H influenzae* by MALDI-TOF MS must have the identification confirmed using conventional biochemical techniques (data not shown[48]).

Table 4
Difficult-to-identify organisms by MALDI-TOF MS

Organism	Challenge
Shigella species	Cannot differentiate from *Escherichia coli*
Streptococcus pneumoniae and viridans group streptococci (α-hemolytic streptococci)	Tends to overcall *S pneumoniae* and has difficulty differentiating species within the viridans group. *Streptococcus anginosus* group streptococci can, however, be differentiated by MALDI-TOF MS.
Haemophilus influenzae	Tends to overcall *H influenzae*; species identification should be confirmed by biochemical methods
Any taxonomically closely related organisms	Examples include *Raoultella* and *Klebsiella*; *Stenotrophomonas maltophilia* and *Pseudomonas hibiscicola*
Species identification of certain Gram-negative rods	Identification to the species level for *Campylobacter*, *Salmonella*, and *Achromobacter* are often incorrect
Anaerobes	Databases still require further development and extraction methods require standardization
Filamentous fungi	Lack of reference spectra in commercially available databases

The primary reason for organism misidentification, failure to yield a valid identification, or the inability to differentiate between closely related species in the literature has generally resulted from either the absence of a given organism in the reference database or an insufficient number of spectral entries for that organism (see **Table 4**). It is predicted that the aforementioned issues with the identification of *S pneumoniae* may be ameliorated with further enhancement of the reference databases. Because of the dynamic nature of the database software and the open source nature of the platform, updates to the database can be made by either the manufacturer or the individual user. However, laboratories choosing to engage in database supplementation must take great pains to ensure accuracy during this process. Finally, certain organisms do not seem to be effectively identified by MALDI-TOF MS without a prior extraction step using a strong organic acid (eg, formic acid). This results in increased use of hazardous materials in the laboratory and a concomitant increase in waste disposal costs. The extraction process itself only adds approximately 6 minutes per sample to the total turnaround time (reduced further by batching).[17] Many laboratories have therefore decided that the increased use of such chemicals is worth the ability to rapidly identify these organisms by MALDI-TOF MS.

POTENTIAL FUTURE APPLICATIONS OF MALDI-TOF MS IN THE CLINICAL MICROBIOLOGY LABORATORY

The application of MALDI-TOF MS to additional aspects of clinical microbiology is an exciting and increasingly realistic prospect. In particular, the identification of organisms directly from positive blood cultures and clinical specimens has been the subject of numerous studies. Even though eliminating the need to isolate organisms in culture would reduce the time to pathogen identification by at least 12 to 48 hours, recovery of the organism in vitro will continue to be required in most cases to perform susceptibility testing to a full complement of antimicrobial agents. For a more in-depth discussion of the topics in this section, see the article by Demarco and Ford elsewhere in this issue.

Direct Organism Identification from Blood Cultures

The identification of organisms directly from positive blood culture bottles by MALDI-TOF MS has garnered much attention in the past several years. The power of this approach stems from the dramatically decreased turnaround time in identifying the causative agent of infection (hours vs days), and the reduced cost compared with molecular-based methods. Because the organism burden during bacteremia and sepsis is far below the limit of detection for MALDI-TOF MS (10–1000 colony forming units [CFU]/mL vs 10^7 CFU/mL),[49] growth in blood culture media is first required. In addition, samples must first be processed to remove interfering blood culture components present before MALDI-TOF MS can be performed (ie, serum proteins, nonbacterial cells, and blood culture broth nutrients). Numerous methods have been evaluated to achieve this including in-house–developed methods (eg, detergent lysis with saponin) and commercially available methods (eg, MALDI Sepsityper kit [Bruker Daltonics] and the MolYsis Basic kit [Molzym (Bremen, Germany)]).[50–60] Most of these previously mentioned methods are rapid and have high positive predictive values for the identification of bacteria directly from positive monomicrobial blood cultures. Sample preparation and identification takes approximately 1 hour and can decrease turnaround times compared with conventional methods by greater than 24 hours.[50,54] However, one major limitation of MALDI-TOF MS for the direct identification of organisms from positive blood cultures is the inability to reliably identify polymicrobial infections.[61] Further studies are required to determine whether the identification of multiple bacterial species from polymicrobial blood cultures is truly feasible.

The clinical impact of organism identification by MALDI-TOF MS directly from positive blood cultures has been addressed in two recent studies. In a prospective analysis of 253 episodes of bacteremia by Vlek and colleagues,[62] 89 episodes were subjected to direct blood culture identification using MALDI-TOF MS. The authors noted an 11.3% increase at 24 hours in the proportion of patients receiving appropriate antimicrobial therapy where MALDI-TOF MS had been performed compared with the nonintervention group.[62] In a more recent study by Clerc and colleagues,[63] the impact of MALDI-TOF MS on the initiation of appropriate therapy in 202 episodes of Gram-negative bacteremia was assessed. The authors observed a modification of empiric therapy in 35.1% of cases overall and in 59.3% of episodes caused by AmpC-producing Enterobacteriaceae (eg, Enterobacter species, Citrobacter species, and so forth). Because of the size and design of both studies, additional outcomes, such as length of stay and mortality, were not evaluated. However, these studies demonstrate that the more timely provision of identification results to physicians in cases of bacteremia positively impacts patient care.

Direct-from-specimen Identification

A limited number of studies have investigated the use of MALDI-TOF MS for the identification of bacteria directly from clinical specimens. Urine, in particular, is believed to be an ideal candidate for such an approach because of the dearth of bacteria and host proteins present in the urine of healthy, uninfected patients.[25] Nevertheless, differential centrifugation of the specimen before MALDI-TOF MS analysis seems to be required to remove leukocytes and other nonbacterial components present in the urine of infected patients. Kohling and colleagues[64] have reported the ability to complete the entire identification procedure from urine specimens (including sample preparation) in 30 minutes.

When urine specimens containing bacterial concentrations greater than 10^5 CFU/mL were subjected to testing by MALDI-TOF MS, 91.8% were identified correctly to the species level compared with conventional methods (culture in conjunction with traditional identification methods).[65] However, in a second study on 107 urine specimens with bacterial concentrations ranging from 10^2 to 10^5 CFU/mL, only 58% of the specimens were correctly identified.[64] This presumably resulted from the wider range of bacterial concentrations being tested, even though the authors reported that MALDI-TOF MS could reliably detect bacteria in urine at concentrations of 10^3 CFU/mL. To our knowledge, no prospective study has been published detailing the performance of MALDI-TOF MS for polymicrobial urine specimens. Even though MALDI-TOF MS is unlikely to be implemented in most clinical microbiology laboratories for direct-from-urine organism identification in its current form, the results of these studies suggest the potential for such an approach in the future with appropriate optimization.

Detection of Antimicrobial Resistance

Antimicrobial resistance is a significant cause of morbidity and mortality. In the United States alone, it is estimated that more than 70% of the 1.7 million hospital-acquired infections that occur annually are caused by resistant organisms.[66] Rapid and accurate detection of antimicrobial resistance is therefore important for patient management and infection prevention. After MALDI-TOF MS was successfully shown to be capable of organism identification, the potential application of this method for the detection of antibiotic resistance became an area of active and intensive investigation. Although the published data regarding whether MALDI-TOF MS can reliably and reproducibly differentiate methicillin-resistant *Staphylococcus aureus* from methicillin-sensitive *S aureus* isolates is conflicting,[67–70] studies suggest that MALDI-TOF MS is capable of distinguishing between vancomycin-resistant and vancomycin-susceptible *Enterococcus faecium* strains.[71]

The ability of MALDI-TOF MS to detect resistance in Gram-negative bacteria has also been investigated. Specifically, the ability of MALDI-TOF MS to differentiate between extended-spectrum β-lactamase and metallo-β-lactamase –producing strains of *E coli*, *Klebsiella pneumoniae*, and *P aeruginosa* was examined. Spectral patterns for β-lactamase–producing isolates tended to be distinct from nonproducing isolates, although an accuracy of only 70% made this method insufficiently reliable for implementation as a clinical test.[72] Nevertheless, MALDI-TOF MS does show particular promise for the detection of β-lactamase activity itself.

The principle of this method lies in the ability of MALDI-TOF MS to detect hydrolysis of the β-lactam by a β-lactamase in antibiotic-bacterial mixtures. As a proof of principle, strains of *E coli* producing β-lactamases were incubated with ampicillin for 3 hours, after which time an observable decrease in intensity of the ampicillin-specific peak was observed. Importantly, this process was specifically inhibited by the addition of a β-lactamase inhibitor (clavulanic acid).[73] Comparable results were obtained for other β-lactam antibiotics including cephalosporins and carbapenems. The results obtained by MALDI-TOF MS correlated well with conventional susceptibility methods with respect to the detection of resistance.[73] Several subsequent studies have shown that the hydrolysis assay coupled with MALDI-TOF MS is also a powerful, rapid, and cost-effective method to detect a variety of clinically relevant carbapenemases including NDM-1, KPC, VIM-1, OXA-48, and OXA-162 enzymes.[74–77] Although sensitivities of this method near 100%, and assay times are as short as 1 to 2.5 hours, this technique is unlikely to be implemented for routine use until such time as standardized procedures and automated software for result interpretation become available.

Strain Typing

The use of MALDI-TOF MS for epidemiologic and infection prevention applications has increasingly been described in recent years. Because MALDI-TOF MS is capable of detecting a wide array of proteins, taxonomic classification is possible using additional functionality present within the MALDI-TOF MS operating software.[78] Currently available methods used to type strains, including pulsed-field gel electrophoresis and multilocus sequence typing, are laborious and expensive to perform.[79] Numerous studies have addressed the use of MALDI-TOF MS as a method for typing methicillin-resistant *S aureus*[67,79–81] and *Listeria monocytogenes* isolates,[82] determination of the epidemiologic relatedness of vancomycin-resistant *E faecium* strains,[71] subtyping of *S pneumoniae* isolates during an outbreak of conjunctivitis,[83] and rapid subspecies determination of *Salmonella* and *Yersinia enterocolitica* isolates.[84–86] The interested reader is referred to the article by Demarco and Ford elsewhere in this issue for more information regarding the application of MALDI-TOF MS to strain typing.

SUMMARY

MALDI-TOF MS is a rapid and reliable method for microbial identification that has been incorporated into the work flow of many clinical microbiology laboratories. Implementation of this method enables laboratories to provide definitive organism identifications to physicians on a time scale that was previously unimaginable. However, the ability of MALDI-TOF MS to more accurately identify microorganisms poses unique opportunities and challenges for physicians and laboratorians. Because of the inadequacies of conventional identification methods, identification of certain organisms to the species level has not routinely been performed. Examples of this include coagulase-negative staphylococci and members of the *Enterobacter cloacae* and *Citrobacter freundii* complexes. With the superior performance of MALDI-TOF MS over conventional methods, identification to the species level in an accurate, easy, and cost-efficient manner is now possible. This affords the opportunity for discovery of unique disease associations with certain microorganisms. Nevertheless, it also raises the possibility for overtreatment with antibiotics by physicians unfamiliar with a species name where a more generalized complex name had heretofore been reported. There are no practice guidelines for either the implementation of MALDI-TOF MS or the reporting of results. The development of such guidelines in a multidisciplinary manner is essential as this technology is increasingly adopted by laboratories and adapted to other areas of clinical microbiology, such as antimicrobial resistance detection.

REFERENCES

1. Gaieski DF, Pines JM, Band RA, et al. Impact of time to antibiotics on survival in patients with severe sepsis or septic shock in whom early goal-directed therapy was initiated in the emergency department. Crit Care Med 2010;38:1045–53.
2. Kumar A, Roberts D, Wood KE, et al. Duration of hypotension before initiation of effective antimicrobial therapy is the critical determinant of survival in human septic shock. Crit Care Med 2006;34:1589–96.
3. Bizzini A, Greub G. Matrix-assisted laser desorption ionization time-of-flight mass spectrometry, a revolution in clinical microbial identification. Clin Microbiol Infect 2010;16:1614–9.
4. Carbonnelle E, Mesquita C, Bille E, et al. MALDI-TOF mass spectrometry for bacterial identification in the clinical microbiology laboratory. Clin Biochem 2011;44:104–9.
5. Seng P, Drancourt M, Gouriet F, et al. Ongoing revolution in bacteriology: routine identification of bacteria by matrix-assisted laser desorption ionization time-of-flight mass spectrometry. Clin Infect Dis 2009;49:543–51.

6. Anhalt JP, Fenselau C. Identification of bacteria using mass spectrometry. Anal Chem 1975;47:219–25.

7. Hillenkamp F, Karas M. Mass spectrometry of peptides and proteins by matrix-assisted ultraviolet laser desorption/ionization. Methods Enzymol 1990;193: 280–95.

8. Karas M, Bachmann D, Hillenkamp F. Influence of the wavelength in high-irradiance ultraviolet laser desorption mass spectrometry of organic molecules. Anal Chem 1985;57:2935–9.

9. Karas M, Bachmann D, Bahr U, et al. Matrix-assisted ultraviolet laser desorption of non-volatile compounds. Int J Mass Spectrom Ion Process 1987;78:53–68.

10. Karas M, Hillenkamp F. Laser desorption ionization of proteins with molecular masses exceeding 10,000 daltons. Anal Chem 1988;60(20):2299–301.

11. Claydon MA, Davey SN, Edwards-Jones V, et al. The rapid identification of intact microorganisms using mass spectrometry. Nat Biotechnol 1996;14:1584–6.

12. Holland RD, Wilkes JG, Rafii F, et al. Rapid identification of intact whole bacteria based on spectral patterns using matrix-assisted laser desorption/ionization with time of flight mass spectrometry. Rapid Commun Mass Spectrom 1996; 10:1227–32.

13. Krishnamurthy T, Ross PL. Rapid identification of bacteria by direct matrix-assisted laser desorption/ionization mass spectrometric analysis of whole cells. Rapid Commun Mass Spectrom 1996;10:1992–6.

14. Welham KJ, Domin MA, Scannell DE, et al. The characterization of micro-organisms by matrix-assisted laser desorption time-of-flight mass spectrometry. Rapid Commun Mass Spectrom 1998;12:176–80.

15. Emonet S, Shah HN, Cherkaoui A, et al. Application and use of various mass spectrometry methods in clinical microbiology. Clin Microbiol Infect 2010;16: 1604–13.

16. Fenselau C, Demirev PA. Characterization of intact microorganisms by MALDI mass spectrometry. Mass Spectrom Rev 2001;20:157–71.

17. Bizzini A, Durussel C, Bille J, et al. Performance of matrix-assisted laser desorption ionization-time of flight mass spectrometry for identification of bacterial strains routinely isolated in a clinical microbiology laboratory. J Clin Microbiol 2010;48:1549–54.

18. Smole SC, King LA, Leopold PE, et al. Sample preparation of gram positive bacteria for identification by matrix assisted laser desorption/ionization time-of-flight. J Microbiol Methods 2002;48:107–15.

19. van Veen SQ, Claas EC, Kuijper EJ. High-throughput identification of bacteria and yeast by matrix-assisted laser desorption ionization-time of flight mass spectrometry in conventional medical microbiology laboratories. J Clin Microbiol 2010;48:900–7.

20. Holland RD, Duffy CR, Rafii F, et al. Identification of bacterial proteins observed in MALDI TOF mass spectra from whole cells. Anal Chem 1999;71:3226–30.

21. Rhyzhov V, Fenselau C. Characterization of the protein subset desorbed by MALDI from whole bacterial cells. Anal Chem 2001;73:746–50.

22. Sun L, Teramoto K, Sato H, et al. Characterization of ribosomal proteins as bio-markers for matrix-assisted laser desorption/ionization mass spectral identification of *Lactobacillus plantarum*. Rapid Commun Mass Spectrom 2006;20: 3789–98.

23. Sogawa K, Watanabe M, Sato K, et al. Rapid identification of microorganisms by mass spectrometry: improved performance by incorporation of in-house spectral data into a commercial database. Anal Bioanal Chem 2012;403:1811–22.

24. Saenz AJ, Petersen CE, Valentine NB, et al. Reproducibility of matrix-assisted laser desorption/ionization time-of-flight mass spectrometry for replicate bacterial culture analysis. Rapid Commun Mass Spectrom 1999;13:1580–5.

25. Wieser A, Schneider L, Jung J, et al. MALDI-TOF MS in microbiological diagnostics-identification of microorganisms and beyond (mini-review). Appl Microbiol Biotechnol 2012;93:965–74.

26. Welker M, Moore ER. Applications of whole-cell matrix-assisted laser-desorption/ionization time of flight mass spectrometry in systematic microbiology. Syst Appl Microbiol 2011;34:2–11.

27. Sogawa K, Watanabe M, Sato K, et al. Use of MALDI BioTyper system with MALDI-TOF mass spectrometry for rapid identification of microorganisms. Anal Bioanal Chem 2011;400:1905–11.

28. Bille E, Dauphin B, Leto J, et al. MALDI-TOF MS Andromas strategy for the routine identification of bacteria, mycobacteria, yeasts, *Aspergillus* spp. and positive blood cultures. Clin Microbiol Infect 2012;18:1117–25.

29. Cherkaoui A, Hibbs J, Emonet S, et al. Comparison of two matrix-assisted laser desorption ionization-time of flight mass spectrometry methods with conventional phenotypic identification for routine identification of bacteria to the species level. J Clin Microbiol 2010;48:1169–75.

30. Carbonnelle E, Grohs P, Jacquier H, et al. Robustness of two MALDI-TOF mass spectrometry systems for bacterial identification. J Microbiol Methods 2012;89: 133–6.

31. Dubois D, Grare M, Prere MF, et al. Performances of the VITEK MS matrix-assisted laser desorption ionization-time of flight mass spectrometry system for rapid identification of bacteria in routine clinical microbiology. J Clin Microbiol 2012;50:2568–76.

32. Farfour E, Leto J, Barritault M, et al. Evaluation of the Andromas matrix-assisted laser desorption ionization-time of flight mass spectrometry system for identification of aerobically growing gram-positive bacilli. J Clin Microbiol 2012;50: 2702–7.

33. Fernandex-Olmos A, Garcia-Castillo M, Morosini MI, et al. MALDI-TOF MS improves routine identification of non-fermenting gram negative isolates from cystic fibrosis patients. J Cyst Fibros 2012;11:59–62.

34. Marko DC, Saffert RT, Cunningham SA, et al. Evaluation of the Bruker Biotyper and Vitek MS matrix-assisted laser desorption ionization-time of flight mass spectrometry systems for identification of nonfermenting gram-negative bacilli isolated from culture from cystic fibrosis patients. J Clin Microbiol 2012;50: 2034–9.

35. Saleeb PG, Drake SK, Murray PR, et al. Identification of mycobacteria in solid-culture media by matrix-assisted laser desorption ionization-time of flight mass spectrometry. J Clin Microbiol 2011;49:1790–4.

36. Veloo AC, Knoester M, Degener JE, et al. Comparison of two matrix-assisted laser desorption ionization-time of flight mass spectrometry methods for the identification of clinically relevant anaerobic bacteria. Clin Microbiol Infect 2011;17:1501–6.

37. Fedorko DP, Drake SK, Stock F, et al. Identification of clinical isolates of anaerobic bacteria using matrix-assisted laser desorption ionization-time of flight mass spectrometry. Eur J Clin Microbiol Infect Dis 2012;31:2257–62.

38. Fournier R, Wallet F, Grandbastien B, et al. Chemical extraction versus direct smear for MALDI-TOF mass spectrometry identification of anaerobic bacteria. Anaerobe 2012;18:294–7.

39. Nagy E, Becker S, Kostrzewa M, et al. The value of MALDI-TOF MS for the identification of clinically relevant anaerobic bacteria in routine laboratories. J Med Microbiol 2012;61:1393–400.

40. Van Herendael BH, Bruynseels P, Bensaid M, et al. Validation of a modified algorithm for the identification of yeast isolates using matrix-assisted laser desorption/ionization time-of-flight mass spectrometry (MALDI-TOF MS). Eur J Clin Microbiol Infect Dis 2012;31:841–8.

41. Dhiman N, Hall L, Wohlfiel SL, et al. Performance and cost analysis of matrix-assisted laser desorption ionization-time of flight mass spectrometry for routine identification of yeast. J Clin Microbiol 2011;49:1614–6.

42. Bader O, Weig M, Taverne-Ghadwal L, et al. Improved clinical laboratory identification of human pathogenic yeasts by matrix-assisted laser desorption ionization time-of-flight mass spectrometry. Clin Microbiol Infect 2011;17:1359–65.

43. Alanio A, Beretti JL, Dauphin B, et al. Matrix-assisted laser desorption ionization time-of-flight mass spectrometry for fast and accurate identification of clinically relevant *Aspergillus* species. Clin Microbiol Infect 2011;17:750–5.

44. De Carolis E, Posteraro B, Lass-Flori C, et al. Species identification of *Aspergillus*, *Fusarium* and *Mucorales* with direct surface analysis by matrix-assisted laser desorption ionization time-of-flight mass spectrometry. Clin Microbiol Infect 2012;18:475–84.

45. Alshawa K, Beretti JL, Lacroix C, et al. Successful identification of clinical dermatophyte and *Neoscytalidium* species by matrix-assisted laser desorption ionization-time of flight mass spectrometry. J Clin Microbiol 2012;50:2277–81.

46. Tan KE, Ellis C, Lee R, et al. Prospective evaluation of a matrix-assisted laser desorption ionization-time of flight mass spectrometry system in a hospital clinical microbiology laboratory for identification of bacteria and yeasts: a bench-by-bench study for assessing the impact on time to identification and cost-effectiveness. J Clin Microbiol 2012;50:3301–8.

47. Gaillot O, Blondiaux N, Loiez C, et al. Cost-effectiveness of switch to matrix-assisted laser desorption ionization-time of flight mass spectrometry for routine bacterial identification. J Clin Microbiol 2011;49:4412.

48. Ikryannikova LN, Filimonova AV, Malakhova MV, et al. Discrimination between *Streptococcus pneumoniae* and *Streptococcus mitis* based on sorting of their MALDI mass spectra. Clin Microbiol Infect 2013. [Epub ahead of print].

49. Christner M, Rohde H, Wolters M, et al. Rapid identification of bacteria from positive blood culture bottles by use of matrix-assisted laser desorption-ionization time of flight mass spectrometry fingerprinting. J Clin Microbiol 2010;48:1584–91.

50. Buchan BW, Riebe KM, Ledeboer NA. Comparison of the MALDI Biotyper system using Sepsityper specimen processing to routine microbiological methods for identification of bacteria from positive blood culture bottles. J Clin Microbiol 2012;50:346–52.

51. Ferroni A, Suarez S, Beretti JL, et al. Real-time identification of bacteria and *Candida* species in positive blood culture broths by matrix-assisted laser desorption ionization-time of flight mass spectrometry. J Clin Microbiol 2010; 48:1542–8.

52. Klein S, Zimmermann S, Kohler C, et al. Integration of matrix-assisted laser desorption/ionization time-of-flight mass spectrometry in blood culture diagnostics: a fast and effective approach. J Med Microbiol 2012;61:323–31.

53. Kok J, Thomas LC, Olma T, et al. Identification of bacteria in blood culture broths using matrix-assisted laser desorption-ionization Sepsityper and time of flight mass spectrometry. PLoS One 2011;6:e23285.

54. Lagace-Wiens PR, Adam HJ, Karlowsky JA, et al. Identification of blood culture isolates directly from positive blood cultures by use of matrix-assisted laser desorption ionization-time of flight mass spectrometry and a commercial extraction system: analysis of performance, cost and turnaround time. J Clin Microbiol 2012;50:3324–8.

55. Loonen AJ, Jansz AR, Stalpers J, et al. An evaluation of three processing methods and the effect of reduced culture times for faster direct identification of pathogens from BacT/ALERT blood cultures by MALDI-TOF MS. Eur J Clin Microbiol Infect Dis 2012;31:1575–83.

56. Martiny D, Dediste A, Vandenberg O. Comparison of an in-house method and the commercial Sepsityper kit for bacterial identification directly from positive blood culture broths by matrix-assisted laser desorption-ionization time of flight mass spectrometry. Eur J Clin Microbiol Infect Dis 2012;31:2269–81.

57. Meex C, Neuville F, Descy J, et al. Direct identification of bacteria from the BacT/ALERT anaerobic blood cultures by MALDI-TOF MS: MALDI Sepsityper kit versus an in-house method for bacterial extraction. J Med Microbiol 2012;61:1511–6.

58. Prod'hom G, Bizzini A, Durussel C, et al. Matrix-assisted laser desorption ionization-time of flight mass spectrometry for direct bacterial identification from positive blood culture pellets. J Clin Microbiol 2010;48:1481–3.

59. Stevenson LG, Drake SK, Murray PR. Rapid identification of bacteria in positive blood culture broths by matrix-assisted laser desorption ionization-time of flight mass spectrometry. J Clin Microbiol 2010;48:444–7.

60. Yan Y, He Y, Maier T, et al. Improved identification of yeast species directly from positive blood culture media by combining Sepsityper specimen procession and Microflex analysis with the matrix-assisted laser desorption ionization Biotyper system. J Clin Microbiol 2011;49:2528–32.

61. La Scola B, Raoult D. Direct identification of positive blood culture bottles by matrix-assisted laser desorption ionisation time-of-flight mass spectrometry. PLoS One 2009;4:e8041.

62. Vlek AL, Bonten MJ, Boel CH. Direct matrix-assisted laser desportion ionization time-of-flight mass spectrometry improves appropriateness of antibiotic treatment of bacteremia. PLoS One 2012;7:e32589.

63. Clerc O, Prod'hom G, Vogne C, et al. Impact of matrix-assisted laser desorption ionization time-of-flight mass spectrometry on the clinical management of patients with Gram-negative bacteremia: a prospective observational study. Clin Infect Dis 2013;56:1101–7.

64. Kohling HL, Bittner A, Muller KD, et al. Direct identification of bacteria in urine samples by matrix-assisted laser desorption/ionization time-of-flight mass spectrometry and relevance of defensins as interfering factors. J Med Microbiol 2012;61:339–44.

65. Ferreira L, Sanchez-Juanes F, Gonzalez-Avila M, et al. Direct identification of urinary tract pathogens from urine samples by matrix-assisted laser desorption ionization-time of flight mass spectrometry. J Clin Microbiol 2010;48:2110–5.

66. Klevens RM, Edwards JR, Richards CL Jr, et al. Estimating health care-associated infections and deaths in U.S. hospitals, 2002. Public Health Rep 2007;122:160–6.

67. Bernardo K, Pakulat N, Macht M, et al. Identification and discrimination of Staphylococcus aureus strains using matrix-assisted laser desorption/ionization-time of flight mass spectrometry. Proteomics 2002;2:747–53.

68. Du Z, Yang R, Guo Z, et al. Identification of Staphylococcus aureus and determination of its methicillin resistance by matrix-assisted laser desorption/ionization time-of-flight mass spectrometry. Anal Chem 2002;74:5487–91.

69. Edwards-Jones V, Claydon MA, Evason DJ, et al. Rapid discrimination between methicillin-sensitive and methicillin-resistant *Staphylococcus aureus* by intact cell mass spectrometry. J Med Microbiol 2000;49:295–300.

70. Lu JJ, Tsai FJ, Ho CM, et al. Peptide biomarker discovery for identification of methicillin-resistant and vancomycin-intermediate *Staphylococcus aureus* strains by MALDI-TOF. Anal Chem 2012;84:5685–92.

71. Griffin PM, Price GR, Schooneveldt JM, et al. Use of matrix-assisted laser desorption ionization-time of flight mass spectrometry to identify vancomycin-resistant enterococci and investigate the epidemiology of an outbreak. J Clin Microbiol 2012;50:2918–31.

72. Schaumann R, Knoop N, Genzel GH, et al. A step towards the discrimination of beta-lactamase-producing clinical isolates of *Enterobacteriaceae* and *Pseudomonas aeruginosa* by MALDI-TOF mass spectrometry. Med Sci Monit 2012; 18:MT71–7.

73. Sparbier K, Schubert S, Weller U, et al. Matrix-assisted laser desorption ionization-time of flight mass spectrometry-based functional assay for rapid detection of resistance against B-lactam antibiotics. J Clin Microbiol 2012;50: 927–37.

74. Burckhardt I, Zimmermann S. Using matrix-assisted laser desorption ionization-time of flight mass spectrometry to detect carbapenem resistance within 1 to 2.5 hours. J Clin Microbiol 2011;49:3321–4.

75. Hrabak J, Walkova R, Studentova V, et al. Carbapenemase activity detection by matrix-assisted laser desorption ionization-time of flight mass spectrometry. J Clin Microbiol 2011;49:3222–7.

76. Hrabak J, Studentova V, Walkova R, et al. Detection of NDM-1, VIM-1, KPC, OXA-48, and OXA-162 carbapenemases by matrix-assisted laser desorption ionization-time of flight mass spectrometry. J Clin Microbiol 2012;50:2441–3.

77. Kempf M, Bakour S, Flaudrops C, et al. Rapid detection of carbapenem resistance in *Acinetobacter baumannii* using matrix-assisted laser desorption ionization-time of flight mass spectrometry. PLoS One 2012;7:e31676.

78. Murray PR. Matrix-assisted laser desorption ionization time-of-flight mass spectrometry: usefulness for taxonomy and epidemiology. Clin Microbiol Infect 2010; 16:1626–30.

79. Wolters M, Rohde H, Maier T, et al. MALDI-TOF MS fingerprinting allows for discrimination of major methicillin-resistant *Staphylococcus aureus* lineages. Int J Med Microbiol 2011;301:64–8.

80. Jackson KA, Edwards-Jones V, Sutton CW, et al. Optimisation of intact cell MALDI method for fingerprinting of methicillin *Staphylococcus aureus*. J Microbiol Methods 2005;62:273–84.

81. Walker J, Fox AJ, Edwards-Jones V, et al. Intact cell mass spectrometry (ICMS) used to type methicillin-resistant *Staphylococcus aureus*: media effects and inter-laboratory reproducibility. J Microbiol Methods 2002;48:117–26.

82. Barbuddhe SB, Maier T, Schwarz G, et al. Rapid identification and typing of *Listeria* species by matrix-assisted laser desorption ionization-time of flight mass spectrometry. Appl Environ Microbiol 2008;74:5402–7.

83. Williamson YM, Moura H, Woolfitt AR, et al. Differentiation of *Streptococcus pneumoniae* conjunctivitis outbreak isolates by matrix-assisted laser desorption-time of flight mass spectrometry. Appl Environ Microbiol 2008;74: 5891–7.

84. Dieckmann R, Helmuth R, Erhard M, et al. Rapid classification and identification of salmonellae at the species and subspecies levels by whole-cell matrix-assisted

laser desorption ionization-time of flight mass spectrometry. Appl Environ Microbiol 2008;74:7767–78.

85. Marinach C, Alanio A, Palous M, et al. MALDI-TOF MS-based drug susceptibility testing of pathogens: the example of *Candida albicans* and fluconazole. Proteomics 2009;9:4627–31.

86. Stephan R, Cernela N, Ziegler D, et al. Rapid species specific identification and subtyping of *Yersinia enterocolitica* by MALDI-TOF mass spectrometry. J Microbiol Methods 2011;87:150–3.

87. Justesen US, Holm A, Knudsen E, et al. Species identification of clinical isolates of anaerobic bacteria: a comparison of two matrix-assisted laser desorption ionization-time of flight mass spectrometry systems. J Clin Microbiol 2011;49: 4314–8.

88. Marklein G, Josten M, Klanke U, et al. Matrix-assisted laser desorption-time of flight mass spectrometry for fast and reliable identification of clinical yeast isolates. J Clin Microbiol 2009;47:2912–7.

89. Stevenson LG, Drake SK, Shea YR, et al. Evaluation of matrix assisted laser deorption ionization-time of flight mass spectrometry for identification of clinically important yeast species. J Clin Microbiol 2010;48:3482–6.

Beyond Identification

Emerging and Future Uses for MALDI-TOF Mass Spectrometry in the Clinical Microbiology Laboratory

Mari L. DeMarco, PhD[a], Bradley A. Ford, MD, PhD[b],*

KEYWORDS

- Antimicrobial susceptibility testing • Bacteremia • Bloodstream infection
- Direct identification • MALDI-TOF • Mass spectrometry • Urinary tract infection
- Machine learning

KEY POINTS

- Matrix-assisted laser desorption/ionization time-of-flight (MALDI-TOF) identification of microorganisms has revolutionized the clinical microbiology laboratory by making identification of microorganisms from culture faster and less expensive.
- Direct identification of microorganisms from urine and blood culture bottles is possible given specimens with sufficient microbial biomass.
- Direct identification methods have the potential to significantly improve turn-around-time and patient care.
- Clinical laboratory MALDI-TOF instruments are capable of distinguishing phenotypic characteristics such as strain types, β-lactamases and other resistance determinants but doing so requires an entirely different approach than that used for routine organism identification.

MALDI-TOF MS IN CLINICAL MICROBIOLOGY

The routine use of matrix-assisted laser desorption/ionization time-of-flight mass spectrometry (MALDI-TOF MS) has revolutionized microorganism identification in the clinical microbiology laboratory. For MALDI-TOF identification, after a patient's specimen is cultured on solid media, an isolated colony is transferred onto a MALDI-target plate for analysis. The MALDI-TOF instrument generates a proteomic

The authors have nothing to disclose.

[a] Department of Pathology and Laboratory Medicine, University of British Columbia, St. Paul's Hospital, Vancouver, BC, V6Z 1Y6, Canada; [b] Department of Pathology, University of Iowa Hospitals and Clinics, 200 Hawkins Drive, C606GH, Iowa City, IA 52242, USA
* Corresponding author.
E-mail address: bradley-ford-1@uiowa.edu

fingerprint (spectrum) from abundant peptides and proteins in the sample (eg, ribosomal peptides). With the commercially available systems, prepackaged software automatically generates identification by comparing the spectrum with a curated database of representative microorganisms. This method presents a significant improvement in turnaround time (TAT) and reduced reagent costs, although it requires visible growth of isolated colonies on solid media. To further improve the TAT of microorganism identification via MALDI-TOF, methods for identification from liquid samples, that is, direct identification methods (also referred to as direct detection methods), are being developed. As the TAT of microorganism identification from body fluids is reduced from days to hours with these new methods, demand has intensified for comparably rapid detection of clinically important phenotypes that cannot be determined from a species name.

Recent reviews have comprehensively covered the state of the MALDI-TOF landscape,[1] and in depth strain typing[2]; the reader is referred to the concurrent review in this issue for an overview of standard MALDI-TOF identification. Herein the authors present practical approaches for laboratorians interested in implementing direct identification processing methods for MALDI-TOF detection of microbes in bloodstream infection (BSI) and urinary tract infection (UTI). In addition, postanalytical approaches for classifying MALDI-TOF spectral data to detect characteristics other and species-level identification (eg, strain-level classification, typing, and resistance mechanisms) are explored.

LIMITATIONS INHERITED FROM DIRECT COLONY TESTING

When considering emerging and future applications of MALDI-TOF, it is helpful to review current standard clinical applications of MALDI-TOF. There are currently 2 systems widely available for clinical use in the United States, the Bruker Biotyper (Bruker Daltonics, Billerica, MA, USA) and the bioMérieux VITEK MS (bioMérieux; Durham, NC, USA). Both systems have demonstrated excellent concordance with conventional methods in determining species-level identification of organisms grown on solid media.[3,4] However, there are a handful of organisms that cannot be resolved with current MALDI-TOF methods, which can result in misidentifications; common examples include *Escherichia coli/Shigella* spp and the *Streptococcus pneumoniae/mitis/oralis* group. Standard clinical laboratory protocols typically include smearing an isolated colony onto a defined spot on a metal target, drying in room air, and overlaying with 1 μl matrix solution composed of saturated α-cyano-4-hydroxycinnamic acid (HCCA) in 50% acetonitrile/2.5% trifluoroacetic acid or similar organic solvent/acid combination.[5–7] Deviations from this protocol are rare, although sinapinic acid matrix has been used for mycobacteria[8] and allows for analysis of higher molecular weight proteins in comparison with HCCA.[9] Of importance is that the choice of matrix, organic solvents, and acids such as trifluoroacetic or formic acid can have dramatic effects on the peak number, peak quality, and mass range obtained from bacterial cells,[10] and that reference microorganism databases are matrix specific.

Mass spectrometers used in clinical microbiology use relatively inexpensive linear-mode MALDI-TOF MS coupled to software that automatically identifies the microorganism present based on the spectra generated from the sample. These instruments have modest mass accuracy, which is entirely suited for their intended clinical application; they also use proprietary scoring algorithms in their microorganism identification software. For this reason nonstandard applications, higher-resolution (more costly) equipment, and/or additional software programs may be required. "Beyond identification" applications of MALDI-TOF are therefore limited by the instrument, the mass range, and the resolution of typical spectra obtained for identification purposes, and by the obstacle of venturing beyond prepackaged processing software. This article first considers cases whereby standard identification may be performed without growth on solid media (direct identification methods), before discussing more complex applications whereby both sample processing and data analysis must be customized.

BLOODSTREAM INFECTION

The diagnosis of BSI relies on inoculation of blood into bottles containing nutrient broth and continuously monitoring for signs of pathogen growth (eg, CO_2 production or O_2 consumption). When a blood-culture bottle is determined to be positive by the instrument, a Gram stain provides some information regarding the identity of the organism; however, definitive identification requires subculture on solid media followed by biochemical characterization. Herein, these methods are referred to as conventional methods (**Fig. 1A**). This process, from culture positivity to pathogen identification, typically takes 18 to 48 hours, excluding susceptibility testing.[11] Providing guidance to physicians regarding selection of antimicrobial therapy is essential in cases of BSI, as rapid administration of appropriate antimicrobial therapy significantly improves patient outcomes.[12–15] Thus, when clinical suspicion of BSI is high enough to draw blood cultures, more rapid and definitive identification of pathogens is desirable (see **Fig. 1B**).

Specimen Processing

A variety of specimen-processing methods for MALDI-TOF have been reported for the identification of pathogens directly from positive blood-culture bottles: differential centrifugation, gel-based separation, biochemical and chemical cell lysis, and chemical protein extraction.[16–22] In general, an aliquot (1–8 mL) from a positive blood-culture bottle is processed to isolate and concentrate microorganisms so that they can be applied to a MALDI-target plate for identification. The analytical performance of direct identification from positive blood-culture bottles varies according to the isolation/extraction method used. For example, a commonly used procedure, the commercial Sepsityper kit (Bruker Daltonics), is performed sequentially as follows: a lysis

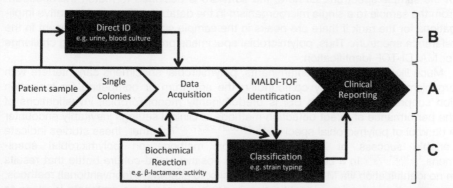

Fig. 1. (A) Standard workflow for bacterial identification by MALDI-TOF. (B) Direct identification (ID) methods bypass the time-consuming step of culture on solid media. (C) Emerging workflows for detecting biochemical activities such as β-lactamase activity, and for extracting spectral information to be used for strain typing, resistance-determinant detection, and other clinically relevant classifications.

solution is added to a 1-mL aliquot of positive blood-culture specimen, the sample is pelleted by centrifugation, the pellet is washed and centrifuged before performing an ethanol–formic acid extraction procedure (involving several pipetting and centrifugation steps), and the final pellet is applied to the MALDI-TOF target. MALDI-TOF direct identification methods from positive blood cultures have demonstrated excellent identification rates of approximately 80% to 90%, and good concordance with conventional methods.[11,23] Direct identification rates are negatively affected in cases where no identification is made or when there is a misidentification. From a clinical standpoint, microorganism misidentifications may have more serious consequences, so laboratories should be aware of groups of microorganisms that are known to yield misidentifications via MALDI-TOF.

Along with the type of extraction procedure used,[24] both the type of blood-culture bottle[25,26] and incubation time affect direct identification rates.[27,28] In a comparison of 7 types of blood-culture bottles, incubated on 3 different automated instruments, identification rates ranged from 62% to 76%.[25] No head-to-head comparisons between bottles and instruments were made for practical reasons. Another source of variability results from the length of time blood-culture bottles are incubated, as spectral quality declines with increasing incubation. Given strains of *Candida albicans* incubated over several days, spectra obtained after 4 days of incubation had fewer and less prominent peaks relative to spectra collected after 2 days of incubation.[28] Likewise for bacteria, increased incubation times (from 1 to 7 days) resulted in lower identification scores.[27] Given a random sampling of clinical blood-culture bottles that will be positive within an 8-day incubation window, approximately 85% become positive within the first 48 hours.[29] Therefore, the negative effects of prolonged incubation time on spectral quality and identification scores may have minimal impact in the clinical laboratory.

Polymicrobial Specimens

One of the major advantages of MALDI-TOF identification is the automated identification process. Matches are reported and ranked according to a score or percentage that indicates the quality of the match. These matching algorithms, while efficient and unbiased, have some limitations. Database matching software is limited by the quality of the database (including the breadth of microorganisms represented), the uniqueness of the proteomic signature of the organism in question, and the quality of the sample spectrum. Of note, the software is designed to match the spectrum from the sample to a single microorganism in the database. There are negative implications for the rank if there are peaks in the sample spectrum that are absent in the reference spectrum. Thus, polymicrobial specimens present an interesting challenge for MALDI-TOF identification.

Much like nonbacterial contaminants, polymicrobial specimens can interfere with organism identification by confounding the spectrum or competing for ionization (ion suppression). Although BSI is predominantly monomicrobial, investigations of the performance of direct detection methods in clinical settings inevitably encounter a handful of polymicrobial specimens.[11,16,21,22,27,30] Together, these studies indicate variable success of direct identification methods on polymicrobial specimens.[11,16,21,27,30] In a clinical laboratory, a positive blood-culture bottle that results in no identification via MALDI-TOF could reflex to alternative (conventional) methods; however, if species-level identification is achieved, are there protocols in place to confirm that the identification is complete (for polymicrobial specimens)? In another scenario, as specimens are often processed in duplicate on MALDI-TOF, what if 2 high-confidence but discrepant identifications are made? As the number of reported clinical polymicrobial specimens tested by direct identification methods is small and the results are variable, there are no clear answers. Confounding matters, studies occasionally exclude polymicrobial specimens when reporting the analytical performance of direct identification methods, yielding falsely elevated sensitivities and omitting the impact of polymicrobial specimens on laboratory workflows.

To implement direct identification methods for positive blood-culture bottles at St Louis Children's Hospital, protocols were devised to account for both monomicrobial and polymicrobial specimens (Winkler, personal communication, 2013). In brief, a preliminary report (released to physicians) from direct identification includes a disclaimer that the positive identification does not rule out the presence of additional microorganisms. Because all positive blood-culture bottles are subcultured onto solid media for antimicrobial susceptibility testing, plates are examined for multiple colony types. A final report is generated after MALDI-TOF identification from solid media is performed, confirming or amending the preliminary report. In the current stage of development, MALDI-TOF direct identification methods from positive blood cultures necessitate safeguards, such as those already described, to account for rare misidentifications and polymicrobial specimens.

Gram-Positive Bacteria

One noticeable trend from studies of direct identification from positive blood cultures is that the performance of MALDI-TOF identification of gram-positive bacteria often lags behind that of gram-negative bacteria.[11,21] In a prospective study of 164 positive blood cultures (100 gram-positive, 45 gram-negative, and 5 yeast), the specimens containing gram-negative bacteria were more likely to yield high-confidence identification (91.1%) than those containing gram-positive bacteria (53.0%).[11] Spectra were analyzed a second time, discarding peaks below 4000 m/z. Of note, the percentage of high-confidence identifications for gram-positives rose from 53.0% to 63.0%, and gram-negatives showed a modest improvement from 91.1% to 95.6%. The discrepancy has been attributed in part to the resistance of the gram-positive cell wall to lysis, and to the similarity of some gram-positive proteomic footprints (resulting in misidentifications). However, the successful strategy of excluding low molecular weight regions of the spectrum[11,19] suggests either that nonbacterial contaminants can convolute the spectra or that growth in liquid versus solid media can result in distinct proteomic fingerprints.

Fungi

Fungi have also been challenging to identify directly from positive blood-culture bottles, which may be due to the sparse representation of fungi in spectral databases and the resistance of their cell wall to lysis. In addition, the biomass in blood-culture broth, when the instrument signals a positive bottle, is lower for yeast than for bacteria. With these limitations in mind, Spanu and colleagues[31] developed a fungi-specific blood-culture processing method. In this method, an 8-mL aliquot of positive blood-culture broth was processed by centrifugation, washing, and treatment with a surfactant and an ethanol–formic acid extraction.[31] Over a 17-month period, 346 positive blood-culture specimens containing fungi and 340 negative blood-culture specimens were collected and analyzed by MALDI-TOF direct identification and conventional methods. All negative blood-culture specimens were also negative by MALDI-TOF. For the positive blood cultures, of which 56% were C albicans, sensitivity was 91.3% (95% confidence interval 87.7–93.9). Low concentrations of fungi in blood-culture bottles were less likely to be identified. This result is consistent with previous MALDI-TOF experiments whereby 10^6 CFU/mL of Candida or 10^8 to 10^9 CFU/mL of bacteria were necessary to generate optimal spectra.[27,28] For direct identification methods, there is a sharp decline in spectral quality and, consequently, identification rates associated with declining concentrations of organisms (**Fig. 2**). In the case of bacteremia, a majority of positive blood cultures tend to fall within 10^7 to 10^9 CFU/mL,[27] a concentration range that is amenable to direct identification methods; however, for fungemia, relatively lower organism concentrations may contribute to the lower identification rates observed.

To the best of the authors' knowledge, there are no reported prospective trials evaluating the use of direct identification methods for filamentous fungi in the clinical laboratory. Recent studies of MALDI-TOF identification from specimens subcultured onto solid media, however, have demonstrated a possible role for MALDI-TOF in the identification of clinically relevant filamentous fungi such as *Penicillium*, *Fusarium*, and *Aspergillus*.[8,32] Because filamentous fungi are underrepresented in commercially available databases, the onus is currently on individual laboratories to develop their

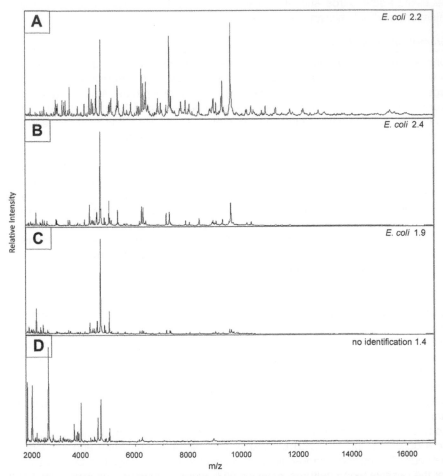

Fig. 2. The microorganism burden of the biological sample is a significant factor in the success of direct identification methods. Spectra are from direct identification using the diafiltration–MALDI-TOF method starting with urine containing (*A*) 10^7, (*B*) 10^6, (*C*) 10^5, and (*D*) 10^4 CFU/mL of *Escherichia coli*. The microorganism identified along with the Biotyper confidence score is noted on each spectrum.

own reference databases. Moreover, the ability of filamentous fungi to display complex phenotypes will likely necessitate tight control of preanalytical variables (culture medium, incubation time, and so forth) to limit phenotypic variation.

A challenge for clinical implementation of direct identification methods is the harmonization of bacterial and fungal processing methods such that all clinical specimens can be processed without a priori knowledge of the infectious organism. With evolving spectral libraries and fine-tuning of processing methods, routine direct identification of BSIs within an hour of the blood-culture bottle becoming positive is on the horizon.

URINARY TRACT INFECTION

Conventional methods for identification of UTI include quantitative culture on solid media, Gram stain of select colonies, and biochemical testing. This process can take 24 to 48 hours before microorganisms are reported to physicians. Direct identification methods from urine therefore have the potential to significantly improve TAT and patient care.

Urine specimens, relative to blood specimens, are more ideally suited for direct identification from the original specimen because thresholds for clinically relevant bacteriuria are set at about 10^5 CFU/mL.[33] This high organism burden should facilitate capture and identification of pathogens via MALDI-TOF (see **Fig. 2**). However, in contrast to blood culture, for which gas consumption or production is a reliable indicator of a positive culture, current UTI screening methods such as point-of-care urine dipsticks have poor analytical sensitivity and specificity, and are therefore unreliable mechanisms for triaging specimens for further analysis by MALDI-TOF. Therefore, direct identification methods must perform well on all urine specimens received in the clinical laboratory, not just a subset of pathogen-containing samples. Direct identification methods for urine require both high sensitivity to capture and identify pathogens present in the specimen and the ability to discriminate between UTI-positive and UTI-negative specimens. Unlike BSI-negative specimens, UTI-negative specimens comprise a more diverse group: specimens with no microorganism growth and with clinically insufficient growth, and contaminated (polymicrobial) specimens. Thus, direct identification methods for urine must strike a careful balance between sensitivity and specificity to avoid reporting false positives for specimens with clinically insignificant amounts of bacteria or for contaminated specimens.

A handful of methods for direct identification of pathogens directly from urine have been presented, and include the centrifugation,[34] filter-paper,[35] and diafiltration[36] methods. In general, 4 to 15 mL of a urine specimen is processed to isolate organisms, and the concentrate is applied to the target plate for analysis. Major challenges for these methods include (1) capture and concentration of pathogens, and (2) purification to reduce ion suppression and interference. Whereas urine from patients with UTIs has a high organism burden relative to other biofluids, spotting urine directly on the target plate at 10^7 CFU/mL or less delivers an insufficient biomass for generation of quality spectra by MALDI-TOF (DeMarco and Burnham, unpublished data). Thus sample concentration is required for detection and identification of organisms at clinically relevant thresholds. Unfortunately, concentrating the specimen can also result in the accumulation of other molecules (salts, proteins, lipids), cells (epithelial cells, white blood cells, and so forth), and particulates. During MS analysis these contaminants can suppress ionization and/or obscure the proteomic fingerprint of the organism of interest. Therefore, the specimen must be subjected to selective concentration and/or purification steps.

To date, no prospective trial of either the centrifugation[34] or filter-paper method[35] has been reported; however, retrospective analyses of the centrifugation and filter-paper methods provides an indication of their clinical utility.[34,35] In brief, for the centrifugation method 4 mL of urine was centrifuged at high speed to pellet (isolate) bacteria for subsequent processing on MALDI-TOF.[34] The filter-paper method used a vacuum filtration device for isolation and concentration of pathogens from 15 mL of urine.[35] Using sterile urine spiked with known quantities of E coli, 2 independent laboratories implementing the centrifugation method achieved reliable detection limits of at least 10^7 CFU/mL.[23,36] Using the same approach, the filter-paper method also achieved a reliable detection limit of 10^7 CFU/mL or higher (DeMarco and Burnham, unpublished data). These detection limits are consistent with findings from retrospective trials of clinical samples comparing these direct identification methods with conventional analysis, whereby high bacterial concentrations were required for high-confidence MALDI-TOF identification.[34,35] In these studies there was no mention of the CFU/mL thresholds or confidence scores at which direct identification results would be clinically reported, prohibiting further analysis of the analytical performance of the centrifugation and filter-paper methods.

For the diafiltration method, urine specimens were desalted, fractionated, and concentrated using a centrifugal filter device.[36] With the diafiltration method, species-level identification was achieved for urine samples with microorganism concentrations 10^5 CFU/mL or greater for gram-negative bacteria and Candida, and at least 10^6 CFU/mL for gram-positive organisms. In a blind prospective trial of 100 clinical specimens the diafiltration method, relative to conventional culture, yielded a sensitivity of 67% and specificity of 100% (DeMarco and Burnham, unpublished data). Although this method could not be used to rule out infection, it has the analytical characteristics (positive predictive value 100%) required to rule in infection in a clinically relevant sampling of urine specimens.

MALDI-TOF direct identification methods from urine are still in the early phases of development, and currently lack the robust detection limits necessary for routine clinical use. Methodological improvements are under way with the aim of lowering detection limits, thus increasing their sensitivity. The methods described herein are amenable to automation, which would facilitate implementation of direct identification workflows for laboratory staff.

BEYOND IDENTIFICATION

As already described, direct identification from matrices such as blood-culture bottles or urine is oriented toward processing steps that isolate organisms or the proteins they contain; in the end, a typical automatic MALDI-TOF species identification is made. This section considers postanalytical approaches to deriving information from MALDI-TOF spectra that reveal microbial characteristics other than their species-level or genus-level identification. Such methods include strain-level classification, typing, and presumptive identification of resistance mechanisms.

Outside the Box

In processing spectra outside the manufacturer's identification system, the clinical microbiologist must select processing software that can perform baseline correction, denoising/smoothing, and peak detection, alignment, and binning (see **Fig. 1C**). The data format of the spectral files for both clinical MS platforms is proprietary, requiring conversion to an open-source format for further analysis (eg, with Bruker's CompassXport tool [Bruker Daltonics] or readBrukerFlexData[37] in the R statistical package).[38]

With quality spectra in hand, data can be imported, processed, and classified using robust software packages such as ClinProTools for Bruker instruments (Bruker Daltonics)[39] along with the associated support vector machine (SVM) classifier plugin (discussed generically below). MALDIquant[37] is a package for the R statistical programming environment that can import Bruker data and has the appeal of being free of charge. It is also associated with other R packages such as MassSpecWavelet for peak finding,[40] speaq for peak alignment,[41] and open-source SVM support in LIBSVM,[42] among many others. A similar set of functions could be assembled in the commercial MATLAB (The MathWorks; Natick, MA, USA) software, but because both R and MATLAB require programming skills, their implementation in the clinical laboratory is challenging.

Classification with Spectral Features

The general goal of these classification strategies is to select a set of peaks that can differentiate 2 or more phenotypic states. Classification can be performed on data generated from whole cells, a biochemical reaction, purified proteins, or other material. With appropriate software selected, the spectral files must first be "cleaned up" to remove noise and find a baseline. In the process, some signal (ie, low intensity peaks) is inevitably also lost. One can then find the tops of peaks and assign an *m/z* value to them (vertical lines in **Fig. 3**A). However, between similar strains or different experiments, which peaks of almost identical mass are indeed identical (ie, they

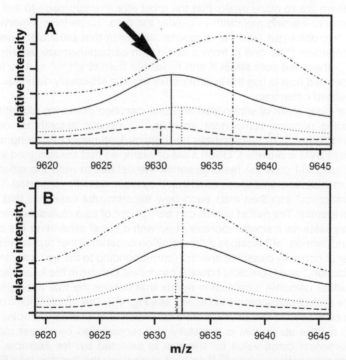

Fig. 3. Postprocessing steps such as calibration are essential for successful classification. (*A*) Four spectral peaks from different *Staphylococcus aureus* reference strains; one (indicated by an *arrow*) is misaligned and might not be grouped with the others. (*B*) A comparison between all 4 spectra allows correction of the misaligned peak by −6 *m/z*; it is now clear that this peak is not useful for classification because it is common to all strains.

presumptively, by virtue of their apparent mass, represent the same underlying analyte)? Hypothetically, peaks from different samples that are identical should have the same m/z value but, as mentioned earlier, clinical-grade instruments are not perfectly accurate and accuracy, as it relates to MS, is a mass-dependent quantity. **Fig.** 3A shows a single identical peak from 4 different strains of *Staphylococcus aureus*. The peak with the greatest offset might be called "different" because its m/z value has the largest deviation from the others. However, by applying a mass accuracy-based m/z tolerance and comparing the m/z values of all peaks in the 4 spectra with each other, the peaks in **Fig.** 3 can be aligned. Peaks common to these 4 strains now have the same m/z value, and distinguishing peaks can be reliably identified (see **Fig.** 3B).

The output of spectral preprocessing is therefore a set of peaks of well-estimated m/z. This information can then be used to cluster spectra into phenotypic groups (eg, strain types, groups with and without carbapenemase activity).

Clustering Algorithms

A brute-force approach to selecting a classification, or clustering, model using MALDI-TOF peaks would yield $\left(\dfrac{n!}{r!(n-r)!} \right)$ potential combinations of peaks, where n is the total number of peaks and r is the number of peaks chosen. Given, for example, 150 peaks of which 4 are informative about a phenotype such as a resistance mechanism, there are more than 20 million combinations to test. In a whole-cell spectrum, therefore, there are so many peaks that the most effective approach to this task is to apply a machine-learning algorithm to cluster the data. To perform supervised clustering, the microbiologist tells the computer algorithm that particular spectra have different properties ("this one is from a strain with carbapenemase activity and that one is not", "these are from strain X and those are from strain Y," and so forth). The algorithm decides how to use the lists of peaks to most effectively distinguish spectra from the defined categories.

There are many types of supervised and unsupervised clustering algorithms available, including principal-component analysis,[43,44] genetic algorithms, neural networks,[45] and SVMs.[46] To demonstrate the general features of clustering analysis, a brief review of SVM is provided. Given a set of examples that are assigned to different categories, an SVM uses the features within the dataset to map the different categories into multidimensional space such that they are maximally separated. This mathematical "machine" can then map each new experimental case into that space to assign it an identity. The model (which can be thought of as a multidimensional panel of laboratory tests, vs a single laboratory test with a cutoff separating the categories "normal" and "abnormal") includes a "recognition capability" that represents the relative number of correctly classified spectra (corresponding to the test's sensitivity) and "cross-validation," which predicts how the model will behave in the future (specificity). One can further calculate a confusion matrix that defines the true and false positive states of the multidimensional classifier (eg, see **Fig.** 4B). The simplest form of a confusion matrix corresponds to that of a 2-state laboratory test whereby samples are associated with a "true state" that is hopefully well represented by a "test state," from which a numerical cutoff value for the test is selected by, for example, receiver-operating characteristic analysis[47,48] to best distinguish the 2 states (see **Fig.** 4A).

Although multiclass machine-learning problems may be intimidating at first glance, they are similar to using several tests to diagnose a patient or determine a risk score (eg, using ultrasonography, α-fetoprotein, unconjugated estriol, human chorionic gonadotropin, and inhibin A to classify fetuses as "probably having Down syndrome"

A

Test State	Disease State	
	Diseased	Healthy
Positive	TP	FP
Negative	FN	TN

B

Predicted Identification	Actual Identification, *Moraxella* species					
	atlantae	*catarrhalis*	*lacunata*	*lincolnii*	*nonliquefaciens*	*osloensis*
atlantae	881	14	0	0	0	116
catarrhalis	2	780	0	0	32	41
lacunata	0	6	874	0	25	12
lincolnii	0	104	5	922	158	121
nonliquefaciens	0	65	70	0	673	23
osloensis	45	8	21	49	10	517

Fig. 4. (*A*) A familiar matrix for calculating the performance of a 2-state laboratory test (P, positive; N, negative; T, true; F, false) is similar to (*B*) a confusion matrix generated by a supervised learning algorithm using simulated biochemical test results (see text), where true results lie on the shaded diagonal. Columns contain 1000 simulated results in total, which the classifier distributes across rows of predictions spanning 72 species (only 6 *Moraxella* species are shown; because of their biochemical similarity the algorithm makes many misidentifications within this group). Replacement of a set of biochemical reactions with a larger set of MALDI-TOF peaks would generate a similar matrix, and species names could be replaced with any phenotype of interest.

or "probably not having Down syndrome"). Analogously, clustering algorithms can be used on a set of spectra to identify key peaks that will help classify the individual samples into groups (eg, carbapenemase activity vs no carbapenemase activity).

As a practical example, consider the confusion matrix in **Fig. 4**B, which is a subsection of a 72-species-by-72-species confusion matrix generated using the probability frequencies of 18 biochemical reactions published in the RapID NF Plus (Remel Thermo Fisher Scientific, Lenexa, KS, USA) package insert. To generate this large table, 1000 simulated RapID NF Plus results per species were generated in silico using PyBact (open source software).[49] These results were classified with LIBSVM[42] and a confusion matrix was generated in WEKA (open source software),[50] a portion of which containing *Moraxella* species is shown in **Fig. 4**B. This confusion matrix helps identify both correct classifications and misclassifications (eg, *Moraxella catarrhalis* is often misidentified as *Moraxella lincolnii*). Returning to MALDI-TOF data, if peaks, like the biochemical reactions in a standard panel, are assigned as being present or absent, the process of classification as well as the tabular result is essentially identical, except for the additional classification power represented by many tens to several hundreds of MALDI-TOF peaks. In this sense, machine-learning algorithms should seem familiar to a technologist who has scored a set of biochemicals, then submitted these to a database that returned an identification, a probability score, and potential alternative identifications.

Whereas the example here uses species names, any known property of the organism that generated the spectrum can be attached to the peak list and classified with equal ease. For example, by training several different classifiers, a single spectrum from a strain of *S aureus* might be classified for methicillin resistance, clonality, and presence or absence of a β-lactamase using a single spectrum that was collected for identification purposes (see **Fig. 1**C).

The inherent danger in applying a clustering algorithm as a black-box warning was widely appreciated after publication of a 2002 article that claimed to find a set of MS peaks to discriminate sera from patients with ovarian cancer from controls.[51] It was soon revealed that the data were contaminated with spurious peaks that were introduced into one group but not the other. The algorithm used to classify the cancer group and controls reliably identified these peaks and used them to separate the two groups.[52] For microorganisms, the application of Koch's molecular postulates[53] can help deter such errors. Classification can be guided by analyzing purified factors of interest, or by knocking in or out genetic determinants of a phenotype and observing appearance or disappearance of a peak or peaks.[54]

CURRENT APPLICATIONS

The principles outlined in the preceding section provide a framework for understanding a rapidly growing body of literature on upcoming clinical uses of MALDI-TOF. Most of these works use machine-learning algorithms like those introduced herein. Examples of a few promising applications are presented below.

Organism Typing

Clustering techniques illustrate the power of using entire spectra and efficient classifiers to identify very similar species or strain types. De Bruyne and colleagues[55] proved that biochemically similar *Leuconostoc*, *Fructobacillus*, and *Lactococcus* species could be identified to species level using an approach similar to that outlined in the foregoing example. Reil and colleagues[56] used a similar approach to identify *Clostridium difficile* ribotypes 001, 027, and 078/126, which, while failing to separate an additional 25 ribotypes, collectively accounted for 80% of isolates in a 355-strain series. Although viridans streptococci are difficult to identify with standard clinical MALDI-TOF software,[17,57] spectral peaks have recently been identified that reliably discriminate *S pneumoniae* from the *S mitis* group, which is otherwise a common misidentification.[45,58]

Clonality and Epidemiology

Spectral features can be used to identify populations of organisms that, because of their clonality or the presence of resistance determinants that result in peaks in MALDI-TOF spectra, presumptively harbor resistance mechanisms. Methicillin-resistant *S aureus* (MRSA), vancomycin-resistant *Enterococcus* (VRE), and strains that carry various β-lactamases are examples of those with the most obvious clinical significance. Griffin and colleagues[59] successfully distinguished *vanB*-containing *Enterococcus faecium* from vancomycin-susceptible isolates in the regular clinical workflow with 96.7% sensitivity and 98.1% specificity (taking 67 isolates that were polymerase chain reaction [PCR]-positive for *vanB* vs 8 isolates that were PCR-negative but vancomycin-resistant, as well as single vanA-positive *E faecium* and *Enterococcus faecalis* strains and 1 non-VRE strain) using 5 MALDI-TOF peaks. MRSA-specific peaks were first identified in 2000,[60] and the ability to identify MRSA by MALDI-TOF has subsequently been confirmed.[61,62] Wolters and colleagues[63] demonstrated that common clonal complexes of hospital-associated MRSA also be discriminated with *spa* typing, as with current laboratory-standard MALDI-TOF hardware. Because of the large number of peaks that must be accurately detected for typing and the assessment of clonality, essentially all studies (including the aforementioned) use a similar ethanol–formic acid extraction procedure[64] that disrupts the cell wall more efficiently,[65] and may remove substances that interfere with matrix crystallization.[62]

Direct Identification of Antibiotic Resistance

Antimicrobial susceptibility testing by MALDI-TOF has recently been reviewed in depth,[66] and a few select applications are reviewed here. Beyond the more common resistance phenotypes in the previous section that can be inferred from strain typing, Wybo and colleagues[67] segregated carbapenem-resistant *Bacteroides fragilis* isolates that contain the *cfiA* gene, such that the MALDI-TOF profile predicted carbapenem resistance (using EUCAST breakpoints) with positive predictive and negative predictive values of 90% and 99.2%. Of 248 strains in the test set, 41 were *cfiA*-positive by PCR, and MALDI-TOF classified all positive and negative strains correctly; by this measure MALDI-TOF was 100% sensitive and specific, but because *cfiA* confers minimum inhibitory concentrations of 2 to more than 32 µg/mL, phenotypic cutoffs were used as a more conservative gold standard. However, because *cfiA* positivity is essentially the only mechanism of carbapenemase resistance in *B fragilis*[68] and both *cfiA*-positive and -negative strains are geographically widespread,[69] a MALDI-TOF approach to detecting presumptive carbapenem resistance in *B fragilis* may be particularly successful.

The straightforward case of *cfiA* illustrates 2 key considerations for the clinical laboratory: the ability of the previously trained MALDI-TOF algorithm to address shifting epidemiology and the necessity to confirm results that indicate presumptive resistance. Clustering algorithms are built using a training set, and may not adequately classify new instances that are not represented in the original training set. However, the ability to assign a presumptive resistance mechanism at the same time as an organism's identification may prevent treatment failures and the spread of resistant organisms in a hospital environment where the clonal epidemiology of isolates is well known and tracked closely. By analogy to the preliminary BSI identification generated by the direct identification protocol at St Louis Children's Hospital (described earlier), the benefits of a speedy result may outweigh any drawbacks if they are carefully anticipated.

Direct detection of protein determinants of resistance is typically limited by the size of the resistance determinant, which is often beyond the 20,000 *m/z* upper limit of typical clinical protocols and also beyond the limit of the commonly used HCCA matrix. However, β-lactamases can be detected indirectly by MALDI-TOF by monitoring for hydrolysis of a β-lactam substrate. This approach requires generation of detectable amounts of hydrolyzed substrate and, as such, the procedure generally takes several hours and requires care to prevent contamination of the in vitro reaction with low molecular weight bacterial components that might obscure the substrate and hydrolysis products. Although this compares unfavorably with long-established methods such as cefinase testing,[70] it has been applied to a wide variety of β-lactam substrates[71] including carbapenems.[72,73] As with strain typing, conventional methods may be required as backups to detect nonhydrolytic resistance[74] or resistance phenotypes that are inducible over a longer time scale,[75] but MALDI-TOF methods are arguably more rapid, more convenient, and as definitive as current confirmatory tests for, for example, extended-spectrum β-lactamases or carbapenemases.

SUMMARY

The "beyond identification" MALDI-TOF literature is expanding at a rapid rate, with simultaneous adoption of MALDI-TOF instruments for standard clinical identification. This development has placed microbiology laboratories at a crossroads where new clinical laboratory skill sets are needed to determine whether novel applications of

MALDI-TOF might be brought into routine use. This review summarizes practical considerations in the identification of organisms directly from urine specimens and positive blood-culture bottles, and has broadly outlined methods by which MALDI-TOF spectra might be processed to characterize isolates of a known species for additional clinically relevant properties.

REFERENCES

1. van Belkum A, Welker M, Erhard M, et al. Biomedical mass spectrometry in today's and tomorrow's clinical microbiology laboratories. J Clin Microbiol 2012;1(50):1513–7.
2. Sandrin TR, Goldstein JE, Schumaker S. MALDI TOF MS profiling of bacteria at the strain level: a review. Mass Spectrom Rev 2013;32(3):188–217.
3. Carbonnelle E, Grohs P, Jacquier H, et al. Robustness of two MALDI-TOF mass spectrometry systems for bacterial identification. J Microbiol Methods 2012;89: 133–6.
4. Benagli C, Rossi V, Dolina M, et al. Matrix-assisted laser desorption ionization-time of flight mass spectrometry for the identification of clinically relevant bacteria. PLoS One 2011;6:e16424.
5. Justesen US, Holm A, Knudsen E, et al. Species identification of clinical isolates of anaerobic bacteria: a comparison of two matrix-assisted laser desorption ionization-time of flight mass spectrometry systems. J Clin Microbiol 2011; 1(49):4314–8.
6. Marko DC, Saffert RT, Cunningham SA, et al. Evaluation of the Bruker Biotyper and Vitek MS matrix-assisted laser desorption ionization-time of flight mass spectrometry systems for identification of nonfermenting gram-negative bacilli isolated from cultures from cystic fibrosis patients. J Clin Microbiol 2012; 1(50):2034–9.
7. Rosenvinge FS, Dzajic E, Knudsen E, et al. Performance of matrix-assisted laser desorption-time of flight mass spectrometry for identification of clinical yeast isolates. Mycoses 2013;56(3):229–35.
8. Bille E, Dauphin B, Leto J, et al. MALDI-TOF MS Andromas strategy for the routine identification of bacteria, mycobacteria, yeasts, *Aspergillus* spp. and positive blood cultures. Clin Microbiol Infect 2012;18:1117–25.
9. Meetani MA, Voorhees KJ. MALDI mass spectrometry analysis of high molecular weight proteins from whole bacterial cells: pretreatment of samples with surfactants. J Am Soc Mass Spectrom 2005;16:1422–6.
10. Williams TL, Andrzejewski D, Lay JO Jr, et al. Experimental factors affecting the quality and reproducibility of MALDI TOF mass spectra obtained from whole bacteria cells. J Am Soc Mass Spectrom 2003;14:342–51.
11. Buchan BW, Riebe KM, Ledeboer NA. Comparison of the MALDI Biotyper system using Sepsityper specimen processing to routine microbiological methods for identification of bacteria from positive blood culture bottles. J Clin Microbiol 2012;1(50):346–52.
12. Leibovici L, Shraga I, Drucker M, et al. The benefit of appropriate empirical antibiotic treatment in patients with bloodstream infection. J Intern Med 1998;244: 379–86.
13. Kollef MH. Inadequate antimicrobial treatment: an important determinant of outcome for hospitalized patients. Clin Infect Dis 2000;31(Suppl 4):S131–8.
14. Dellinger RP, Levy MM, Rhodes A, et al. Surviving Sepsis Campaign. Crit Care Med 2013;41:580–637.

15. Weinstein MP, Reller LB, Murphy JR, et al. The clinical significance of positive blood cultures: a comprehensive analysis of 500 episodes of bacteremia and fungemia in adults. I. Laboratory and epidemiologic observations. Clin Infect Dis 1983;1(5):35–53.

16. Stevenson LG, Drake SK, Murray PR. Rapid identification of bacteria in positive blood culture broths by matrix-assisted laser desorption ionization-time of flight mass spectrometry. J Clin Microbiol 2010;1(48):444–7.

17. Prod'hom G, Bizzini A, Durussel C, et al. Matrix-assisted laser desorption ionization-time of flight mass spectrometry for direct bacterial identification from positive blood culture pellets. J Clin Microbiol 2010;48:1481–3.

18. La Scola B, Raoult D. Direct identification of bacteria in positive blood culture bottles by matrix-assisted laser desorption ionisation time-of-flight mass spectrometry. PLoS One 2009;4(11):e8041.

19. Ferroni A, Suarez S, Beretti JL, et al. Real-time identification of bacteria and *Candida* species in positive blood culture broths by matrix-assisted laser desorption ionization-time of flight mass spectrometry. J Clin Microbiol 2010; 48:1542–8.

20. Marinach-Patrice C, Fekkar A, Atanasova R, et al. Rapid species diagnosis for invasive candidiasis using mass spectrometry. PLoS One 2010;5(1):e8862.

21. Meex C, Neuville F, Descy J, et al. Direct identification of bacteria from BacT/ALERT anaerobic positive blood cultures by MALDI-TOF MS: MALDI Sepsityper kit versus an in-house saponin method for bacterial extraction. J Med Microbiol 2012;61:1511–6.

22. Fothergill A, Kasinathan V, Hyman J, et al. Rapid identification of bacteria and yeasts from positive BacT/ALERT blood culture bottles by using a lysis-filtration method and MALDI-TOF mass spectrum analysis with SARAMIS database. J Clin Microbiol 2013;51(3):805–9.

23. Croxatto A, Prod'hom G, Greub G. Applications of MALDI-TOF mass spectrometry in clinical diagnostic microbiology. FEMS Microbiol Rev 2012;36: 380–407.

24. Loonen AJ, Jansz AR, Stalpers J, et al. An evaluation of three processing methods and the effect of reduced culture times for faster direct identification of pathogens from BacT/ALERT blood cultures by MALDI-TOF MS. Eur J Clin Microbiol Infect Dis 2012;31:1575–83.

25. Romero-Gómez MP, Gómez-Gil R, Paño-Pardo JR, et al. Identification and susceptibility testing of microorganism by direct inoculation from positive blood culture bottles by combining MALDI-TOF and Vitek-2 Compact is rapid and effective. J Infect 2012;65:513–20.

26. Szabados F, Michels M, Kaase M, et al. The sensitivity of direct identification from positive BacT/ALERTTM (bioMérieux) blood culture bottles by matrix-assisted laser desorption ionization time-of-flight mass spectrometry is low. Clin Microbiol Infect 2011;1(17):192–5.

27. Christner M, Rohde H, Wolters M, et al. Rapid identification of bacteria from positive blood culture bottles by use of matrix-assisted laser desorption-ionization time of flight mass spectrometry fingerprinting. J Clin Microbiol 2010;48: 1584–91.

28. Qian J, Cutler JE, Cole RB, et al. MALDI-TOF mass signatures for differentiation of yeast species, strain grouping and monitoring of morphogenesis markers. Anal Bioanal Chem 2008;392:439–49.

29. Reisner BS, Woods GL. Times to detection of bacteria and yeasts in BACTEC 9240 blood culture bottles. J Clin Microbiol 1999;37:2024–6.

30. Lagacé-Wiens PR, Adam HJ, Karlowsky JA, et al. Identification of blood culture isolates directly from positive blood cultures by use of matrix-assisted laser desorption ionization-time of flight mass spectrometry and a commercial extraction system: analysis of performance, cost, and turnaround time. J Clin Microbiol 2012;50:3324–8.

31. Spanu T, Posteraro B, Fiori B, et al. Direct MALDI-TOF mass spectrometry assay of blood culture broths for rapid identification of *Candida* species causing bloodstream infections: an observational study in two large microbiology laboratories. J Clin Microbiol 2012;50:176–9.

32. Santos C, Paterson RR, Venâncio A, et al. Filamentous fungal characterizations by matrix-assisted laser desorption/ionization time-of-flight mass spectrometry. J Appl Microbiol 2010;108:375–85.

33. Kwon JH, Fausone MK, Du H, et al. Impact of laboratory-reported urine culture colony counts on the diagnosis and treatment of urinary tract infection for hospitalized patients. Am J Clin Pathol 2012;137:778–84.

34. Ferreira L, Sánchez-Juanes F, González-Avila M, et al. Direct identification of urinary tract pathogens from urine samples by matrix-assisted laser desorption ionization-time of flight mass spectrometry. J Clin Microbiol 2010;48: 2110–5.

35. Köhling HL, Bittner A, Müller KD, et al. Direct identification of bacteria in urine samples by matrix-assisted laser desorption/ionization time-of-flight mass spectrometry and relevance of defensins as interfering factors. J Med Microbiol 2012;61:339–44.

36. DeMarco ML, Burnham CD. Direct identification of microbes in urine specimens using mass spectrometry. Clin Chem 2012;58(S10):A137.

37. Gibb S, Strimmer K. MALDIquant: a versatile R package for the analysis of mass spectrometry data. Bioinformatics 2012;1(28):2270–1.

38. Ihaka R, Gentleman RR. A language for data analysis and graphics. J Comput Graph Stat 1996;5:299–314.

39. Ketterlinus R, Hsieh SY, Teng SH, et al. Fishing for biomarkers: analyzing mass spectrometry data with the new ClinProTools software. Biotechniques 2005;(Suppl): 37–40.

40. Du P, Kibbe WA, Lin SM. Improved peak detection in mass spectrum by incorporating continuous wavelet transform-based pattern matching. Bioinformatics 2006;1(22):2059–65.

41. Vu T, Valkenborg D, Smets K, et al. An integrated workflow for robust alignment and simplified quantitative analysis of NMR spectrometry data. BMC Bioinformatics 2011;20(12):405.

42. Chang CC, Lin CJ. LIBSVM: a library for support vector machines. ACM Trans Intell Syst Technol 2011;2(27):1–27.

43. Chen P, Lu Y, Harrington PB. Biomarker profiling and reproducibility study of MALDI-MS measurements of *Escherichia coli* by analysis of variance-principal component analysis. Anal Chem 2008;1(80):1474–81.

44. Seibold E, Maier T, Kostrzewa M, et al. Identification of *Francisella tularensis* by whole-cell matrix-assisted laser desorption ionization-time of flight mass spectrometry: fast, reliable, robust, and cost-effective differentiation on species and subspecies levels. J Clin Microbiol 2010;1(48):1061–9.

45. Ikryannikova LN, Filimonova AV, Malakhova MV, et al. Discrimination between *S. pneumoniae* and *S. mitis* based on sorting of their MALDI mass spectra. Clin Microbiol Infect 2012. [Epub ahead of print]. http://dx.doi.org/10.1111/ 1469-0691.12113.

46. Barla A, Jurman G, Riccadonna S, et al. Machine learning methods for predictive proteomics. Brief Bioinform 2008;1(9):119–28.

47. Centor RM. Signal detectability the use of ROC curves and their analyses. Med Decis Making 1991;1(11):102–6.

48. Provost F. The case against accuracy estimation for comparing induction algorithms. Proceeding ICML '98 Proceedings of the Fifteenth International Conference on Machine Learning. San Francisco (CA): Morgan Kaufmann Publishers Inc; 1998. p. 445-53.

49. Nantasenamat C, Preeyanon L, Isarankura-Na-Ayudhya C, et al. PyBact: an algorithm for bacterial identification. EXCLI J 2011;10:240–5.

50. Hall M, Frank E, Holmes G, et al. The WEKA data mining software: an update. SIGKDD Explor Newsl 2009;11:10–8. Available at: http://citeseerx.ist.psu.edu/viewdoc/summary?doi=10.1.1.163.817.

51. Petricoin EF III, Ardekani AM, Hitt BA, et al. Use of proteomic patterns in serum to identify ovarian cancer. Lancet 2002;16(359):572–7.

52. Check E. Proteomics and cancer: running before we can walk? Nature 2004; 3(429):496–7.

53. Falkow S. Molecular Koch's postulates applied to microbial pathogenicity. Rev Infect Dis 1988;1(10):S274–6.

54. Gagnaire J, Dauwalder O, Boisset S, et al. Detection of staphylococcus aureus delta-toxin production by whole-cell MALDI-TOF mass spectrometry. PLoS One 2012;6:7.

55. De Bruyne K, Slabbinck B, Waegeman W, et al. Bacterial species identification from MALDI-TOF mass spectra through data analysis and machine learning. Syst Appl Microbiol 2011;34:20–9.

56. Reil M, Erhard M, Kuijper EJ, et al. Recognition of *Clostridium difficile* PCR-ribotypes 001, 027 and 126/078 using an extended MALDI-TOF MS system. Eur J Clin Microbiol Infect Dis 2011;1(30):1431–6.

57. Davies AP, Reid M, Hadfield SJ, et al. Identification of clinical isolates of α-haemolytic streptococci by 16S rRNA gene sequencing, MALDI TOF MS by MALDI Biotyper and conventional phenotypic methods—a comparison. J Clin Microbiol 2012;50(12):4087–90.

58. Werno AM, Christner M, Anderson TP, et al. Differentiation of *Streptococcus pneumoniae* from nonpneumococcal streptococci of the *Streptococcus mitis* group by matrix-assisted laser desorption ionization–time of flight mass spectrometry. J Clin Microbiol 2012;1(50):2863–7.

59. Griffin PM, Price GR, Schooneveldt JM, et al. The use of MALDI-TOF MS to identify vancomycin resistant enterococci and investigate the epidemiology of an outbreak. J Clin Microbiol 2012;50(9):2918–31.

60. Edwards-Jones V, Claydon MA, Evason DJ, et al. Rapid discrimination between methicillin-sensitive and methicillin-resistant *Staphylococcus aureus* by intact cell mass spectrometry. J Med Microbiol 2000;1(49):295–300.

61. Jackson KA, Edwards-Jones V, Sutton CW, et al. Optimisation of intact cell MALDI method for fingerprinting of methicillin-resistant *Staphylococcus aureus*. J Microbiol Methods 2005;62:273–84.

62. Du Z, Yang R, Guo Z, et al. Identification of staphylococcus aureus and determination of its methicillin resistance by matrix-assisted laser desorption/ionization time-of-flight mass spectrometry. Anal Chem 2002;1(74):5487–91.

63. Wolters M, Rohde H, Maier T, et al. MALDI-TOF MS fingerprinting allows for discrimination of major methicillin-resistant *Staphylococcus aureus* lineages. Int J Med Microbiol 2011;301:64–8.

64. Freiwald A, Sauer S. Phylogenetic classification and identification of bacteria by mass spectrometry. Nat Protoc 2009;4:732–42.
65. Smole SC, King LA, Leopold PE, et al. Sample preparation of Gram-positive bacteria for identification by matrix assisted laser desorption/ionization time-of-flight. J Microbiol Methods 2002;48:107–15.
66. Hrabák J, Chudáčková E, Walková R. Matrix-assisted laser desorption ionization-time of flight (MALDI-TOF) mass spectrometry for detection of antibiotic resistance mechanisms: from research to routine diagnosis. Clin Microbiol Rev 2013;1(26):103–14.
67. Wybo I, Bel AD, Soetens O, et al. Differentiation of cfiA-negative and cfiA-positive *Bacteroides fragilis* isolates by matrix-assisted laser desorption ionization-time of flight mass spectrometry. J Clin Microbiol 2011;1(49):1961–4.
68. Livermore DM, Woodford N. Carbapenemases: a problem in waiting? Curr Opin Microbiol 2000;3:489–95.
69. Podglajen I, Breuil J, Casin I, et al. Genotypic identification of two groups within the species *Bacteroides fragilis* by ribotyping and by analysis of PCR-generated fragment patterns and insertion sequence content. J Bacteriol 1995;1(177): 5270–5.
70. O'Callaghan CH, Morris A, Kirby SM, et al. Novel method for detection of β-lactamases by using a chromogenic cephalosporin substrate. Antimicrob Agents Chemother 1972;1(1):283–8.
71. Sparbier K, Schubert S, Weller U, et al. Matrix-assisted laser desorption ionization-time of flight mass spectrometry-based functional assay for rapid detection of resistance against B-lactam antibiotics. J Clin Microbiol 2012; 1(50):927–37.
72. Burckhardt I, Zimmermann S. Using matrix-assisted laser desorption ionization-time of flight mass spectrometry to detect carbapenem resistance within 1 to 2.5 hours. J Clin Microbiol 2011;1(49):3321–4.
73. Hrabák J, Walková R, Študentová V, et al. Carbapenemase activity detection by matrix-assisted laser desorption ionization-time of flight mass spectrometry. J Clin Microbiol 2011;1(49):3222–7.
74. Delcour AH. Outer membrane permeability and antibiotic resistance. Biochim Biophys Acta 2009;1794:808–16.
75. Dunne WM, Hardin DJ. Use of several inducer and substrate antibiotic combinations in a disk approximation assay format to screen for AmpC induction in patient isolates of *Pseudomonas aeruginosa*, *Enterobacter* spp., *Citrobacter* spp., and *Serratia* spp. J Clin Microbiol 2005;1(43):5945–9.

Bacterial Strain Typing

Duncan MacCannell, PhD

KEYWORDS

- Bacterial typing techniques • Molecular epidemiology • Multilocus sequence typing
- DNA sequence analysis • Pulsed-field gel electrophoresis • Genomics

KEY POINTS

- Rapid advancements in molecular microbiology have contributed to a wealth of fragment- and sequence-based techniques for bacterial strain typing.
- For many bacterial species, pulsed-field gel electrophoresis (PFGE) remains the definitive gold standard strain-typing method for outbreak investigations and surveillance, although with limited throughput.
- The advent of cost-effective whole-genome sequencing and other high-throughput, data-intensive laboratory technologies is fundamentally changing the field of public health microbiology.
- These technologies offer unparalleled resolution, accuracy, and precision for strain typing and characterizing bacterial isolates, but will require significant attention to data management, bioinformatics and workforce development.

INTRODUCTION

The identification and subtyping of pathogenic microorganisms is an essential component of modern public health infectious disease surveillance and outbreak response. Timely and accurate strain typing data enables the rapid detection of outbreak clusters, improves the definition of cases and at-risk populations, informs ongoing infection control and public health response activities, and guides the development of prevention strategies to prevent future outbreaks from occurring.

During the early part of the twentieth century, bacterial identification was focused primarily on taxonomic classification, and rarely extended beyond the species or subspecies level. In cases in which more detailed identifications were required, bacterial strain types were typically assigned on the basis of serology, or measurable phenotypic differences in the growth requirements, characteristics, or kinetics of the isolate, or differences in antimicrobial susceptibility, phage resistance, or metabolic function.[1]

The author has no disclosures.
The findings and conclusions in this report are those of the author, and do not necessarily represent the views of the Centers for Disease Control and Prevention.
National Center for Emerging and Zoonotic Infectious Diseases, Centers for Disease Control and Prevention, 1600 Clifton Road Northeast, MS-C12, Atlanta, GA 30333, USA
E-mail address: dmaccannell@cdc.gov

In the late 1970s, the development of laboratory techniques for the analysis of proteins and nucleic acid sequences established molecular microbiology as a new paradigm for public health, enabling unprecedented tools for the molecular-based identification and characterization of bacteria; a greater understanding of infectious disease ecology, bacterial diversity, and population dynamics; and laboratory-based surveillance for the emergence of clinically important new strains or pathotypes. In the decades that followed, continued and rapid advances in molecular protocols and technologies have revolutionized the practice of public health microbiology, and have fundamentally changed the nature, accuracy, and timeliness of laboratory data for outbreak investigation and response.

Today, laboratory methods for molecular epidemiology are at another important point of inflection, as methods transition between gel-based fragment analysis and techniques that derived from increasingly cost-effective high-throughput sequencing. Whole-genome sequencing, and other high-throughput laboratory technologies are becoming an increasingly feasible for near real-time, high-resolution strain typing, characterization, and comparative analyses of bacterial pathogens. However, the tremendous volume and complexity of the data that are generated by these approaches requires parallel investments in high-performance computing, data storage, and workforce development, with careful consideration of how these data will be organized, integrated, accessed, and shared.

PERFORMANCE CHARACTERISTICS AND SELECTION CRITERIA

Molecular strain typing methods for bacteria can generally be divided into 2 main categories: (1) general purpose techniques, which can be easily or directly applied to many different types of bacteria without significant modification; and (2) target-specific techniques, which leverage discriminatory features of a family, genus, or species of microorganisms. Both approaches have significant advantages and disadvantages, and the selection of an appropriate method depends on the experimental context and granularity of information that is required. General purpose approaches include broadly applicable strain typing techniques, such as plasmid profiling, restriction fragment length polymorphism (RFLP), random amplification of polymorphic DNA (RAPD)/ arbitrarily primed polymerase chain reaction (AP-PCR), repetitive element PCR (rep-PCR), PCR-ribotyping, and whole-genome sequencing.[2–5] Although these techniques differ in their genetic targets and their use of conserved or nonspecific primers, they can all be directly or easily applied to a range of microorganisms to generate reproducible strain type information. Other approaches require detailed understanding of the target microorganism, and are tailored and optimized for specific applications. Examples include variable number tandem repeat (VNTR, multiple locus VNTR analysis [MLVA]), clustered regularly interspersed palindromic repeats (CRISPRs), spacer oligotyping (spoligotyping), single nucleotide polymorphism (SNP) analysis, microarrays, sequence-based or multilocus sequence typing (MLST), and comparative genomic analysis, among others.[6–12]

A number of key performance characteristics are used for the development, selection, and validation of molecular typing approaches (**Table 1**). The first consideration is often the discriminatory power of the assay, or its ability to distinguish between unrelated isolates. Conventional metrics, such as sensitivity and specificity, can be used to evaluate the accuracy of clustering relative to other data; however, diversity statistics, such as Simpson's index of diversity (SID), are typically used to quantify the discriminatory power and resolution of the assay. The reproducibility of the assay is also an important consideration, particularly during the development, implementation, and validation of new typing methods. Inconsistent or unstable results introduce subjectivity into the interpretation of typing data, and may seriously limit the usefulness of a given assay. A similar concept is the typability of the assay, or its ability to generate useful strain typing data from most organisms under consideration. These factors contribute to the relevance of the typing data, and their correlation with epidemiologic findings, and are an important consideration in the selection of an appropriate typing platform or assay.

There are also a number of practical considerations about how the assay is implemented, and how the data will be used. These factors include the speed, cost, and throughput of the assay platform; sustainability in terms of isolate volumes, robustness, complexity, and generalizability; capacity to type without an isolate; ability to be deployed to the field; the ease with which data can be interpreted and shared; and the availability of consistent standards and baseline comparator data. All of these factors must be considered and weighed in the development or selection of a new strain typing method, and balanced against consensus from the literature and international research community.

PULSED FIELD GEL ELECTROPHORESIS

For many bacteria, pulsed-field gel electrophoresis (PFGE) remains the definitive gold standard strain typing method for outbreak investigation and surveillance applications. PFGE was first developed nearly 3 decades ago for the analysis of yeast artificial chromosomes, and separates large (50 kb–10 Mb) fragments of genomic DNA through an agarose gel using an algorithmically controlled, switching electrical field.[13] In general, samples are prepared for electrophoresis by suspending the bacteria in agarose and lysing them with enzymes and detergents in situ, to prevent degradation or mechanical shearing of the chromosome during the extraction process. Slices of these agarose genomic plugs are then digested with one or more carefully selected, rare-cutting restriction endonucleases, such as *Xba*I, *Avr*II, *Sma*I, or *Spe*I, and separated on a gel with a high molecular weight marker or universal reference strain, such as *Salmonella* serotype Braenderup H9812 (ATCC BAA-664), as a size standard for normalization.[14] There are several different PFGE separation modes, but the most commonly used is contour-clamped homogeneous electric field (CHEF) electrophoresis, which incorporates a constant electrical field gradient that runs parallel to the intended path of DNA migration, and alternating pulses of current from secondary electrodes that are oriented at opposing 60° angles to the direction of travel. The result of this arrangement is a periodically switching electric field vector that causes the large fragments of DNA to sift or zig-zag through pores in the agarose matrix, separating in an approximate log size-dependent manner over the course of a 15-hour to 30-hour electrophoresis run.[15] The resulting band patterns are normalized with specialized image analysis software, such as BioNumerics (Applied Maths, Austin TX), and compared against a local or networked database of comparator patterns, using band-based or curve-based similarity statistics (**Fig. 1**).

PFGE is a highly discriminatory strain-typing approach that can be used to generate reproducible patterns from a wide range of bacteria, even those in which a thorough, a priori understanding of the molecular biology of the organism may be lacking. In general, sample preparation protocols are similar, although many bacteria require some degree of parameter adjustment to optimize the lysis, restriction, or electrophoresis conditions.

Standardized PFGE protocols have been developed for many high-priority bacterial pathogens, and form the foundation for international consensus standards and

Table 1
Performance characteristics of common bacterial strain typing techniques

	Typing Mechanism	Discriminatory Power	Typability	Reproducibility	Throughput	Generalizability (Other Bacteria)	Labor Intensity	Analytical Complexity	Suggested Applications
AFLP	Fragment	+++	+++	+++	++	Yes	++	++	Outbreak investigation
MLST	Sequence	++	++++	++++	++	Yes	+++	+	Molecular evolution, phylogenetics, characterization
MLVA	Fragment (h)	++++	+++	+++	++++	No	++	+	Outbreak investigation, forensics
PCR-Ribotyping (Clostridium difficile)	Fragment (h)	+++	++++	+++	+++++	Yes	++	+	Outbreak investigation, surveillance
PFGE	Fragment	+++	++++	++++	+	Yes	++++	++++	Outbreak investigation, surveillance
Plasmid profiling	Fragment	Variable	++	++	++	Yes	+	++	Characterization
RAPD/AP-PCR	Fragment	++	+++	+	+++	Yes	++	+++	Outbreak investigation
Rep-PCR	Fragment	++	+++	++	++++	Yes	++	+	Outbreak investigation, surveillance
Gene/Target sequencing	Sequence								
Spa typing (Staphylococcus aureus)		++	++++	++++	++++	No	++	+	Surveillance
Emm typing (Streptococcus pyogenes)		++	++++	++++	++++	No	++	+	Surveillance

	Sequence				Application
Whole-genome sequencing	+++++	++++++	+		
Whole-genome SNP typing	++++	+++++	+	Yes	Outbreak investigation, phylogenetics, forensics, attribution
k-mer–based SNP typing	++++	++++	++	Yes	Outbreak investigation, phylogenetics, forensics, attribution
CRISPRs	++++	+++	++	Yes	Outbreak investigation, surveillance, characterization
SuperMLST	++++	++++	++	Yes	Outbreak investigation, phylogenetics, molecular evolution
Binary typing	Variable	+++	++	Yes	Characterization, surveillance

Bold items are discussed in detail in the text.

Performance characteristics ranged from +, which is poor, to +++++, which is exceptional.

Abbreviations: AFLP, amplified fragment length polymorphism; AP-PCR, arbitrarily primed PCR; CRISPRs, clustered regularly interspersed palindromic repeats; MLST, multilocus sequence typing; MLVA, multiple locus variable number tandem repeat analysis; PCR, polymerase chain reaction; PFGE, pulsed-field gel electrophoresis; RAPD, random amplification of polymorphic DNA; Rep-PCR, repetitive element PCR; SNP, single nucleotide polymorphism.

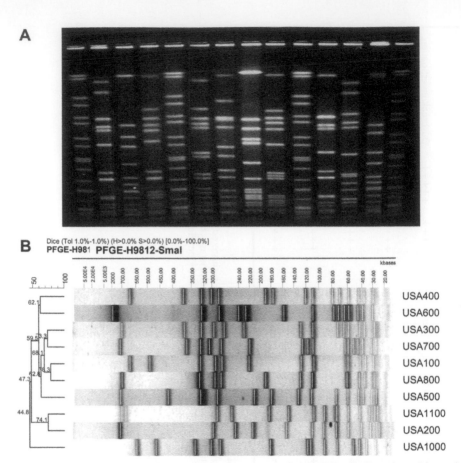

Fig. 1. (*A*) PFGE gel image of MRSA-type strains, visualized with ethidium bromide and short-wave ultraviolet light. The universal standard strain, *Salmonella* serotype Braenderup H9812, is restricted with *Xba*I and run in lanes 1, 5, 10, and 15. The MRSA sample lanes are restricted with *Sma*I. (*B*) Dendrogram of the above PFGE gel, using Dice/UPGMA clustering and a 1% band position tolerance. Gels are normalized in software using the relative migration of H9812 reference bands. MRSA patterns are typically assigned to a USA type on the basis of 80% PFGE pattern similarity, and the overall consistency of other molecular characteristics.

large-scale surveillance programs. The best known among these is PulseNet, which was established in 1996 to improve surveillance and outbreak detection for a number of bacterial foodborne pathogens.[16] It implemented standardized PFGE protocols, analytics, training, and a quality assurance program for participating public health laboratories across the United States, and integrated the data from this network of laboratories through centrally managed pattern databases.

Today, PulseNet includes more than 85 participating state, local, and federal laboratories across the country, and with 7 affiliated PulseNet International surveillance networks in countries and regions throughout the world (eg, PulseNet Asia Pacific, Europe, Latin America), the PulseNet program is a critical component of global food security, and arguably one of the most successful laboratory-based molecular surveillance programs in the history of public health.[17] Through the PulseNet program, and its affiliates, standardized PFGE protocols have been developed for *Salmonella*, *Escherichia*, *Shigella*, *Cronobacter*, *Enterococci*, *Staphylococci*, *Clostridia,* and nontuberculous *Mycobacteria*, among others.[18–21] The growing availability of high-quality genomic sequence data has made enzyme selection, and the development and validation of protocols, significantly easier for organisms in which consensus parameters or standardized methods have yet to be established. However, factors such as DNA methylation and genomic secondary structure often limit the accuracy of in silico prediction of PFGE fragment patterns.[22]

Although PFGE is a robust and proven strain-typing technology, it has a number of important disadvantages and limitations. First among these is throughput: PFGE is extremely time and labor intensive, requiring 1 to 2 days of hands-on time for sample preparation and digestion, and another 1 to 2 days for electrophoresis, imaging, and analysis. Most protocols specify the use of a 10-well or 15-well gel format, limiting the maximum throughput to 11 or 12 isolates per instrument per day under optimal laboratory conditions.[20] More important, perhaps, are potential issues with resolution and the consistent interpretation of agarose gel patterns. Comparison of PFGE patterns and the assignment of strain types rely on the analysis of normalized gel images, and require specialized software, procedures, and standards for consistent analysis, with extensive training and quality control. Minor protocol differences or changes to electrophoresis parameters can result in incompatible data, and in the absence of networked pattern databases, laboratories may require a common reference isolate collection to assign strain-type identifiers that are consistent with literature or community consensus.

For most applications, the resolution of PFGE is exceptional and well-correlated to epidemiologic data, but it is important to note that the underlying patterns are based on genomic macrodigestion, and that the resulting fragment sizes range from larger than 1 megabase to tens of kilobases over a reverse logarithmic size/distance scale. For some highly clonal bacterial species, limited genomic rearrangements (eg, indels, recombination) also reduce the overall diversity of PFGE patterns, and limit its usefulness. As such, PFGE is often poorly suited to identify granular genomic changes, and may not have sufficient resolution to accurately resolve outbreak-associated isolates from a background of sporadic cases. Analysis methods may interject an additional layer of subjectivity, since clustering and pattern assignment are typically based on manual or software-driven band-based comparisons (eg, Dice coefficient), with a small degree of positional tolerance (typically ± 1.0%–1.5% of total run length). Without appropriate quality control, this tolerance range and the subjectivity of band assignment can contribute to the clustering of visibly dissimilar patterns, or the gradual drift of core patterns as minute differences in band size accumulate over time. Position tolerance settings may also limit the effective resolution of PFGE to a minor degree, resulting in fewer than 50 possible band positions for pairwise comparisons. In general, this is not an issue, as most PFGE protocols are intended to resolve between 15 and 30 bands, and resolution can be augmented by re-running samples with a secondary restriction enzyme, resulting in a composite set of patterns (eg, *E coli* is typically digested with both *Xba*I and *Bln*I/*Avr*II).

Despite these challenges, laboratory-based programs, such as PulseNet, have implemented PFGE surveillance across large networks of participating public health laboratories, and have resulted in vast improvements in food safety and public health. PFGE is an important foundation for these efforts, but its technological limitations are driving the development of the next generation of strain-typing technologies, which will build on, enhance, and supplement existing surveillance infrastructure, with improved resolution and capabilities, lower cost, and higher throughput. An important step in the development of new methods is a careful validation, using an established and diverse set of well-characterized, retrospective reference isolates to determine the performance characteristics of the assay, and its overall concordance with PFGE and epidemiologic data. These assays are also run prospectively, in parallel with conventional methods, to evaluate real-world performance.

HIGH-RESOLUTION FRAGMENT ANALYSIS

In recent years, a number of fragment-based approaches have been developed that take advantage of high-resolution fragment sizing using capillary gel electrophoresis (CGE). Most PCR-based assays can be adapted to sequencer-based separation and multiplexed across multiple targets, with only minor adjustment or optimization of conventional primers and the incorporation of appropriate fluorophors. Although a number of approaches have been developed or adapted for CGE, 2 examples highlighted here are MLVA and PCR-ribotyping.

The first of these techniques is MLVA, which targets sets of short tandem repeats (microsatellites) across the bacterial genome. Sequencing has identified scores of VNTR loci in bacteria and archaea, with repeat units that range in size between 6 base pairs (bp) and several kilobases.[23] In MLVA, typically 6 to 8 different VNTR loci are targeted using fluorescently labeled flanking primers, and the resulting amplicons are then separated and sized using high-resolution capillary electrophoresis. Assignment of alleles from the electropherogram is relatively straightforward, and analytical tools are incorporated into several different software packages, including BioNumerics and Geneious Pro (BioMatters, Auckland NZ). Flanking sequences are deducted from the observed peak sizes, and the remaining fragment is divided by the expected length of the tandem repeat at each locus to determine how many repeat units are present (eg, 54-bp fragment/6-bp repeat sequence = 9.0 tandem repeats). The evolutionary clock speed can differ significantly at each locus, and although some VNTRs evolve too quickly to be useful as epidemiologic markers, most MLVA typing schemes incorporate loci with both fast and slow clocks to balance the stability and discriminatory power of the assay.[24,25] Although the inclusion of fast-evolving loci helps to improve the overall resolving power of a new MLVA typing scheme, these loci can also introduce important subjectivity into data interpretation, as they may change over the course of an outbreak. Candidate VNTRs should therefore be validated extensively against a large database of epidemiologically verified sporadic and outbreak-associated isolates, to establish quantifiable guidelines for data interpretation.

Another approach, which has been recently adapted to capillary sequencer platforms, is PCR-ribotyping (ribospacer PCR) for *Clostridium difficile*. PCR-ribotyping uses conserved primers to amplify the intergenic spacer region between the 16S and 23S ribosomal genes. Depending on the number and configuration of rDNA operons in the cell, different ribopatterns will result from PCR amplification, which had conventionally been visualized using agarose gel electrophoresis. More than 250 different PCR ribotypes have been described since the primers were first published in 1999, and are the basis for large reference collections.[5,26] However, conventional PCR-ribotype agarose gel patterns are difficult to interpret, and the move to CGE-based separation has allowed for accurate, consistent, and easily comparable patterns, with peaks between 100 and 700 bp. Even so, CGE PCR-ribotyping remains unstandardized, and comparisons between institutions is difficult. A standardized international consensus method for CGE PCR-ribotyping of *Clostridium difficile* is currently under development (**Fig. 2**).

High-resolution fragment analysis has a number of important advantages. Foremost among these are cost and throughput. Sample preparation is typically a simple

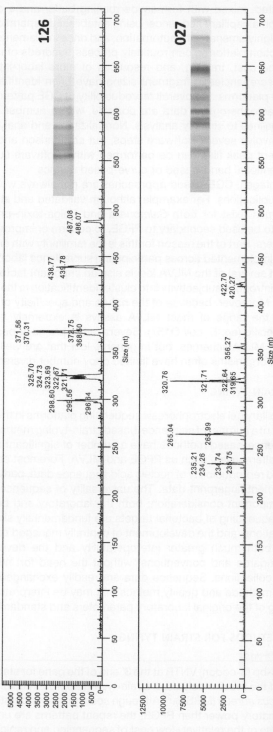

Fig. 2. CGE PCR-ribotyping of *Clostridium difficile*, with conventional agarose gel results for each isolate inset. The top electrophoretic pattern is from an NAP7/126 strain, whereas the bottom panel is an NAP1/027 epidemic strain. Of additional note: CGE PCR-ribotyping reactions may be multiplexed with other fragment-based methods, including the assessment of major deletions to the *tcdC* toxin regulator gene, as demonstrated in the bottom panel (*green trace*).

genomic extraction, followed by quantification and PCR in a 96-well plate format. The products are then diluted, mixed with formamide running buffer and a commercial sizing ladder, and run on a capillary sequencer using established separation parameters. This workflow is highly amenable to automation, and once implemented, modern sequencers and extraction platforms can routinely process hundreds of isolates per day at a fraction of the cost, training, and resources of more labor-intensive approaches. Although discrepancies in fragment sizing have been identified between certain electrophoresis platforms, the overall reproducibility of CGE patterns is generally quite high, and electopherogram data are portable, with a number of different software tools and pipelines to simplify analysis. Normalization and analysis of CGE PCR-ribotyping data involve several software steps, but comparison and clustering of the exported fragment peak files can be performed within software such as BioNumerics, using conventional band-based or curve-based metrics.

Despite these advantages, CGE-based approaches are not always well suited for primary surveillance applications. For example, although validated and standardized PulseNet MLVA schemes exist for both *Salmonella* and Shiga-toxin–producing *E. coli* (STEC), they tend to be used secondary to PFGE, to confirm or improve the resolution of outbreak clusters. Part of the reason for this is the familiarity with and extent to which PFGE has been implemented across participating surveillance laboratories, but high allelic variability at several of the MLVA loci is also an important factor, since hypervariable alleles can introduce subjectivity into cluster identification in the absence of other supporting data. Moreover, because of the nature and specificity of the VNTRs that they interrogate, the range of most MLVA assays is extremely narrow, and many are serotype-specific (eg, *E. coli* O157). Several attempts have been made to design broad/universal MLVA schemes, but in general, loci that are well conserved across a wide range of organisms often have limited copy number diversity.[27]

SEQUENCE-BASED STRAIN TYPING

The introduction of capillary gel electrophoresis sequencing platforms in the late 1990s led to the development of a number of sequence-based strain-typing methods for pathogenic bacteria. Sequence-based methods have a number of significant advantages over fragment-based alternatives, such as PFGE and MLVA. Foremost among these is the nonambiguity and reproducibility of nucleic acid sequence data, particularly relative to gel-based fragment/fingerprint data. The universality of sequence-based approaches is also an important consideration: both the laboratory and bioinformatic methods for Sanger sequencing of bacterial targets are fundamentally similar across a wide range of applications, and the development of centrally managed sequence repositories allows for both much greater interoperability and the development of consensus typing standards and conventions, without the need for independently maintained reference collections. Sequence data are readily exchanged, with well-established analytical methods and quality metrics that may be interpreted without a detailed understanding of the original laboratory parameters and standards.

GENE SEQUENCING METHODS FOR STRAIN TYPING
spa Typing

spa typing targets a 24-bp (8-codon) VNTR at the 3′ end of the gene for staphylococcal protein A and is one of the most widely used strain-typing approaches for methicillin-resistant *Staphylococcus aureus* (MRSA).[28] Although *spa* typing is understood to have slightly lower discriminatory power than PFGE, the repeat patterns are unambiguous and stable, and because of the relatively low cost of sequencing and rapid turnaround time, *spa* typing is an attractive option for large-scale or routine laboratory-based surveillance of MRSA diversity and circulating strain types, particularly when paired with additional markers or confirmatory tests.[29–31]

emm Typing

An important target for sequence-based strain typing among Group A beta-hemolytic streptococci (GAS) is the Lancefield M protein gene (*emm*), which encodes an important surface antigen and virulence factor.[32] The sequence of the *emm* gene determines the M serotype of *Streptococcus pyogenes*, and sequencing is able to reliably identify more than 150 different serovars without the need for conventional serology, making this sequence target important for both strain typing and antigenic prediction.[33,34] The sequencing assay uses a set of highly conserved primers to amplify the 5′ junction of the *emm* gene, and the resulting amplicon includes more than 45 bp of the upstream membrane export signal sequence, and up to 750 bp of the gene itself. For the purpose of typing, a 180-bp segment of this amplicon is used, which includes 30 bp of the signal sequence, and the first 150 bp of the gene. Trimmed sequences are then queried against a database of reference *emm* sequence types using BLAST,[35] to assign an *emm* type and subtype (eg, *emm*3.4). As with *spa*, MLST, and other centrally managed typing schemes, novel *emm* sequences and chromatograms can be submitted to the database curator for verification, review, and subsequent inclusion.

MLST

MLST involves the sequencing and analysis of 400-bp to 500-bp segments of 6 to 8 housekeeping genes that encode essential functional or metabolic proteins.[11] The MLST typing scheme for *Neisseria*, for example, includes loci in the following 7 housekeeping genes, which are essential to signal transduction, membrane translocation, and carbohydrate metabolism: *abcZ* (putative ABC transporter), *adk* (adenylate kinase), *aroE* (shikimate dehydrogenase), *fumC* (fumarate hydratase), *gdh* (glucose-6-phosphate dehydrogenase), *pdhC* (pyruvate dehydrogenase subunit), and *pgm* (phosphoglucomutase).[11] For each isolate that is to be strain typed by MLST, all 7 loci are sequenced, typically using capillary Sanger sequencing. The data are then trimmed, assembled, and queried against an authoritative online database of known sequence variants. Each allele is assigned an individual sequence type based on a perfect sequence match against the database, and the resulting MLST profile is expressed as a series of numbers, indicating the sequence type at each of the 7 loci (eg, 2, 3, 4, 3, 8, 4, 6), and each profile is, in turn, assigned an MLST sequence type (eg, ST-11). As MLST typing schemes mature, and the relationships between STs become more clearly defined, individual STs are grouped into larger clonal complexes on the basis of evolutionary proximity.

Consensus MLST typing schemes have been developed for many important bacterial species, and 2 separate Web portals have been established at Oxford[36] and Imperial College London (UK)[37] to provide centralized access to MLST protocols, sequence analysis tools, databases of reference sequences, and lists of allelic profiles and STs.[11,38–40] At present, the 2 Web sites include databases and resources for more than 55 different clinically important genera or species, including bacteria and eukaryotes. For a number of species, including *Listeria*, *Chlamydophila*, and *Vibrio*, multiple virulence locus sequence typing (MVLST), has been proposed as a derivative of MLST. These schemes typically include a smaller number of core housekeeping genes (typically 3 or 4), with the balance of remaining loci selected from among well-conserved genes associated with pathogenesis.[41–43]

MLST produces unambiguous and reproducible sequence-based results, which can be used to establish high-level molecular evolutionary context for strains from many different bacterial species. MLST is a highly portable global standard for many bacterial pathogens, and is well supported by most commercially available software packages and open source sequence analysis tools, with excellent online resources for analysis and database comparisons. Despite these advantages, MLST is poorly suited for most outbreak investigations and routine surveillance applications. Because mutations in bacterial housekeeping genes accumulate with a relatively slow molecular clock, MLST often has insufficient resolution to accurately distinguish between isolates that are outbreak-associated and a background of sporadic cases, unless they are genetically distant. Although some MVLST schemes have been shown to have higher discriminatory power and reproducibility than PFGE, results have varied.[42] Cost and complexity are also important considerations, as MLST typically requires more than a dozen Sanger sequencing reactions for each isolate. Even in laboratories in which appropriate bioinformatics software and training for processing and analysis are available, the routine assembly, analysis, and integration of MLST sequences can be difficult to maintain.

For some bacteria, specialized tools have been developed, such as the Meningococcus Genome Informatics Platform (MGIP) to bridge this gap and to streamline and simplify the analysis of MLST data for specific surveillance needs.[44,45] Next-generation sequencing has also been explored as a means to provide a more cost-effective approach for high-throughput MLST sequence typing, and may make large-scale efforts more feasible in the future.[46] In the meantime, MLST profiles are often extracted from whole-genome sequence (WGS) data to correlate with other genomic features or WGS-based phylogenetics.[47,48] With a growing abundance of WGS data, MLST schemes are no longer limited by the cost of Sanger sequencing, and recently scalable, Web-based databases and analytical tools have been developed to handle larger datasets, which may incorporate upwards of 25 different loci.[49]

WHOLE-GENOME SEQUENCING

Less than a decade ago, the introduction of next-generation sequencing technologies based on massively parallel pyrosequencing sparked technological advance in high-throughput sequencing, resulting in a logarithmic decline in the per-base cost of sequencing, and a concomitant increase in sequence output. Today, major hardware platforms in this sphere include Life Technologies IonTorrent (Guilford, CT), Roche 454 (Branford, CT), Illumina (San Diego, CA), and Pacific BioSciences RS (Menlo Park, CA). The underlying technology and performance characteristics of these instruments varies tremendously, with read lengths, sequence outputs, runtimes, and error rates that may differ by several orders of magnitude.[50,51] Applications to laboratory-based public health surveillance are now being realized: for example, a recent investigation of MRSA in a neonatal intensive care unit underscored the utility and feasibility of WGS-based strain typing during ongoing outbreak investigations. Of equal importance, perhaps, was the observation that the costs associated with WGS for the investigation were less than $150/isolate, which the investigators noted was comparable to the 2, real-time PCR-based diagnostic tests that are typically used to confirm MRSA carriage or infection.[52] As remarkable as this is, WGS platforms, consumables, and chemistries are a rapidly evolving technology space, and per-isolate costs for sequencing is expected to decline as the technology matures and sequence output, quality, and sample throughput continue to increase.

The greatest challenge to the use of WGS for outbreak investigations lies not in the cost or complexity of implementation, but in the massive volumes of data that it generates. For example, an outbreak investigation involving just 10 patients could easily produce 50 to 100 gigabytes of raw sequence data that must be analyzed, assembled, interpreted, and compared. Given the nature of these data, similarity statistics based on direct sequence alignments and comparisons are not as tractable as they would be with shorter sequences. Therefore, strain-typing approaches based on WGS data tend to focus on specific or distilled elements, such as polymorphisms, and differences in gene complement. As genomic outbreak detection and molecular epidemiology become more definitively established as a field, the development of international consensus standards for data quality, sequence-associated meta-data, storage and compression, transmission, and analytical methods will be critical to ensure the universality of WGS-derived strain typing data for global disease detection and response.

WHOLE-GENOME SNP TYPING

In WGS SNP genotyping approaches, raw whole-genome sequence data from each query isolate are assessed, trimmed, and mapped against an established internal or external reference genome. This reference is typically a closely related, finished genome from public repositories or other sources, but for outbreak investigations and other specialized applications, high-quality de novo assemblies from epidemiologically-important isolates may also be used (eg, from the putative index case). The selection of an appropriate reference sequence depends on the context of the investigation, specific hypotheses to be tested, and the underlying genomic diversity of the organism.[52,53]

Once each query sequence has been mapped against the selected reference, the focus turns to variant detection and evaluation, typically on the basis of SNPs in the mapped reads relative to the reference. Depending on the genomic size, diversity, and the quality of sequence data, the initial pool of candidate SNPs may number in the tens or hundreds of thousands. These are then filtered according to sequence quality scores and confidence; the distribution of SNPs across the reference genome; and the functional implications of each variant position (genic/nongenic, synonymous/nonsynonymous). Additional screening is performed at the population level, and most SNP typing approaches include steps to limit both homoplastic alleles (eg, convergent acquisition of a given allele among evolutionarily unrelated strains), and linkage disequilibrium or redundancy. The latter consideration, in particular, may result in significant data reduction, as many SNP alleles cosegregate or have nonrandom population-level associations due to selective pressure, horizontal gene transfer, or other evolutionary factors. At the end of this selective process, the number of SNPs is greatly reduced, and the panel of remaining SNPs is generally composed of parsimoniously informative loci from the core bacterial genome (eg, high confidence core SNPs).

The identification of parsimoniously informative tag SNPs and the consequent strain typing based on these variations can both be done relatively quickly, given sufficient computational resources and laboratory/bioinformatics staff who are appropriately experienced and trained. Thus, whole-genome SNP genotyping is well suited for near real-time high-resolution investigation of outbreaks of bacterial disease, where the number of isolates is not overwhelming. Once a well-validated panel of informative SNPs has been identified for a given set of organisms, however, it can be used as the foundation for standardized and high-throughput SNP-based surveillance typing assays on a variety of platforms, such as real-time PCR, multiplex sequencing, DNA mass spectrometry, and solid/liquid phase microarrays.[54]

Whole-genome SNP typing also has important limitations and caveats to consider, which are particularly related to its dependence on reference mapping. In species with high genomic plasticity or diversity, such as *Neisseria* or *Burkholderia* spp, mapping sequencing reads against historical reference sequences may not be relevant to contemporary isolates because of significant genomic rearrangement and divergence. In other species, such as *Bacillus* spp, the higher degree of genomic stability makes whole-genome SNP typing approaches far more tractable. Similarly, in organisms in which extrachromosomal or mobilizable genetic elements are understood to play an important role in evolution and pathogenesis, strain typing based on the core chromosomal genome of the organism may give an incomplete assessment of strain relatedness. One solution has been to use a composite reference sequence for read mapping, which includes the bacterial chromosome, with major plasmid and transposon sequences appended. This composite approach has important limitations, however, as these extrachromosomal sequences can be gained or lost over a relatively short evolutionary time frame, and the SNPs that they contain are likely to be under different selective pressures than chromosomal loci.

K-MER–BASED APPROACHES

In recent years, the use of k-mers has been put forth as a potential approach for computationally efficient variant detection and strain typing. In this approach, genomic sequences or unassembled reads are exploded into large sets of k-mers, or oligonucleotide sequences of length "k," based on a suffix array type approach.[9] For many bacteria, a typical value for k falls between 21 and 25 bp. The sets of k-mers are sorted, de-duplicated and compared, to identify those that may contain SNPs at the central base position, and trees are then built from these putative sequence-based comparisons.

Unlike traditional SNP typing approaches, which often take into consideration the genomic context and sequence quality at each locus, the current crop of k-mer–based analysis methods consider only the SNP and the 10 or 12 bp of upstream and downstream sequence that surrounds it. This approach imposes clear limitations on the ability of k-mer–based methods to reliably detect closely spaced SNPs or indels, and remains vulnerable to sequencing errors. However, these tradeoffs are balanced by significant advantages for large-scale genomic molecular epidemiology, primarily with respect to speed and resolution. Because k-mer–based approaches do not require initial assembly or alignment, they are uniquely well suited for the rapid analysis of short-read whole-genome sequence data, and may be applied directly to large sets of raw genomic data. The algorithms and capabilities of these methods continue to improve, and current analysis pipelines can assess for horizontal gene transfer and annotate SNP positions based on reference sequences. As such, k-mer–based SNP analysis is an excellent choice as an initial screening tool for genomic comparison and clustering, and the findings may be used to corroborate, support, or guide the application of more resource-intensive downstream analyses and comparisons.[9]

CLUSTERED, REGULARLY INTERSPERSED SHORT PALINDROMIC REPEATS

Clustered, regularly interspaced short palindromic repeats (CRISPRs) are found in many bacterial and archaeal genomes, and are believed to play an important role in limiting horizontal gene transfer, and as a resistance mechanism against lysogenic bacteriophage.[55,56] CRISPRs are complex and highly variable genomic structures, which include an AT-rich leader sequence, followed by a series of short (24–48 bp) viral-derived or plasmid-derived spacer sequences, with flanking or interleaved palindromic repeats.[55,57] Transcription of this region serves as an adaptive "immune" response to the incursion of foreign nucleic acids, and responses are mediated and chaperoned by a modular set of upstream CRISPR-associated (Cas) proteins, which are highly conserved across a wide range of bacterial and archaeal species.[58]

Because CRISPRs include both conserved structural motifs and highly variable spacer sequences, they would seem to present an ideal target for sequence-based bacterial identification, strain typing, and characterization. Recent studies have investigated the use of CRISPRs in a wide range of bacterial species, and with the increasing availability of high-quality whole genome sequence data, CRISPRs continue to be explored, both as a tool for strain typing and to better understand the role that these sequences play in bacterial responses to evolutionary and microecological pressures.[7,55–59] Because of their size and repetitive structure, however, CRISPRs are generally not well suited for routine molecular surveillance using next-generation sequencing. Short-read sequencing platforms are currently unable to consistently assemble and resolve differences in large, highly repetitive genomic structures without additional sequencing, bioinformatic efforts, and cost. Thus, for large numbers of strains, accurate assembly and analysis of CRISPR sequences may not be feasible or cost-effective, relative to alternative WGS-based strain-typing approaches.

Although this technological limitation affects the usefulness of CRISPRs for large-scale or high-throughput molecular surveillance, CRISPRs are nonetheless well suited to directed studies of smaller groups of organisms, in which hybrid sequencing and assembly techniques are more feasible. For some bacterial species, such as *Salmonella* serovar Enteritidis and *E coli*, the development and validation of real-time PCR-based assays against CRISPR sequences has proven to be an effective and highly scalable strategy for routine surveillance, although these assays have yet to be broadly evaluated or applied.[60,61] Among the *Mycobacteria*, spacer oligotyping (spoligotyping) assays, which involve hybridization against 43 different CRISPR spacer sequences, have been widely used for surveillance and epidemiologic investigations for more than a decade.[8,59]

BINARY TYPING AND "SUPERMLST"

With the advent of next-generation sequencing, binary typing has expanded beyond the consideration of the presence (1) or absence (0) of a handful of genes or genetic markers. BLAST score ratios (BSR), for example, provide a holistic approach and simplified metric for comparing strain similarity using a pairwise comparison of open reading frames.[12] Differences in gene complement can be attributed to plasmids, transposons, phage, or other horizontal gene transfers, and as such, this comparative analysis can identify important changes in resistance determinants or virulence factors. This pairwise approach is effectively an in-silico hybridization microarray, and indeed, genic or marker-based strain typing approaches can be drawn directly from the WGS data, as described here, or used as the basis for targeted assays designed for comparative microarrays or massively multiplexed PCR.[62]

A similar concept was mentioned earlier, in the discussion of MLST. With the growing availability of high-quality WGS data, it is possible to define and query large numbers of MLST loci (eg, "SuperMLST"), using publically available frameworks and tools, such as BIGSdb.[49,63] Depending on how loci are defined, these extended MLST approaches can be used to capture important characteristic information, such as the qualitative presence or absence of marker sequences; (minor) allelic differences, such as SNPs and indels; and mutations associated with specific functional or phenotypic changes (eg, *gyrA* point mutations associated with fluoroquinolone resistance).

As the cost and availability of genomic sequencing continues to improve, these genic or locus-based WGS comparisons will play an increasingly important role in characterizing and classifying pathogenic bacteria. There are, however, some important factors that may limit their effectiveness for routine surveillance, namely (1) their requirement of high-quality assemblies; and (2) their emphasis on the carriage of known genes or markers. The first of these is especially problematic, given the nature of modern short-read next-generation sequencers, which typically result in draft genomic assemblies of 30 to 100 contigs, and are subject to a number of variables related to reference mapping or de novo assembly. To compare multiple loci in a meaningful and consistent manner, all genomes under consideration must be successfully sequenced, assembled, and a set of complete and accurate open reading frames or marker sequences must be extracted from each genomic sequence under consideration. Given the complexity of this work flow, and the current limitations and costs associated with next-generation sequencing technologies, the typability and reproducibility of locus-based WGS genotyping approaches may limit their usefulness as a primary strain-typing technique, at least for large-scale investigations. However, these approaches can be used in combination with SNP or k-mer-based strain-typing information, often without the need for additional sequencing or laboratory effort, where they can provide important corollary information (**Fig. 3**).

One important and practical application of binary typing is not in the direct comparison of isolates, but in their interrogation for known resistance and virulence factors. Curated databases, such as the Antibiotic Resistance Genes Database (ARDB), the Comprehensive Antibiotic Resistance Database (CARD), and the Virulence Factors Database (VFDB) contain thousands of validated and documented genes and marker sequences that are associated with antimicrobial resistance and pathogenesis.[64–66] For example, WGS sequence data from a bacterial outbreak can be quickly queried

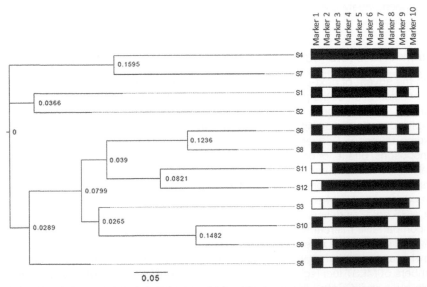

Fig. 3. k-mer–based whole genome sequence typing of an outbreak of *Klebsiella pneumoniae*. This dendrogram was generated using a 25-mer sequence length, from a rough de novo assembly of the 12 isolates. The genomic sequences were subsequently screened against a database of more than 1500 resistance markers to identify a binary resistance type. (Only 10 targets are included here.)

against ARDB and CARD, to provide a rapid, qualitative assessment of the presence or absence of more than 1500 different antimicrobial resistance genes. These data can then be used to corroborate functional testing (eg, antibiogram), to identify or confirm underlying mechanisms of resistance, or to identify important sources of horizontal transmission that may refine outbreak clusters, or have important bearing on investigation or prevention strategies.

FUTURE CHALLENGES
Changing Workforce and Bioinformatics Demands

The advent of next-generation sequencing and other high-throughput laboratory technologies represents an important paradigm shift for public health microbiology. The tremendous volume and complexity of the data that are generated by these approaches also requires parallel investments in high-performance computing, storage, and specialized staffing, with careful consideration of how these data will be organized, integrated, accessed, and shared.[67] Raw genomic sequence data for a bacterial genome represents several gigabytes worth of data, and large surveillance programs would quickly accumulate hundreds of terabytes of sequence.

Incorporating the next generation of data-intensive strain-typing technologies into laboratory practice also underscores the emerging role of bioinformatics in public health. An important priority is to ensure that public health laboratories have the necessary training, resources, and staff to leverage genomics and other emerging technologies effectively, and to apply these advances to the surveillance and investigation of infectious diseases. This transition will require training in molecular biology and bioinformatics for existing staff, and the incorporation of bioinformaticists and data scientists into the public health workforce. Formal training in bioinformatics, genomics, and other "-omics" has already been incorporated into many academic microbiology training programs, and future graduates are likely to be well suited to meet these challenges as the workforce evolves.

Culture-Independent Diagnostic Testing

The ever-increasing importance of culture-independent diagnostic testing (CIDT) in clinical microbiology laboratories throughout the world presents a double-edged sword for public health. On the one hand, at the patient level, CIDT offers a more rapid, reliable, detailed, and cost-effective diagnosis, which may directly improve case detection, patient care, and local infection control practices. On the other, the widespread adoption of culture-independent testing has already begun to stem the number of isolates available for public health surveillance, as routine culture and isolation are no longer required for many clinical diagnostic work flows.[68]

Unchecked, this disruption in the availability of timely, culture-based molecular surveillance data will have an important and immediate effect on our ability to develop reliable estimates of the burden of bacterial illnesses; on our capacity to monitor trends in strain type diversity and emerging pathogens; on our ability to perform functional testing, such as antimicrobial susceptibility testing; and on the cost and complexity of maintaining effective public health surveillance. Reliance on cultures may be addressed by reflexive culture of CIDT-positive specimens, either by clinical or public health laboratories, or by the development of new, culture-independent subtyping and characterization assays based on advanced molecular technologies. The latter option will require concerted research and development efforts, retraining, and the implementation of new laboratory and informatics infrastructure. Despite steady progress on next-generation subtyping, until assays are finalized, validated, and implemented, a wholesale reduction in the availability of bacterial cultures due to CIDT could have a potentially devastating or costly effect on many surveillance programs.[68]

SUMMARY

The current state of the art for bacterial strain typing includes a solid foundation of proven and widely adopted conventional sequence- and fragment-based molecular methods, such as MLST and PFGE, and an emerging set of techniques based on whole-genome sequence data. Regardless of the state of the technology, interpretation of molecular epidemiologic data requires an understanding of the underlying population dynamics of the pathogen, including geospatial distribution, host and environmental factors, and the influence of microbial ecology. Strain-typing results must always be interpreted in the proper context, and molecular data alone cannot take the place of a sound epidemiologic investigation. That said, the application of a new strain-typing approaches based on whole-genome sequencing and other advanced molecular technologies offers unparalleled resolution and synergism, and will certainly improve the accuracy, speed, and cost of outbreak investigations and routine infectious disease surveillance alike. Adapting to and incorporating these new molecular technologies, and responding to changes in clinical diagnostic work flows, will be important challenges and opportunities for public health microbiology in the years to come, and will fundamentally change its capabilities and the nature of its practice.

REFERENCES

1. Van Belkum A, Tassios PT, Dijkshoorn L, et al. Guidelines for the validation and application of typing methods for use in bacterial epidemiology. Clin Microbiol Infect 2007;13(Suppl 3):1–46.
2. Kamerbeek J, Schouls L, Kolk A, et al. Simultaneous detection and strain differentiation of *Mycobacterium tuberculosis* for diagnosis and epidemiology. J Clin Microbiol 1997;35(4):907–14.
3. Akopyanz N, Bukanov NO, Westblom TU, et al. DNA diversity among clinical isolates of *Helicobacter pylori* detected by PCR-based RAPD fingerprinting. Nucleic Acids Res 1992;20(19):5137–42.
4. Versalovic J, Koeuth T, Lupski R. Distribution of repetitive DNA sequences in eubacteria and application to fingerprinting of bacterial genomes. Nucleic Acids Res 1991;19(24):6823–31.
5. Bidet P, Barbut F, Lalande V, et al. Development of a new PCR-ribotyping method for *Clostridium difficile* based on ribosomal RNA gene sequencing. FEMS Microbiol Lett 1999;175(2):261–6.
6. Van Belkum A. Tracing isolates of bacterial species by multilocus variable number of tandem repeat analysis (MLVA). FEMS Immunol Med Microbiol 2007; 49(1):22–7.
7. Díez-Villaseñor C, Almendros C, García-Martínez J, et al. Diversity of CRISPR loci in *Escherichia coli*. Microbiology 2010;156(Pt 5):1351–61.
8. Driscoll JR. Spoligotyping for molecular epidemiology of the *Mycobacterium tuberculosis* complex. Methods Mol Biol 2009;551:117–28.
9. Gardner S, Slezak T. Scalable SNP analyses of 100+ bacterial or viral genomes. J Forensic Res 2010;1(2):107.
10. Garaizar J, Rementeria A, Porwollik S. DNA microarray technology: a new tool for the epidemiological typing of bacterial pathogens? FEMS Immunol Med Microbiol 2006;47(2):178–89.

11. Maiden MC, Bygraves JA, Feil E, et al. Multilocus sequence typing: a portable approach to the identification of clones within populations of pathogenic microorganisms. Proc Natl Acad Sci U S A 1998;95(6):3140–5.
12. Rasko DA, Myers GS, Ravel J. Visualization of comparative genomic analyses by BLAST score ratio. BMC Bioinformatics 2005;6:2.
13. Schwartz DC, Cantor CR. Separation of yeast chromosome-sized DNAs by pulsed field gradient gel electrophoresis. Cell 1984;37(1):67–75.
14. Hunter SB, Vauterin P, Lambert-Fair MA, et al. Establishment of a universal size standard strain for use with the PulseNet standardized pulsed-field gel electrophoresis protocols: converting the national databases to the new size standard. J Clin Microbiol 2005;43(3):1045–50.
15. Herschleb J, Ananiev G, Schwartz DC. Pulsed-field gel electrophoresis. Nat Protoc 2007;2(3):677–84.
16. Swaminathan B, Barrett TJ, Hunter SB, et al. PulseNet: the molecular subtyping network for foodborne bacterial disease surveillance, United States. Emerg Infect Dis 2001;7(3):382–9.
17. Cooper KL, MacCannell DR, Ribot EM. Pulsenet: a program to detect and track food contamination events. Wiley Handbook of Science and Technology for Homeland Security [Internet]. John Wiley & Sons, Inc; 2008. Available at:. http://onlinelibrary.wiley.com/doi/10.1002/9780470087923.hhs414/abstract. Accessed November 15, 2012.
18. Brengi SP, O'Brien SB, Pichel M, et al. Development and validation of a PulseNet standardized protocol for subtyping isolates of *Cronobacter* species. Foodborne Pathog Dis 2012;9(9):861–7.
19. Pichel M, Brengi SP, Cooper KL, et al. Standardization and international multicenter validation of a PulseNet pulsed-field gel electrophoresis protocol for subtyping *Shigella flexneri* isolates. Foodborne Pathog Dis 2012;9(5):418–24.
20. Ribot EM, Fair MA, Gautom R, et al. Standardization of pulsed-field gel electrophoresis protocols for the subtyping of *Escherichia coli* O157:H7, *Salmonella*, and *Shigella* for PulseNet. Foodborne Pathog Dis 2006;3(1):59–67.
21. Zelazny AM, Root JM, Shea YR, et al. Cohort study of molecular identification and typing of *Mycobacterium abscessus, Mycobacterium massiliense*, and *Mycobacterium bolletii*. J Clin Microbiol 2009;47(7):1985–95.
22. Bikandi J, San Millán R, Rementeria A, et al. In silico analysis of complete bacterial genomes: PCR, AFLP-PCR and endonuclease restriction. Bioinformatics 2004;20(5):798–9.
23. MLVA - Multiple Loci VNTR Analysis databases and software [Internet]. Available at: http://minisatellites.u-psud.fr/. Accessed January 14, 2013.
24. Danin-Poleg Y, Cohen LA, Gancz H, et al. Vibrio cholerae strain typing and phylogeny study based on simple sequence repeats. J Clin Microbiol 2007;45(3):736–46.
25. Lindstedt BA, Vardund T, Aas L, et al. Multiple-locus variable-number tandem-repeats analysis of *Salmonella enterica* subsp. enterica serovar Typhimurium using PCR multiplexing and multicolor capillary electrophoresis. J Microbiol Methods 2004;59(2):163–72.
26. Stubbs SL, Brazier JS, O'Neill GL, et al. PCR targeted to the 16S-23S rRNA gene intergenic spacer region of *Clostridium difficile* and construction of a library consisting of 116 different PCR ribotypes. J Clin Microbiol 1999;37(2):461–3.
27. Lindstedt BA, Brandal LT, Aas L, et al. Study of polymorphic variable-number of tandem repeats loci in the ECOR collection and in a set of pathogenic *Escherichia coli* and *Shigella* isolates for use in a genotyping assay. J Microbiol Methods 2007;69(1):197–205.

28. Frénay HM, Bunschoten AE, Schouls LM, et al. Molecular typing of methicillin-resistant *Staphylococcus aureus* on the basis of protein A gene polymorphism. Eur J Clin Microbiol Infect Dis 1996;15(1):60–4.

29. Tang YW, Waddington MG, Smith DH, et al. Comparison of protein A gene sequencing with pulsed-field gel electrophoresis and epidemiologic data for molecular typing of methicillin-resistant *Staphylococcus aureus*. J Clin Microbiol 2000;38(4):1347–51.

30. Golding GR, Campbell JL, Spreitzer DJ, et al. A preliminary guideline for the assignment of methicillin-resistant *Staphylococcus aureus* to a Canadian pulsed-field gel electrophoresis epidemic type using spa typing. Can J Infect Dis Med Microbiol 2008;19(4):273–81.

31. Koreen L, Ramaswamy SV, Graviss EA, et al. spa typing method for discriminating among *Staphylococcus aureus* isolates: implications for use of a single marker to detect genetic micro- and macrovariation. J Clin Microbiol 2004; 42(2):792–9.

32. Lancefield R. Current knowledge of type-specific M antigens of group A streptococci. J Immunol 1962;89:307–13.

33. McGregor KF, Spratt BG, Kalia A, et al. Multilocus sequence typing of *Streptococcus pyogenes* representing most known *emm* types and distinctions among subpopulation genetic structures. J Bacteriol 2004;186(13):4285–94.

34. Steer AC, Law I, Matatolu L, et al. Global *emm* type distribution of group A streptococci: systematic review and implications for vaccine development. Lancet Infect Dis 2009;9(10):611–6.

35. *Streptococcus pyogenes emm* sequence database [Internet]. Available at: http://www.cdc.gov/ncidod/biotech/strep/strepblast.htm. Accessed January 14, 2013.

36. PubMLST.org [Internet]. Available at: http://pubmlst.org/. Accessed January 14, 2013.

37. MLST.NET [Internet]. Available at: http://www.mlst.net. Accessed January 14, 2013.

38. Chan MS, Maiden MC, Spratt BG. Database-driven multi locus sequence typing (MLST) of bacterial pathogens. Bioinformatics 2001;17(11):1077–83.

39. Jolley KA, Chan MS, Maiden MC. mlstdbNet - distributed multi-locus sequence typing (MLST) databases. BMC Bioinformatics 2004;5:86.

40. Aanensen DM, Spratt BG. The multilocus sequence typing network: mlst.net. Nucleic Acids Res 2005;33(Web Server issue):W728–33.

41. Teh CS, Chua KH, Thong KL. Genetic variation analysis of *Vibrio cholerae* using multilocus sequencing typing and multi-virulence locus sequencing typing. Infect Genet Evol 2011;11(5):1121–8.

42. Zhang W, Jayarao BM, Knabel SJ. Multi-virulence-locus sequence typing of *Listeria monocytogenes*. Appl Environ Microbiol 2004;70(2):913–20.

43. Yousef Mohamad K, Roche SM, Myers G, et al. Preliminary phylogenetic identification of virulent *Chlamydophila pecorum* strains. Infect Genet Evol 2008; 8(6):764–71.

44. Katz LS, Bolen CR, Harcourt BH, et al. Meningococcus genome informatics platform: a system for analyzing multilocus sequence typing data. Nucleic Acids Res 2009;37(Web Server issue):W606–11.

45. Meningococcus Genome Informatics Platform [Internet]. Available at: http://mgip.biology.gatech.edu/home.php. Accessed January 14, 2013.

46. Boers SA, Van der Reijden WA, Jansen R. High-throughput multilocus sequence typing: bringing molecular typing to the next level. PLoS One 2012;7(7):e39630.

47. Larsen MV, Cosentino S, Rasmussen S, et al. Multilocus sequence typing of total-genome-sequenced bacteria. J Clin Microbiol 2012;50(4):1355–61.

48. Lomonaco S, Verghese B, Gerner-Smidt P, et al. Novel epidemic clones of *Listeria monocytogenes*, United States, 2011. Emerg Infect Dis 2013;19(1):147–50.

49. Jolley KA, Maiden MC. BIGSdb: scalable analysis of bacterial genome variation at the population level. BMC Bioinformatics 2010;11:595.

50. Loman NJ, Constantinidou C, Chan JZ, et al. High-throughput bacterial genome sequencing: an embarrassment of choice, a world of opportunity. Nat Rev Microbiol 2012;10(9):599–606.

51. Chan JZ, Pallen MJ, Oppenheim B, et al. Genome sequencing in clinical microbiology. Nat Biotechnol 2012;30(11):1068–71.

52. Stucki D, Malla B, Hostettler S, et al. Two new rapid SNP-typing methods for classifying *Mycobacterium tuberculosis* complex into the main phylogenetic lineages [Internet]. PLoS One 2012;7(7). Available at:. http://www.ncbi.nlm.nih.gov/pmc/articles/PMC3401130/. Accessed January 14, 2013.

53. Price LB, Stegger M, Hasman H, et al. *Staphylococcus aureus* CC398: host adaptation and emergence of methicillin resistance in livestock. MBio 2012; 3(1). pii:e00305-11.

54. Van Gent M, Bart MJ, Van der Heide HG, et al. SNP-based typing: a useful tool to study *Bordetella pertussis* populations [Internet]. PLoS One 2011;6(5). Available at:. http://www.ncbi.nlm.nih.gov/pmc/articles/PMC3103551/. Accessed January 14, 2013.

55. Brouns SJ, Jore MM, Lundgren M, et al. Small CRISPR RNAs guide antiviral defense in prokaryotes. Science 2008;321(5891):960–4.

56. Marraffini LA, Sontheimer EJ. CRISPR interference limits horizontal gene transfer in staphylococci by targeting DNA. Science 2008;322(5909):1843–5.

57. Barrangou R, Fremaux C, Deveau H, et al. CRISPR provides acquired resistance against viruses in prokaryotes. Science 2007;315(5819):1709–12.

58. Makarova KS, Haft DH, Barrangou R, et al. Evolution and classification of the CRISPR-Cas systems. Nat Rev Microbiol 2011;9(6):467–77.

59. Abadia E, Zhang J, Dos Vultos T, et al. Resolving lineage assignation on *Mycobacterium tuberculosis* clinical isolates classified by spoligotyping with a new high-throughput 3R SNPs based method. Infect Genet Evol 2010;10(7):1066–74.

60. Liu F, Kariyawasam S, Jayarao BM, et al. Subtyping *Salmonella enterica* serovar enteritidis isolates from different sources by using sequence typing based on virulence genes and clustered regularly interspaced short palindromic repeats (CRISPRs). Appl Environ Microbiol 2011;77(13):4520–6.

61. Delannoy S, Beutin L, Burgos Y, et al. Specific detection of enteroaggregative hemorrhagic *Escherichia coli* O104:H4 strains by use of the CRISPR locus as a target for a diagnostic real-time PCR. J Clin Microbiol 2012;50(11):3485–92.

62. Carrillo CD, Kruczkiewicz P, Mutschall S, et al. A framework for assessing the concordance of molecular typing methods and the true strain phylogeny of *Campylobacter jejuni* and *C. coli* using draft genome sequence data [Internet]. Front Cell Infect Microbiol 2012;2. Available at:. http://www.ncbi.nlm.nih.gov/pmc/articles/PMC3417556/. Accessed January 14, 2013.

63. Bacterial Isolate Genome Sequence Database (BIGSdb) [Internet]. Available at: http://pubmlst.org/software/database/bigsdb/. Accessed January 14, 2013.

64. ARDB - Antibiotic Resistance Genes Database [Internet]. Available at: http://ardb.cbcb.umd.edu/. Accessed January 14, 2013.

65. The Comprehensive Antibiotic Resistance Database [Internet]. Available at: http://arpcard.mcmaster.ca/. Accessed January 14, 2013.

66. VFDB: Virulence Factors Database [Internet]. Available at: http://www.mgc.ac. cn/VFs/. Accessed January 14, 2013.

67. Aarestrup FM, Brown EW, Detter C, et al. Integrating genome-based informatics to modernize global disease monitoring, information sharing, and response. Emerg Infect Dis 2012;18(11):e1.

68. Cronquist AB, Mody RK, Atkinson R, et al. Impacts of culture-independent diagnostic practices on public health surveillance for bacterial enteric pathogens. Clin Infect Dis 2012;54(Suppl 5):S432–9.

Diagnostic Assays for Identification of Microorganisms and Antimicrobial Resistance Determinants Directly from Positive Blood Culture Broth

Morgan A. Pence, PhD, Erin McElvania TeKippe, PhD,
Carey-Ann D. Burnham, PhD, D(ABMM)*

KEYWORDS

- Blood culture • Molecular diagnostics • *Staphylococcus aureus* • MRSA
- Rapid pathogen detection • Bacteremia

KEY POINTS

- The detection of bloodstream infections is one of the critical functions of the clinical microbiology laboratory.
- With traditional culture techniques, the typical turnaround time for organism identification and susceptibility testing is 1–3 days after the blood culture signals positive for growth.
- Diagnostic assays have been developed to reduce the interval to organism identification and/or susceptibility testing for positive blood cultures.
- Many of the diagnostic assays for direct identification/susceptibility testing from blood culture broth are targeted at identification of *Staphylococcus aureus* and/or methicillin resistance.

INTRODUCTION: BLOOD CULTURE OVERVIEW

One of the most important functions of the clinical microbiology laboratory is the detection of bloodstream infections.[1–3] Practices have evolved away from manual methods, using solid media, toward continuously monitored automated systems and broth-based culture media.[4,5]

Disclosures: C.A. Burnham has received research funding from Cepheid, Accelr8, bioMérieux and Luminex Molecular Diagnostics. The other authors have no potential conflicts of interest to report.
Division of Laboratory and Genomic Medicine, Department of Pathology and Immunology, Washington University School of Medicine, Washington University in St Louis, 660 South Euclid Avenue, Campus Box 8118, St Louis, MO 63110, USA
* Corresponding author.
E-mail address: cburnham@path.wustl.edu

Clin Lab Med 33 (2013) 651–684
http://dx.doi.org/10.1016/j.cll.2013.03.010
0272-2712/13/$ – see front matter © 2013 Elsevier Inc. All rights reserved.

Three automated blood culture systems are now commercially available. The BacT/ALERT system (bioMérieux, Durham, NC, USA) was the first automated system to be introduced in the early 1990s. Although this system has undergone modification and updates, the principle of microbial detection is still based on the incorporation of a carbon dioxide sensor into the base of the blood culture bottle. This sensor is separated from the broth/blood mixture by a semipermeable membrane, and as microbial growth occurs in the bottle, the CO_2 concentration changes, resulting in a change in the sensor that is perceived by the instrument. The instrument then signals positive, alerting the laboratory of a positive blood culture. The BACTEC FX and 9000 series automated blood culture systems (BD, Franklin Lakes, NJ, USA) detect microbial growth using a principle that is similar to the BacT/ALERT system. In contrast, the VersaTREK blood culture system (ThermoFisher Scientific, Waltham, MA, USA) detects microbial growth using an alternative principle; the bottles are monitored for changes in headspace pressure (either production or consumption of gasses by microorganisms) over time to produce growth curves. Once instrumentation algorithms reach a threshold, the instrument signals the presence of a positive blood culture. Each of the automated blood culture systems has a variety of different media options available for purchase.

Using conventional techniques, once automated blood culture systems signal positive (typically within 48 hours of incubation for most bacterial pathogens), the blood culture broth is Gram stained and then subcultured to solid medium. Once isolated colonies grow on this medium, identification and susceptibility testing is performed. This procedure typically takes 24 to 48 hours after the bottle initially signals positive.

The Wampole Isolator (Alere, Waltham, MA, USA), a lysis centrifugation blood culture system, is also available, but is not typically used for the detection of most bacteria and yeast that are readily recovered in blood culture broth. The main strength of the Isolator system is recovery of specific filamentous fungi, such as *Histoplasma capsulatum*, and mycobacteria from blood and bone marrow specimens.[3] Most of the rapid diagnostic methods described in this article are performed using positive blood culture broth, not from colonies growing on agar-based medium, and thus blood cultures performed using the Isolator are not specifically discussed in this text.

To date, there are no laboratory methods that rival automated blood culture systems for detection of the causative agent of sepsis. That said, blood cultures in their current form are far from perfect. A large proportion of blood cultures submitted to the laboratory do not grow pathogens. There are a variety of reasons for this, including several preanalytical factors that contribute to the outcome of blood cultures.[3,6–8] The first is the collection of an adequate volume of blood for culture. Depending on a variety of patient factors (such as age, comorbidities, and immune status) as well as the type of organism, the number of colony forming units of organism per milliliter of blood may be very low (in some cases, less than 1 CFU/mL). Failure to collect an adequate volume of blood can result in false-negative blood cultures, and this has been documented as a being a particular problem in pediatric patients.[6–9] It is generally accepted that for blood cultures collected from adult patients, 20 mL of blood should be obtained per blood culture set.[2] Even if organisms are detected, the time to culture positivity can be prolonged if suboptimal blood volume is collected, delaying the result.[10]

The successful outcome of a blood culture depends on several additional preanalytical factors, including the number of blood culture sets collected, the type of blood culture medium used, the length of incubation, and attention to proper technique during the collection process to minimize contamination of the culture.[3,6,7,9–12] It has been demonstrated that most cases of bacteremia are captured if 3 or 4 blood culture sets are drawn during a 24-hour period and the blood culture bottles are incubated for a total of 5 days.[3,13] The addition of anaerobic media to a blood culture set increases the yield of certain organisms, and specific patient populations, such as the immunocompromised, are at risk for bacteremia with anaerobic organisms. These organisms may not be recovered if only aerobic blood culture broth is used.

The issue of blood culture contaminants is important. These contaminants are costly and confusing, especially now, in the era of indwelling medical devices, prosthetic joints, and other medical hardware, and in patients who are profoundly immunosuppressed.[3,14,15] Organisms that historically could almost always be ruled "contaminants" are important causes of bacteremia in the patient populations listed above. Attention to proper blood culture collection procedures and accelerated pathogen identification becomes even more paramount in this context. For example, a positive blood culture with a Gram stain exhibiting Gram-positive cocci in clusters can be a clinical conundrum—this morphology could represent a coagulase-negative *Staphylococcus*, which is frequently a contaminant, or it could represent a blood culture with *Staphylococcus aureus*, a potent pathogen; this is in contrast to some alternative Gram stain morphologies, such as Gram-negative bacilli, which from blood cultures are almost always clinically significant. In addition, with rates of methicillin resistance in *S. aureus* approaching 60% (or greater) in many medical centers in the United States, a Gram stain of Gram-positive cocci in clusters often obligates empiric therapy with vancomycin. The large number of bloodstream infections attributed to *S. aureus* represents a significant burden on the health care system.[16] Thus, it is not surprising that many of the methods for rapid identification of pathogens discussed in this article focus on rapid discrimination of *S. aureus* from coagulase-negative staphylococci and detection of methicillin resistance.

It has been well established that sepsis is a clinical emergency and that mortality increases for every hour in which appropriate antimicrobial therapy is delayed for patients with sepsis.[1,2] In addition, a study by Munson and colleagues[17] demonstrated that a large proportion of decisions regarding initiation of antimicrobial therapy are made either at the time of phlebotomy or when a telephone call is made to the patient's provider reporting a positive Gram stain result from a blood culture bottle; this can be attributed to the delay between the report of a positive Gram stain result and definitive organism identification and susceptibility profile using traditional methods. It is therefore not surprising that many resources have been devoted to developing methods to minimize the interval between blood culture positivity and clinically actionable results.[18] This article describes the methods that have been developed to date to expedite identification of organisms in positive blood culture specimens.

NUCLEIC ACID DETECTION/AMPLIFICATION-BASED METHODS
Rapid Detection of Staphylococci

GeneXpert MRSA/SA
The GeneXpert MRSA/SA blood culture assay (Cepheid, Sunnyvale, CA, USA) is a rapid assay performed on positive blood cultures containing Gram-positive cocci in clusters. The assay uses real-time polymerase chain reaction (PCR) to detect 3 gene targets: *S. aureus* protein A (*spa*), which identifies an organism as *S. aureus*; staphylococcal cassette chromosome mec (*SCCmec*) near the *S. aureus* chromosomal *attB* insertion site; and *mecA* for detection of the methicillin resistance gene. Amplification of all 3 genes is required for the identification of methicillin-resistant *S. aureus* (MRSA). The GeneXpert MRSA/SA assay consists of a self-contained cartridge in which extraction, amplification of nucleic acids, and detection PCR products occur. The closed system for nucleic acid amplification greatly reduces the chance for

amplicon contamination. Testing requires minimal hands-on time, and only 1 drop of blood from a positive blood culture bottle is required for analysis. The GeneXpert instrumentation is modular and can be purchased in groupings of 1, 2, 4, 16, 28, and 80 modules. Each module is random access, allowing any of the GeneXpert tests — including testing for infectious and noninfectious agents — to be run simultaneously. In approximately 1 hour, the assay identifies methicillin-susceptible *S. aureus* (MSSA) or MRSA, if present in positive blood cultures. The assay has a sensitivity of 97% or more and a specificity of 98% or more in blood specimens from pediatric and adult patients.[19–21] However, one study has suggested that the GeneXpert MRSA/SA assay has reduced sensitivity and specificity for detection of vancomycin-intermediate *S. aureus* (VISA), with only 84.6% of VISA and 80% of heterogeneous VISA isolates correctly identified as MRSA.[22]

During routine clinical use, some customers noted that the GeneXpert MRSA/SA assay occasionally reported a result of MSSA on an isolate that was later identified as MRSA by routine susceptibility testing. In 2010, Cepheid released a statement of corrective action for the assay.[23] The company recommended that isolates identified as MSSA be reported as indeterminate while susceptibility to methicillin is verified by another laboratory method. The GeneXpert MRSA/SA assay was later withdrawn from the market and is currently undergoing redevelopment but is expected to return to the market.

Staph ID/R Blood Culture Panel

Staph ID/R Blood Culture Panel (Great Basin Diagnostics, Salt Lake City, UT, USA) uses an isothermal, helicase-dependent method of nucleic acid amplification (HAD). Helicases are used to unwind double-stranded DNA as opposed to heat denaturation, which is used in PCR reactions. Multiplex PCR by HAD can be problematic because nonspecific binding at cooler temperatures causes primer artifacts.[24] To prevent primer artifacts, the Staph ID/R Blood Culture Panel amplification reaction contains DNA primers that contain a single RNA nucleotide, which prevents amplification at cooler temperatures. At temperatures greater than 50°C, a thermostable RNase cleaves the RNA nucleotide and allows transcription to proceed. After amplification, nucleic acids are detected by species-specific probes bound to a silicon chip and visualized by the addition of enzymatic substrate. Staph ID/R Blood Culture Panel requires minimal hands-on time. All processing occurs in a disposable cartridge, and results are obtained using a benchtop analyzer (**Fig. 1**). *S. aureus* from positive blood cultures as well as *mecA* resistance can be detected in approximately 75 minutes. Only one cartridge can be run at a time, but the system can be used for other Great Basin pathogen assays including *Clostridium difficile*, nasal MRSA detection, and identification of *Candida* species from positive blood culture bottles.

The Staph ID/R Blood Culture Panel detects *tuf,* which encodes the polypeptide elongation factor Tu in bacteria. This species-variable gene is used for identification of *S. aureus* and other *Staphylococcus* species. In addition, the assay detects *mecA* for prediction of methicillin resistance in *S. aureus*. A study by Pasko and colleagues[25] tested 104 positive blood cultures from a Chicago area hospital. Of the 99 bottles with Gram-positive cocci in clusters, Staph ID/R identified 19 MSSA, 6 MRSA, 67 coagulase-negative staphylococci, and 7 non-staphylococcal isolates to group or species level with a sensitivity of greater than 98.5%. The assay was also highly specific, showing no cross-reactivity with other genera that can be morphologically similar to *Staphylococcus* species on Gram stain, notably *Enterococcus*, *Micrococcus*, and *Streptococcus* species. Despite these promising results, there are little data available about the performance of Staph ID/R in the clinical laboratory.

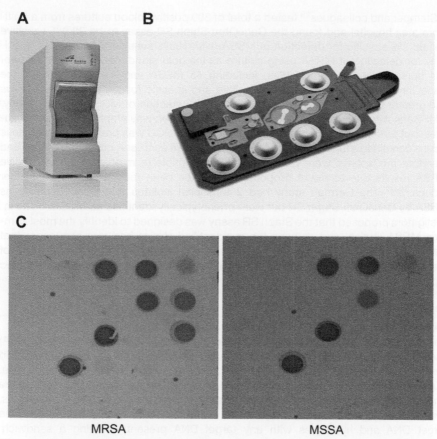

Fig. 1. Staph ID/R blood culture panel (*A*) instrumentation, (*B*) cartridge, and (*C*) optical results. Nucleic acids are detected by species-specific probes bound to a silicon chip and visualized by the addition of enzymatic substrate. Detection of methicillin-resistant *Staphylococcus aureus* (MRSA) and methicillin-sensitive *Staphylococcus aureus* (MSSA) are shown in (*C*). (*Courtesy of* Great Basin Diagnostics, Salt Lake City, UT; with permission.)

GeneOhm StaphSR

The GeneOhm Staph SR (BD) is a PCR-based assay for identification of MSSA and MRSA from positive blood cultures.[26] The assay uses molecular beacon technology to amplify a proprietary species-specific target for detection of *S. aureus*. *SCCmec*, near the chromosomal *orfX* junction, is targeted for detection of MRSA. GeneOhm Staph SR is performed on the SmartCycler System (Cepheid, Sunnyvale, CA, USA), a random access instrument with a capacity to run 16 individual assays simultaneously. Because this assay relies on manual nucleic acid extraction, the GeneOhm Staph SR assay requires hands-on time and technical expertise and has a turnaround time of approximately 2 hours. To reduce the hands-on time and technical expertise requirements, BD has recently launched the BD MAX System.[27] It is a fully automated nucleic acid extraction and PCR method compatible with several commercially available BD GeneOhm assays; it is also an open system so that laboratories can design their own PCR assays. At the time of preparation of this article, Group B *Streptococcus* and MRSA screening assays (from the nares), but not Staph SR for positive blood cultures, are US Food and Drug Administration (FDA) approved for the BD Max System.

Stamper and colleagues[28] tested a total of 300 positive blood cultures from a Baltimore area hospital and found the GeneOhm Staph SR assay to be 98.9% sensitive and 96.7% specific for detection of MSSA, with 100% sensitivity and 98.4% specificity for detection of MRSA using culture as the gold standard. A German study of 134 spiked blood culture bottles, including 45 MSSA and 45 MRSA, found the GeneOhm Staph SR to be 100% sensitive and specific for detection of *S. aureus* and greater than 95% sensitive and specific for detection of MRSA.[29] In this study, 3 MSSA isolates were misidentified as MRSA. *SCCmec* was amplified in these 3 isolates, but further analysis showed that, although the SCC was present, none of these strains contained a functional *mecA* gene (also known as "*mecA* dropout" strains), and therefore the isolates were phenotypically susceptible to methicillin. False-positive MRSA results due to *mecA* dropouts have since been reported by several other groups.[30–32] The German study had 2 additional isolates that were identified as MRSA by GeneOhm Staph SR but were phenotypically identified as MSSA.[29] The investigators proposed that the Staph SR assay was designed to identify the most common MRSA strains, and perhaps the misidentified strains had rare sequences that were not targeted by the assay.[33] Other groups have reported that the sensitivity of the GeneOhm Staph SR can be as low as 50% depending on the prevailing *SCCmec* types present locally.[33–36]

Beyond Staphylococcus aureus Detection

Verigene Gram-Positive (BC-GP) Blood Culture Nucleic Acid Test

Verigene BC-GP Blood Culture Nucleic Acid Test (Nanosphere, Northbrook, IL, USA) uses nanogold technology to detect bloodstream pathogens without nucleic acid amplification. Pathogen-specific capture probes are immobilized on a glass side. Nucleic acids extracted from a positive blood culture are incubated with the capture probes, and hybridization occurs if the target DNA is present. A second set of probes, which are conjugated to gold nanoparticles, contains complimentary sequences to the target DNA and hybridizes with any target DNA present, creating a sandwich. Elemental silver, deposited onto the gold particle through a catalytic process, greatly amplifies the signal produced by each gold nanoparticle and allows detection of bound nucleic acids.[37,38] Nanogold technology is approximately 2 to 3 times more sensitive than enzyme-linked immunosorbent assay (ELISA)-based methods and eliminates the need for amplification of target DNA before hybridization.[37] The technology is also very specific, as hybridization of target DNA to both the capture and detection probes occurs only if in the presence of an exact match.[37] Verigene BC-GP detects staphylococci, streptococci, enterococci, and *Listeria* from positive blood culture broth. In addition, the Verigene BC-GP detects *mecA* for reporting of methicillin resistance in staphylococci as well as *vanA* and *vanB* for detection of vancomycin resistance in enterococci (**Table 1**). The assay has been FDA cleared for all blood culture media intended for use in adults, for all of the continuously monitored blood culture systems currently on the market.

Verigene BC-GP Blood Culture Nucleic Acid Test requires minimal hands-on time, and results are obtained in less than 3 hours. Verigene instrumentation consists of a processing module in which all testing is performed and an analyzer, which reads and records the test results (**Fig. 2**). A typical laboratory setup contains several processing modules, each running 1 sample at a time, and 1 analyzer. Each module is random access, and therefore, different assays can be performed simultaneously. Verigene offers other assays for infectious agent detection such as respiratory virus detection, enteric pathogens, and *C. difficile*, as well as noninfectious cardiac, human genetic, and pharmacogenetic testing.

Table 1
Verigene Gram-positive (BC-GP) blood culture assay targets

Genus-Level	Species-Level	Antibiotic Resistance
Staphylococcus spp	*Staphylococcus aureus*	*mecA*
Streptococcus spp	*Staphylococcus epidermidis*	*vanA*
Micrococcus spp	*Staphylococcus lugdunensis*	*vanB*
Listeria spp	*Streptococcus pneumoniae*	
	Streptococcus pyogenes	
	Streptococcus agalactiae	
	Streptococcus anginosus group	
	Enterococcus faecalis	
	Enterococcus faecium	

To date, no peer-reviewed studies have been published on the efficacy of Verigene BC-GP for detection of blood culture pathogens, but several abstracts presented at national meetings show a sensitivity and specificity of 97% to 100%, consistent with numbers published by Nanosphere.[39–42] These unpublished reports show 99% to 100% sensitivity and specificity for identification of MRSA and vancomycin-resistant *Enterococcus* (VRE) resistance genes compared with routine antimicrobial susceptibility testing. Nanosphere also offers a Gram-negative counterpart to its Gram-Positive Blood Culture Nucleic Acid Test. The Verigene BC-GN assay detects 8 genera and 6 antibiotic resistance genes (**Table 2**). Although the Verigene BC-GP assay is FDA approved, the Verigene BC-GN assay is under development and currently classified as research use only. No data are available about its performance.[40]

FilmArray Blood Culture Identification Panel

The FilmArray Blood Culture Identification (BCID) panel (BioFire Diagnostics, Salt Lake City, UT, USA) is a multiplex PCR, which assays positive blood culture bottles for the presence of 15 genus-level and 11 species-specific organisms including Gram-positive bacteria, Gram-negative bacteria, and yeast (**Table 3**).[43] In addition, the FilmArray BCID panel detects antimicrobial resistance genes: *mecA* in *S. aureus,* *vanA* and *vanB* in enterococci, and *bla*$_{KPC}$ in *Enterobacteriaceae.*

To perform the assay, an aliquot from a positive blood culture is added to the FilmArray reagent pouch. The pouch is a self-contained system in which nucleotide extraction, real-time PCR amplification, and pathogen detection are performed. The

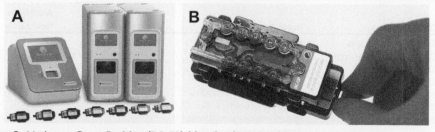

Fig. 2. Verigene Gram-Positive (BC-GP) blood culture nucleic acid test (*A*) instrumentation and (*B*) test cartridge. Nanogold technology is used to amplify the signal produced in the presence of target DNA. One instrument module and an analyzer can easily fit in 2 ft × 2 ft area of bench space. (*Courtesy of* Nanosphere, Northbrook, IL; with permission.)

Table 2
Verigene Gram-negative (BC-GN) blood culture assay targets (in development)

Genus-Level	Species-Level	Antibiotic Resistance
Acinetobacter spp	*Escherichia coli / Shigella* spp	bla_{KPC}
Proteus spp	*Klebsiella pneumoniae*	bla_{NDM}
Citrobacter spp	*Klebsiella oxytoca*	bla_{CTx-M}
Enterobacter spp	*Pseudomonas aeruginosa*	bla_{VIM}
	Serratia marcescens	bla_{IMP}
		bla_{OxA}

multiplex PCR is nested to increase assay sensitivity while maintaining specificity. The initial round of PCR amplifies 200 to 500 bp segments. A second round of PCR contains primer targets within the original PCR product, resulting in amplification of shorter amplicons.

The FilmArray BCID panel requires minimal hands-on time, and results are obtained in approximately 1 hour. In addition, only 1 FilmArray pouch can be run at a time per instrument. BioFire also offers FilmArray test panels for respiratory and gastrointestinal pathogens, both of which use the same instrumentation as the BCID panel.

A retrospective study of 102 clinical blood cultures by Blaschke and colleagues[44] found the FilmArray BCID panel to be 83% to 100% sensitive and greater than 99% specific depending on the pathogen identified. The FilmArray BCID panel missed detecting *Streptococcus pyogenes, S. aureus, Escherichia coli*, and 2 isolates of coagulase-negative staphylococci. MSSA and MRSA were correctly identified in all 14 cultures in which these pathogens were present, but 1 vancomycin-susceptible *Enterococcus* isolate was incorrectly identified as VRE. A prospective study of 89 isolates tested by culture and FilmArray BCID panel found a sensitivity of 88% to 100% and a specificity of greater than 98%.[44] Organisms that grew in the clinical blood cultures but were missed by the FilmArray BCID panel included coagulase-negative staphylococci, *Serratia marcescens, Enterobacteriaceae*, and several cultures of yeast. Although the results of this study are favorable, a small number of specimens were tested in comparison to the large number of bacterial and fungal targets present in the FilmArray BCID panel multiplex PCR. This result was especially of concern for infrequently identified pathogens and the detection of organisms harboring antibiotic resistance genes. The study also found a low level of background contaminants in the

Table 3
FilmArray blood culture identification (BCID) panel targets

Gram-Positive	Gram-Negative	Fungal	Antibiotic Resistance
Staphylococcus spp	*Klebsiella pneumoniae*	*Candida albicans*	*mecA*
Staphylococcus aureus	*Klebsiella oxytoca*	*Candida tropicalis*	*vanA/B*
Streptococcus spp	*Serratia* spp	*Candida parapsilosis*	bla_{KPC}
Streptococcus pneumoniae	*Proteus* spp	*Candida krusei*	
Streptococcus pyogenes	*Haemophilus influenzae*	*Candida glabrata*	
Streptococcus agalactiae	*Neisseria meningitidis*		
Enterococcus spp	*Pseudomonas aeruginosa*		
	Enterobacteriaceae		
	Escherichia coli		
	Enterobacter cloacae complex		
	Acinetobacter baumannii		

pouch, which amplified at high cycle thresholds. These contaminants, which seemed to be lot dependent, would severely complicate the evaluation of positive results. Based on the data to date, it seems that extensive validation in the clinical laboratory would need to be completed before the FilmArray BCID panel could be used clinically.

Pyrosequencing

Pyrosequencing detects the release of a pyrophosphate on nucleotide incorporation as opposed to Sanger sequencing, which detects chain-terminating dideoxynucleotides. In contrast to conventional sequencing, pyrosequencing is restricted to the analysis of short DNA regions (in the range of 10–60 bases). Because of the short length of sequence generated, pyrosequencing is more rapid and cost-effective than traditional Sanger sequencing, and time to results can be approximately 4 hours, including 1 hour of hands-on time. Pyrosequencing of bacteria and *Candida* species from positive blood cultures has been investigated, but to date, no FDA-approved system for this approach exists.

The accuracy of pyrosequencing for microbial identification depends on the region analyzed and the length of the sequence determined. The first study of pyrosequencing directly from blood cultures targeted a 15 bp region of the 16S rRNA gene but was only able to identify bacteria to the genus level or to a classification of "enteric bacteria."[45] Later studies analyzed slightly longer regions of 30 bp in differing variable regions of the 16S rRNA gene and have had more success identifying bacteria to the species level.[46,47] In the study in which the 16S method was the most successful, 102 blood cultures were evaluated, and 84.3% were correctly identified to the genus level, whereas only 64.7% were correctly identified to the species level, with 10.9% remaining unidentified.[47] Another study involved the P3 and P9 regions of the *rnpB* gene, encoding the RNA subunit of RNase P, with the goal of improved accuracy for differentiation of streptococci.[48] The investigators were able to identify 39 species and 2 species pairs (*Streptococcus mitis/Streptococcus oralis* and *Streptococcus anginosus/Streptococcus constellatus*). A third target, the 23S rRNA gene, has also been evaluated, with an overall accuracy of 97.8% compared with standard culture methods, which included 98.8% agreement for monomicrobial and 89.3% agreement for polymicrobial samples.[49] Sequencing of the 23S rRNA gene provided improved ability to differentiate enteric Gram-negative bacteria and streptococcal species compared with 16S rRNA sequencing. For identification of *Candida* species directly from positive blood culture bottles, sequencing of 18S rRNA resulted in 100% agreement compared with standard culture methods.[50]

Pyrosequencing requires DNA extraction, PCR, and sequencing. This technique is labor intensive and requires specialized, expensive instrumentation. It is unlikely that pyrosequencing of positive blood culture broth will become part of the mainstream workflow of clinical laboratories in the near term.

PCR-Electrospray Ionization Mass Spectrometry

PCR combined with electrospray ionization mass spectrometry (PCR-ESI MS) is a method that can identify numerous pathogens from positive blood cultures. After DNA extraction from the blood culture broth, the initial PCR is set up using a set of broad-range and species- or strain-specific primers. The PCR products are subsequently analyzed by ESI MS, which measures the mass/charge (*m/z*) ratio of the amplicons to deduce the nucleotide composition of the PCR product. The nucleotide composition is compared with a database maintained by Abbott Molecular Diagnostics (Des Plaines, IL, USA) to determine the identification of the organism, with results delivered in 6 to 8 hours. No FDA-approved platform for this testing is available at the time of this publication. This instrumentation initially existed as the Ibis T5000 prototype, was acquired by Abbott and improved, and is now known as the PLEX-ID system. The use of PCR-ESI MS directly on blood cultures demonstrated 94% to 98.7% agreement at the genus level compared with standard methods and 86% to 96.6% concordance at the species level.[51,52] In addition, PCR-ESI MS has the ability to detect antimicrobial resistance genes, although these studies have been performed on bacterial isolates and not directly on blood cultures.[53–55]

PCR-ESI MS is a complex procedure involving DNA extraction, PCR, desalting, and mass spectrometry, which requires costly reagents and technical expertise. Although data evaluating the analytical performance characteristics of this method are promising, this technique may be difficult to work into the standard workflow of many clinical laboratories.

Rapid Blood Culture Testing Methods Available Outside of the United States

LightCycler SeptiFast M^GRADE test

SeptiFast (Roche Diagnostics, Mannheim, Germany) is able to detect 25 common bloodstream pathogens, including Gram-positive and Gram-negative bacteria, as well as fungi (**Table 4**). Unlike the other assays mentioned, SeptiFast detects pathogens directly from whole blood without any need for prior incubation. Real-time PCR reactions, performed on the LightCycler, target the ribosomal internal transcribed spacer region.[56] DNA is amplified in 3 parallel, multiplex, real-time PCR assays for detection of Gram-positive, Gram-negative, and fungal pathogens. Labeled probes are added and hybridized to internal sequences of the amplified DNA. Probe-DNA melting temperature analysis is used to differentiate bloodstream pathogens. The melting temperature of a specific organism is based on fragment length, nucleotide composition, and amount of homology between the amplified target and the hybridization probe. SeptiFast Identification Software analyzes the melting curves and reports the presence of bloodstream pathogens. The SeptiFast assay is complex, requires a large amount of hands-on time, and can be completed in approximately 6 hours.

A study by Lehmann and colleagues[57] found that blood cultures spiked with 3 CFU/mL achieved a sensitivity of 0% to 100% depending on the organism. Sensitivities for detection of Gram-negative organisms ranged from 50% to 100%, whereas sensitivities for Gram-positive organisms were much lower, ranging from 0% to 85% (with the majority having sensitivities <50%). Fungal pathogen detection was approximately 70% sensitive. This result seems to be inadequate sensitivity for clinical specimens, especially considering that the typical bacterial burden for bacteremic

Table 4		
LightCycler SeptiFast M^GRADE targets		
Gram-Positive	**Gram-Negative**	**Fungal**
Staphylococcus aureus	Escherichia coli	Candida albicans
Staphylococcus epidermidis	Klebsiella pneumoniae	Candida tropicalis
Staphylococcus haemolyticus	Klebsiella oxytoca	Candida parapsilosis
Streptococcus pneumoniae	Serratia marcescens	Candida krusei
Streptococcus pyogenes	Enterobacter cloacae	Candida glabrata
Streptococcus agalactiae	Enterobacter aerogenes	Aspergillus fumigatus
Streptococcus mitis	Proteus mirabilis	
Enterococcus faecium	Pseudomonas aeruginosa	
Enterococcus faecalis	Acinetobacter baumannii	
	Stenotrophomonas maltophilia	

adults is 1 to 5 organisms per milliliter of blood, and can often be less than 1 organism per milliliter of blood.[58–60] Children were thought to have much higher organism burdens in the blood during bacteremia, but with changing epidemiology in the postvaccine era, most bacteremic children also have less than 10 organisms per milliliter of blood.[61]

Not surprisingly, studies using SeptiFast have reported low sensitivities and specificities in clinical settings. A study by Rath and colleagues[62] of patients who underwent liver transplant found SeptiFast to be 80.9% sensitive and 70.0% specific compared with culture. Control patients who underwent major abdominal surgery had a lower sensitivity and similar specificity of 57.3% and 70.0%, respectively, indicating that imunocompromised patients may have higher bacterial burden in their bloodstream, resulting in somewhat improved SeptiFast sensitivity. Another study of 208 immunocompetent patients with community-onset bloodstream infections found that SeptiFast was 12% to 67% sensitive depending on the organism isolated.[63] In addition, high numbers of discrepant results between culture and SeptiFast have been reported in studies of infective endocarditis, adults with solid malignancies, and children with sepsis.[64–69] Although the rapid identification of blood culture pathogens without the need for culture is enticing, the low sensitivity and specificity of SeptiFast makes its clinical utility dubious.

Prove-it Sepsis
Prove-it Sepsis (Mobidiag, Helsinki, Finland) uses multiplex PCR to detect more than 50 Gram-positive, Gram-negative, and fungal pathogens from positive blood cultures.[70] Amplified DNA undergoes hybridization with sequence-specific capture probes attached to a solid support or microarray. Hybridized DNA is detected by the addition of enzymatic substrate, which produces a visible color signal. Analysis is performed using Prove-it Advisor software. The Prove-it Sepsis assay requires a moderate amount of hands-on time, as DNA extraction must be performed manually. The assay has a turnaround time of approximately 3.5 hours, excluding DNA extraction.

A study in the United Kingdom and Finland of 2107 positive blood cultures found that 86% of bacteria isolated from blood culture were detected on the Prove-it Sepsis multiplex PCR.[71] The assay had a sensitivity of 94.7% and a sensitivity of 98.9% compared with culture. Identification of MRSA was 100% sensitive and specific, but the assay was less accurate in identifying *Stenotrophomonas maltophilia*, *Enterobacteriaceae*, and coagulase-negative staphylococci.

Hyplex BloodScreen PCR ELISA
Hyplex BloodScreen PCR ELISA (Amplex BioSystems, Giessen, Germany) detects 10 common Gram-positive and Gram-negative bacteria from positive blood culture bottles, as well as the *mecA* gene for detection of MRSA. PCR amplification targeting the 16S ribosome is performed separately for Gram-positive and Gram-negative bacteria. The amplified DNA is then added to microtiter plate wells coated with capture probes specific for different bacteria. A hybridization ELISA is performed using the amplified DNA as the target, and the presence of bacteria is detected by the addition of an enzymatic substrate, which produces a visible color signal. The Hyplex BloodScreen PCR ELISA is moderately complex to perform, requiring manual DNA extraction before initiating PCR. DNA isolation, PCR amplification, and hybridization can be performed in 4.5 to 6 hours.

An article by Wellinghausen and colleagues[72] evaluated 482 positive blood cultures from a German hospital and found the Hyplex BloodScreen to be 100% sensitive and 92.5% to 100% specific for detection of Gram-negative bacteria, 96.6% to 100%

sensitive and 97.7% to 100% specific for detection of Gram-positive bacteria, and 100% sensitive and specific for detection of MRSA.

SepsiTest

SepsiTest (Molzym, Bremen, Germany) is a broad-range PCR-based assay that targets conserved areas of 16S and 18S rRNA for bacterial and fungal DNA amplification. After amplification, the amplicons are sequenced for organism identification. SepsiTest can detect 345 bacteria and fungi from positive blood cultures in approximately 8 hours.[73] A German study of 342 positive blood samples found SepsiTest to be 87% sensitive and 85.8% specific compared with culture methods.[74] Seven samples tested positive by culture but negative by SepsiTest, including 5 blood culture specimens with coagulase-negative staphylococci and 2 containing E. coli. In this study, 31 patients had 41 samples that tested positive by SepsiTest but negative by culture. Samples from 13 patients had organisms whose presence could not be attributed to probable infection or probable contamination, so it is unclear if these isolates represented infections or contamination. Of the 13 patients, 8 had received prior antibiotic treatment, making detection of nonviable bacteria possible. Another German study of infectious endocarditis found SepsiTest to be 85% sensitive.[75]

The strength of the SepsiTest is its ability to identify nearly any bacteria or fungi from blood culture. However, this assay requires a high degree of both hands-on time and technical expertise. DNA extraction, detection of PCR products, and sequence analysis are all performed manually, which is unrealistic for routine use in most clinical laboratories. Based on the workflow requirements, the clinical laboratory may have organism identification complete using conventional methods in a time frame comparable to the molecular assay.

FDA approval

At present, 2 DNA-based assays are FDA-approved for pathogen detection directly from positive blood culture bottles: the BD GeneOhm, StaphSR Assay and Verigene BC-GP test. The FilmArray BCID panel is undergoing clinical trials, and the company plans to submit data for FDA approval in 2013. Light Cycler SeptiFast, Prove-it Sepsis, Hyplex BloodScreen PCR-ELISA, and SepsiTest assays are not available in the United States. A summary of the nucleic acid methods for detection of pathogens from blood culture is presented in **Table 5**.

NON-PCR–BASED METHODS
"Traditional" Phenotypic Methods

For many years, clinical laboratories have sought techniques and methodologies to expedite identification of microorganisms in blood culture specimens. Many of these techniques are technically demanding and costly, and other approaches have included the application of traditional biochemical tests to positive blood culture broths. One example of this is the direct tube coagulase test. This test is a modification of the traditional coagulase test for identification of S. aureus and provides results in 2 hours. Sensitivities of 79.5% to 96% and specificities of 100% have been reported,[76–81] although one study reported a low 34% sensitivity with 65% specificity at 4 hours.[82] The accuracy of this test may vary depending on the operator performing and interpreting the test, and in addition, anticoagulants have been reported to interfere with the test, leading to false-negative results.[83] The anticoagulant effect may be reduced if the blood is diluted 1:10 before performing the test.[83] Due to the variability in the performance of this approach, this testing method has not been widely adopted by clinical laboratories.

Table 5

Summary of nucleic acid amplification–based methods for microorganism identification and antimicrobial resistance directly from positive blood culture broth

Assay	Methodology	Organisms Detected	Resistance Genes Detected	Ease of Use	Turnaround Time	FDA Cleared	Comments
Xpert MRSA/SA BC	PCR	Staphylococcus aureus	mecA (MRSA vs MSSA)	Easy	1 h	No	
Staph ID/R	Isothermal, helicase-dependent amplification	S. aureus	mecA (MRSA vs MSSA)	Easy	75 min	No	
GeneOhm StaphSR	PCR	S. aureus	mecA	Complex	2 h	Yes	
FilmArray	Multiplex PCR	27 bacterial and fungal pathogens	mecA, vanB, bla$_{KPC}$	Easy	~1 h	No	
Verigene BP-GP	Hybridization array	Gram-positive cocci and Listeria	mecA, vanA, vanB	Moderate	<3 h	Yes	
Verigene BP-GN	Hybridization array	Gram-negative pathogens	bla$_{KPC}$, bla$_{NDM}$, bla$_{CTX-M}$, bla$_{VIM}$, bla$_{IMP}$, bla$_{OXA}$	Moderate	<3 h	No	Under development, research use only
PCR-ESI MS	PCR/mass spectrometry	Numerous	mecA, vanA/B, bla$_{KPC}$	Complex	6–8 h	No	
Pyrosequencing	Sequencing	Numerous	None (potentially numerous)	Complex	4 h	No	
Light Cycler SeptiFast Test M^{GRADE}	PCR/melting curve analysis	25 bacterial and fungal pathogens	mecA	Complex	6 h	No	Blood directly from patients, not blood bottles with positive results; Not available in the United States
Prove-it Sepsis	Multiplex PCR/microarray hybridization	>50 bacterial and fungal pathogens	mecA	Moderate	3.5 h	No	Not available in the United States
Cepheid Hyplex	Multiplex PCR/ELISA	10 bacterial pathogens	mecA	Moderate	4.5–6 h	No	Not available in the United States
SepsiTest	16S rRNA PCR/sequencing	>350 bacterial and fungal pathogens	None	Complex	8 h	No	Not available in the United States

The thermostable DNase test can also be used for the rapid identification of *S. aureus*. The modification is performed using agar diffusion, whereby boiled blood culture broth is added to wells created in toluidine blue DNase media. Studies have reported sensitivities of 85% to 100% and specificities of 93% to 100%.[80,84–88] Results are available in 2 hours, although they are often positive at 1 hour.[84,85]

The direct bile solubility test is also a modification of a traditional test for the identification of *Streptococcus pneumoniae*. One drop of blood culture broth is mixed with one drop of 2% deoxycholate or water, allowed to air dry, Gram stained, and the number of organisms in each spot quantified. Lysis of 100% of the organisms indicates *S. pneumoniae*. The assay has a reported sensitivity of 100% and specificity of 98.9%.[89] Alternatively, the test can be performed in a tube; blood culture broth is mixed with either saline or deoxycholate, and after incubation, the tubes are observed for the absence or presence of turbidity. Clearing of the tube with deoxycholate is consistent with organism lysis and identification of *S. pneumoniae*.

Streptococcal antigen testing has also been used for the identification of β-hemolytic streptococci directly on blood culture broth. In both the studies evaluating this approach, *S. pneumoniae* was found to cross-react with the group C antigen, necessitating a direct bile solubility test on isolates positive for the group C antigen. When the agglutination test was combined with direct solubility testing in one study,[90] this method achieved a sensitivity of 95.2% and a 100% specificity for pure cultures, whereas a second study reported 97% sensitivity and 98% specificity.[91] The sensitivity decreased to 83% for polymicrobial cultures.[90]

Adaptations of conventional biochemical and/or agglutination methods to positive-testing blood culture broth are inexpensive and easy to perform. However, because these methods are limited to the identification of a small subset of organisms and in many cases have suboptimal performance characteristics, they are not widely used in clinical laboratories.

Direct Identification of Pathogens in Blood Culture Broth Using Automated Systems

As the VITEK 2 (bioMérieux) and Phoenix (BD) automated identification systems have become more widely used, many groups have begun to evaluate them for their use in identification directly from positive blood cultures, although this assay modification is not FDA approved. In general, this approach is not widely used across clinical laboratories, especially in the era where nucleic acid–based tests are often available for identification of *S. aureus* and methicillin resistance.

Most studies evaluating direct inoculation of identification panels with positive blood culture broth require a primary preparatory step before inoculating the blood culture broth into the panel. Although variation exists in the preparatory methods, those most commonly used include centrifugation of the sample and/or the use of serum separator tubes. Three studies included an incubation step with a detergent, saponin, before addition of the blood culture broth to serum separator tubes, which seemed to increase the accuracy of identification.[92–94] Most of the studies evaluating this approach used the BACTEC blood culture media, whereas a small subset of studies evaluated BacT/ALERT blood culture broth.

Both automated identification systems evaluated in these studies demonstrated higher accuracy for identification of Gram-negative bacteria compared with Gram-positive bacteria, and antimicrobial susceptibility categorical agreement was typically in the 90th percentile. Concordance for the VITEK 2 with standard methods ranged from 62% to 100% for Gram-negative rods and 0% to 89% for Gram-positive bacteria.[92,94–99] Antimicrobial susceptibility testing categorical agreement ranged from 69% to 99.2%, with most between 95% and 99.2%.[92,94,95,98,100] Agreement with standard procedures for studies using the Phoenix ranged from 91.8% to 97% for Gram-negative rods and 43.8% to 89.1% for Gram-positive isolates. Antimicrobial susceptibility testing categorical agreement ranged from 77% to 99.5%, with most between 92.7% and 99.5%.[93,98,101–103] An extensive range of identification cards and antimicrobial susceptibility testing panels were used in the studies; it is probable that the card variation and differing preparatory methods contribute to the wide ranges of agreement.

Oxacillin and meropenem are often used as indicators of acquired drug resistance; the 2 antimicrobials tested well using the automated system approach. Oxacillin agreement in Gram-positive cocci ranged from 93.6% to 100%.[93,94,98,101,102] Major error rates of 1% and 3.6% were reported in 2 of the 5 studies, with no major errors observed.[94,102] For Gram-negative rods, meropenem agreement was 98% to 100%.[94,95,98,99,102,103] The percent agreement was lower in a study limited to nonfermenters, which demonstrated 91.3% agreement.[101] A single major error (1%) was reported in one study, and no major errors were observed.[94]

Direct identification of isolates in positive blood cultures by automated systems may be an attractive option for laboratories that already use the VITEK 2 or Phoenix systems, as no additional equipment is needed, but the reported results are variable.

Identification of Pathogens and/or Antimicrobial Resistance Using Chromogenic Agar

Chromogenic agar (**Fig. 3**) has been used to identify MRSA and *Candida* species directly from positive blood cultures. Agars used to detect MRSA contain selective agents, such as cefoxitin, to select for MRSA isolates, and the color of recovered MRSA varies depending on the brand of chromogenic agar used. Several different chromogenic MRSA media are commercially available, although most are FDA approved only for screening cultures from the nares. Most of these media are evaluated at 24 hours of incubation, although prolonged incubation at 48 hours may enhance sensitivity. Several different studies have evaluated an adaptation of these media whereby positive blood cultures are plated directly for expedited detection of MRSA strains. In these studies, blood cultures were plated to MRSA chromogenic agar when Gram-positive cocci or Gram-positive cocci in clusters were seen on Gram stain except for one study evaluating MRSA ID (now chromID MRSA, bioMérieux), where all positive blood cultures were plated to MRSA agar.[104] Sensitivities and specificities ranged from 96% to 100% and 98.5% to 100%, respectively; results are summarized in **Table 6**.

Candida chromogenic agar plates also contain selective agents, such as chloramphenicol, to inhibit bacteria and can recover virtually all species of *Candida,* although only a subset are specifically identified by their color and colony characteristics. Two types of media, CHROMagar Candida (CHROMagar, Paris, France) and Chromogenic Candida Agar (CCA) (now Brilliance Candida Agar, Oxoid, Basingstoke, UK) have been studied in the diagnosis of positive blood cultures.

CHROMagar Candida readily distinguishes *Candida albicans*, *Candida krusei*, and *Candida tropicalis*. Two studies using CHROMagar Candida reported sensitivities of 100% for the 3 species.[105,106] Tan and Peterson[106] analyzed 51 samples (41 *C. albicans*, 9 *C. tropicalis*, and 1 *C. krusei*) from BACTEC Plus and BACTEC Lytic/10 bottles, whereas Murray and colleagues[105] evaluated 137 samples (species breakdown not available) directly from patient blood specimens.

A third study evaluated CCA. There was an agreement of 88% for CCA and routine media, although this included all species of *Candida*, not just those readily identified by color.[107] The study included 42 *Candida* isolates from BACTEC Plus bottles, including 21 *C. albicans*, 4 *C. tropicalis*, and 3 *C. krusei*.

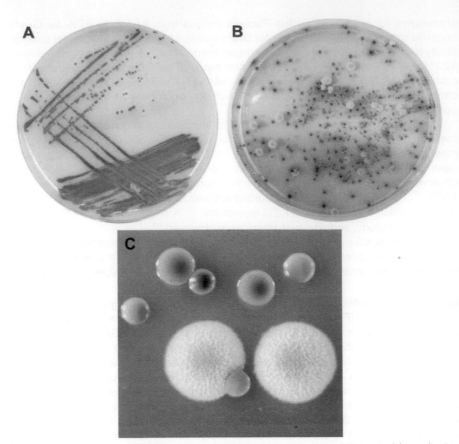

Fig. 3. Spectra MRSA and CHROMagar Candida chromogenic agars. (*A*) Denim blue colonies on Spectra MRSA agar indicate MRSA. (*B, C*) CHROMagar Candida differentiates 3 species based on colony characteristics: *Candida albicans* (green), *Candida tropicalis* (metallic blue) and *Candida krusei* (pink with a rhizoid edge). (*Courtesy of* Remel, Lenexa, KS; with permission and CHROMagar, Paris; with permission.)

To evaluate a method of rapid detection of fluconazole-resistant isolates, one study placed a 25-µg fluconazole disk in the primary inoculum when the positive-testing blood culture broth was applied to CHROMagar Candida.[106] This study evaluated 95 cultures with positive results, with a species breakdown of 41 *C. albicans*, 23 *Candida glabrata*, 20 *Candida parapsilosis*, 9 *C. tropicalis*, 1 *C. krusei*, and 1 *Candida lusitaniae*. Of these, 8 were fluconazole resistant. An 86% agreement was found between this rapid method and the gold standard of minimum inhibitory concentration (MIC) in Mueller-Hinton supplemented with glucose and methylene blue. There were 2 major errors at 24 hours; 2 isolates, one *C. glabrata* and one *C. parapsilosis*, were reported as susceptible but found to be resistant by standard methods. However, these major errors were resolved at 48 hours.

Chromogenic agar is inexpensive and requires no special equipment or training. However, the main drawback is that results are not available until after overnight incubation, in contrast to many of the other "rapid" methods, which provide results in minutes to hours.

Table 6
Summary of the studies evaluating MRSA chromogenic media on positive blood cultures

Media	Manufacturer	Blood Culture Systems Evaluated	n	Sensitivity (24 h) (%)	Specificity (24 h) (%)	Sensitivity (48 h) (%)	Specificity (48 h) (%)	References
CHROMagar MRSA	CHROMagar	BacT/ALERT BACTEC	263, 882	96–97.6	99.9–100	ND	ND	146,147
CHROMagar MRSA II	BD	BacT/ALERT BACTEC VersaTREK	688	100	100	ND	ND	148
MRSA ID	bioMerieux	BACTEC	837	97.8	99.7	100	99.6	104
MRSASelect	Bio-Rad	BacT/ALERT VersaTREK	652	99	99	99	99	149
Spectra MRSA	Remel	BacT/ALERT BACTEC VersaTREK	629	96	99.4	99.4	98.5	150

Abbreviation: ND, not done.

BinaxNOW Staphylococcus aureus and PBP2a

The BinaxNOW *Staphylococcus aureus* assay (Alere, Waltham, MA, USA) is an FDA-cleared immunochromatographic lateral flow method for use on positive blood culture broth in which the Gram stain demonstrates Gram-positive cocci in clusters. Binax-NOW *S. aureus* uses a polyclonal antibody to capture a proprietary *S. aureus*–specific protein and results can be obtained in as little as 30 minutes. The manufacturer reports a sensitivity of 93.3% and a specificity of 99.6%.[108] The test is approved for all auto-mated blood culture systems but was validated using the BacT/ALERT standard aerobic and anaerobic bottles.

BinaxNOW PBP2a (Alere) is also an FDA-approved immunochromatographic lateral flow assay that uses monoclonal antibodies to detect PBP2a. It is approved for use only on positive blood culture broths that have been first identified as *S. aureus*, either by the BinaxNOW *S. aureus* or an equivalent assay, and has currently not yet been released. One study reported a sensitivity of 95.24% and a specificity of 100%.[109]

The major advantage of the BinaxNOW assays is that no additional instrumentation or technical expertise is required, and the assay is inexpensive, making it accessible for almost any size laboratory to implement. A drawback is that the performance characteristics of this assay in co-infections have not been well established.[108]

Keypath MRSA/MSSA Blood Culture Assay

The Keypath MRSA/MSSA Blood Culture Test (MicroPhage, Longmont, CO, USA) uses bacteriophage amplification to detect the presence of *S. aureus* and the *mecA* gene. Bacteriophage are viruses that infect bacteria by attaching and injecting their nucleic acid. The phage replicate inside the bacteria, which eventually results in lysis and release of large amounts of phage. The assay indirectly detects *S. aureus* and *mecA* through detection of biologically amplified phage proteins in an immunoassay (**Fig. 4**). The MRSA/MSSA assay was FDA approved in 2011 for BACTEC Plus blood culture media, and clinical trials for the BacT/ALERT system are currently underway.[110]

To perform the assay, blood is added to 2 tubes containing *S. aureus*–specific phage. In the first tube, if *S. aureus* is present, the phage attaches to the cells and replicates rapidly. The second tube tests for MRSA by using a cefoxitin screen. A set amount of cefoxitin is included in the tube with the *S. aureus*–specific phage. If the isolate is susceptible, there is no growth and therefore no phage amplification. If the isolate is resistant, growth occurs and subsequent phage replication takes place. After 5 minutes of hands-on time to set up the assay, the tubes are incubated for 5 hours, and subsequently, detection occurs via a lateral flow immunoassay in 20 to 30 minutes. Two independent studies reported sensitivities of 91.8% and 90.1% for detection of *S. aureus* from BACTEC and BacT/ALERT blood culture broths with specificities of 98.3% and 100%.[111,112] For detection of MSSA and MRSA specifically, the sensitivities were 82% to 88% and 84% to 93%, respectively, and specificities were 98% to 99% and 99%, respectively. A study by the manufacturer further demonstrated that the assay correctly identified 46/48 isolates with partial, nonfunctional SCCmec elements (also known as *mecA* dropout strains) as MSSA, whereas the isolates were identified as MRSA by GeneOhm MRSA (BD) and Xpert MRSA (Cepheid) PCR assay.[113]

Time to detection for this assay is longer at 5.5 hours than most other assays, but only 5 minutes of hands-on time is required. The assay is simple to perform, requiring minimal training and no special supplies.

Peptide Nucleic Acid Fluorescent In Situ Hybridization

The FDA-approved peptide nucleic acid fluorescent in situ hybridization assay (PNA FISH; AdvanDx, Woburn, MA, USA) uses PNA probes for identification of bacteria

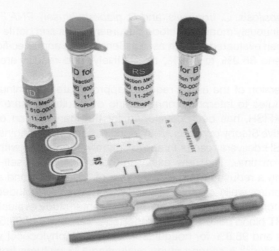

Fig. 4. Keypath MRSA/MSSA assay. Blood culture broth is added to tubes containing phage and incubated for 5 hours to allow phage amplification. The reaction is subsequently transferred to the corresponding color-coded window on the lateral flow immunoassay cartridge. The ID side detects *S. aureus*, whereas the RS side detects cefoxitin resistance. (*Courtesy of* MicroPhage, Longmont, CO; with permission.)

and *Candida* species directly in positive blood culture broth. PNA probes are composed of DNA in which the phosphate backbone has been replaced by a noncharged peptide backbone; this results in rapid binding to the target as the probes do not have to overcome electrostatic repulsion.[114,115] The PNA probes hybridize to target rRNA when present in the sample, with detection of a fluorescent signal in 90 minutes (**Fig. 5**). A variety of PNA FISH assays are available to differentiate *S. aureus*/coagulase-negative staphylococci, *Enterococcus faecalis*/other enterococci, *E. coli/Klebsiella pneumoniae/Pseudomonas aeruginosa*, and *Candida* species

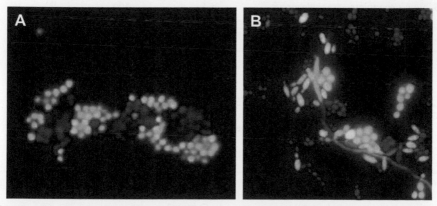

Fig. 5. PNA FISH assays. (*A*) *Staphylococcus aureus*/coagulase-negative staphylococci. *S. aureus* appears green, whereas red indicates coagulase-negative staphylococci. (*B*) Yeast Traffic Light assay demonstrating *Candida albicans/Candida parapsilosis* in green, *Candida tropicalis* in yellow, and *Candida glabrata/Candida krusei* in red. (*Courtesy of* AdvanDx, Woburn, MA; with permission.)

(*C. albicans/parapsilosis*, *C. tropicalis*, and *C. glabrata/krusei*). PNA FISH is approved for all major continuously monitored blood culture systems and bottle types, but not all systems have been evaluated in each assay. Sensitivities and specificities range from 94% to 100% and 86.9% to 100%, respectively, and results are summarized in **Table 7**.

The original version of the assay required approximately 10 minutes of hands-on time and 90 minutes to interpretation/reporting of results. A more rapid version of the assay, *Quick*FISH, has been developed for the identification of *S. aureus* and coagulase-negative *Staphylococcus*. With modifications of the original 90-minute procedure, *Quick*FISH delivers results in approximately 30 minutes with less than 5 minutes of hands-on time. The new assay introduces a novel self-reporting probe design, facilitating a reduced hybridization time of 15 minutes and does not require a wash step. Control wells containing fixed organisms are included on each slide, and therefore batching is not a necessity. A multicenter study evaluating 722 cultures from BacT/ALERT blood culture bottles reported a sensitivity of 99.5% for identification of *S. aureus* and 98.8% for coagulase-negative staphylococci with a combined specificity of 89.5%.[116] A second study evaluating 173 cultures from BACTEC Plus bottles demonstrated that for detection of *S. aureus*, the sensitivity and specificity were both 100%, and for coagulase-negative staphylococci, the sensitivity and specificity were 98.5% and 100%.[76]

The rapid turnaround time of this assay is highly attractive. Multiple studies have evaluated the impact and economic benefit of PNA FISH compared with standard culture practices and found that incorporation of the assay into clinical practice resulted in reduced mortality rates, length of hospital stay, time on antimicrobials, and time to sterilization of blood cultures.[117–121] The main drawback to PNA FISH is that a fluorescent microscope with a special AdvanDx filter is required to analyze the slides, and laboratory staff must be trained in interpretation of fluorescence microscopy. Thus,

Table 7
Sensitivities and specificities of PNA FISH assays on positive blood culture broths

Assay	Species Detected	Sensitivity (%)	Specificity (%)	References
S. aureus/coagulase-negative staphylococci	*Staphylococcus aureus* (green)	96.5	100	151
	Coagulase-negative staphylococci (red)	96.6	96.8	
Enterococcus faecalis/other enterococci	*Enterococcus faecalis* (green)	100	100	152
	Enterococcus faecium, other enterococci (red)			
Gram-negative rod Traffic Light	*Escherichia coli* (green)	100	98.2 (combined)	153
	Klebsiella pneumoniae (yellow)	99.1		
	Pseudomonas aeruginosa (red)	95.8		
Yeast Traffic Light	*Candida albicans* & *Candida parapsilosis* (green)	100 (*C. albicans*, *C. glabrata*, *C. krusei*)	86.9 (combined)	154
	Candida tropicalis (yellow)	94 (*C. parapsilosis*, *C. tropicalis*)		
	Candida glabrata & *Candida krusei* (red)			

this method may not be feasible to adopt in small laboratories. In addition, *Quick*FISH cannot be used with bottles containing charcoal or VersaTREK Redox2 anaerobic bottles.

BACcel

The BACcel system (Accelr8, Denver, CO, USA) is currently under development and uses microscopic analysis of single cells for bacterial identification and antimicrobial susceptibility testing. In the prototypic assays under development, the time to organism identification is approximately 2 hours, with a resistance profile generated in approximately 4 to 6 hours. An initial sample cleanup is required, and the sample is placed in a 32-flowcell cassette and subsequently exposed to multiple test conditions. Time lapse images are analyzed to provide identification and antibiotic susceptibilities. A pilot study of 33 simulated blood samples, containing *S. aureus* at a concentration of approximately 5 CFU/mL, revealed a sensitivity and specificity of 100% compared with nonspiked samples.[122] Detection of resistance to cefoxitin and clinidamycin (*n* = 10) demonstrated sensitivities of 80% and 100%, respectively, and specificities of 100%.

Matrix-Assisted Laser Desorption Ionization Time-of-Flight Mass Spectrometry

Matrix-assisted laser desorption ionization time-of-flight (MALDI-TOF) MS is becoming a popular method to identify pathogens. MALDI-TOF MS uses proteomic profiling to assign identification. The MALDI BioTyper system (Bruker-Daltonics, Bremen, Germany) and the VITEK MS are the commercially available MALDI-TOF MS instrumentation/database platforms for microorganism identification. Most studies evaluating MALDI-TOF MS have focused on identification of organisms growing on solid media; other studies have evaluated MALDI-TOF MS analysis on positive-testing blood culture broth. For use on blood culture broth, an initial extraction is required to eliminate interfering substances, including blood and broth. Correct identification rates vary, based on which extraction method is used but seem most optimized with the use of a commercially available Sepsityper kit (Bruker-Daltonics) or saponin.[123–127] Most studies have evaluated the Bruker Biotyper for this analysis.

MALDI-TOF MS has been shown to be more effective at identifying Gram-negative organisms compared with Gram-positive organisms in positive blood culture broth. For Gram-negative bacteria, the percentage of correctly identified organisms ranges from 68% to 99%, with most studies reporting rates from 90% to 99%.[123,126,128–132] For Gram-positive bacteria, the rate varies from 37% to 89%, with most studies reporting identification rates of 60% to 70%.[123,126,128–130] Studies have demonstrated a specific problem with identifying streptococci (this was also observed with direct colony testing and is not exclusive to blood culture broth). In particular, the Bruker system commonly identifies *S. mitis* as *S. pneumoniae*, and it has been suggested that users should perform a bile solubility test on all isolates identified as *S. pneumoniae* to determine the correct identification.[128,133] For the identification of *Candida* species, one study showed concordance rates of 95.9% for *C. albicans* and 86.5% for non-*albicans* species.[134]

A study with the VITEK MS analyzed all positive blood cultures and was able to identify 73% of positive cultures to species level (including instances were one organism in a polymicrobial infection was identified).[135] This article reported a novel lysis-filtration sample preparation method.

In a study comparing the 3 most common types of blood culture systems, BACTEC (aerobic and anaerobic bottles; *n* = 956), BacT/ALERT (standard aerobic (SA), standard anaerobic (SN), and pediatric FAN (PF) bottles; *n* = 2226), and VersaTREK

(Redox1 and Redox2 bottles; $n = 269$), no significant difference was seen in the percentage of correct identifications.[130] However, in a separate study comparing BACTEC (Plus Aerobic bottles; $n = 103$) and BacT/ALERT (SA and FAN aerobic (FA) bottles; $n = 103$), the researchers found that correct identification was achieved more frequently when using the BACTEC system.[136] A study comparing 2 MS approaches, MALDI-TOF MS and PCR-ESI MS, evaluated PCR-ESI MS specimens directly from blood culture broth, whereas isolates were subcultured before performing MALDI-TOF MS.[137] Thus, a follow-up study analyzing the use of both methods directly on blood cultures is needed to more accurately compare the two.

MALDI-TOF MS is capable of identifying numerous bacteria and yeasts, and time to identification directly from positive blood culture broth ranges from 30 minutes to 2 hours, depending on the method used. One drawback is that MALDI-TOF cannot accurately identify multiple species in polymicrobial blood culture, although it frequently identifies the predominant organism from mixed cultures.[128,129,133,138] In addition, the initial purchase of the instrumentation is a significant expense, and training of laboratory personnel on MALDI-TOF MS operation and sample preparation is required. However, once the instrument is purchased, the ongoing consumable costs are minimal. Neither of the commercially available systems is cleared by the FDA, so laboratories must perform extensive validation studies before implementation of this method, which may be an additional barrier to adoption of this technique by many laboratories at this point in time. A summary of MALDI-TOF MS and the other non-PCR methods is presented in **Table 8**.

CLINICAL IMPACT OF RAPID TECHNIQUES FOR PATHOGEN AND ANTIMICROBIAL RESISTANCE DETECTION IN POSITIVE BLOOD CULTURES

Most the methods described herein for expedited identification of organisms and/or antimicrobial resistance from positive blood cultures have analytical performance characteristics (such as sensitivity, specificity, and turnaround time) that are favorable. However, many of these tests are expensive, so the broad question is, does the information garnered from this analysis translate into improved patient outcomes, such as a reduction in morbidity or morality, a decrease in use of toxic therapy, or a reduction in patient length of stay or health care costs? For many of these technologies, that is still an unresolved question.[139] One reason for this is that it is difficult to study this question accurately. However, for some of the assays, studies to evaluate clinical significance/impact have been conducted.

Candida species are a common cause of health care–associated bloodstream infections.[16] Studies have demonstrated that the incorporation of PNA FISH for identification of *C. albicans/parapsilosis*, *C. tropicalis*, and *C. glabrata/krusei* does result in improved turnaround time for patients to receive targeted treatment and is cost-effective.[117,140] In a study by Heil and colleagues,[119] the impact of PNA FISH for *Candida* in the context of an antimicrobial stewardship program was evaluated. These investigators found that post-PNA FISH implementation, time to targeted therapy was significantly reduced, there was a significant improvement in culture clearance, and even when the cost of the testing was factored in, there was an overall cost savings with implementation of this technology.

Bauer and colleagues[141] evaluated the clinical and economic impact of the GeneXpert MRSA/SA blood culture assay in a single medical center. The findings were striking—post assay implementation, the mean length of stay for patients with *S. aureus* bacteremia was reduced by 6.2 days, the mean reduction in hospital costs was $21,387, and the time to optimization of therapy for MSSA was

Table 8
Summary of non-PCR–based methods for microorganism identification and antimicrobial resistance directly from positive blood culture broth

Assay	Methodology	Organisms Detected	Resistance Genes Detected	Ease of Use	Turnaround Time	Accuracy (%)	References
Tube coagulase	Biochemical	Staphylococcus aureus	None	Easy	2–4 h	34–96	76–82
Bile solubility	Biochemical	Streptococcus pneumoniae	None	Easy	30 min	100	89
DNase test	Colorimetric	S. aureus	None	Easy	2–4 h	85–100	80,84–88
Streptococcal antigen test	Latex agglutination	β-Hemolytic streptococci	None	Easy	30 min	95–97	90,91
Automated systems (VITEK 2/Phoenix)	Biochemical	Numerous	None (but AST can be performed)	Moderate	3–5 h (ID) 13–19 h (AST)	Variable	92–103
Chromogenic agar	Growth/color	MRSA Candida spp	mecA	Easy	24 h	88–100	104–107,146–150
BinaxNOW S. aureus	Immunoassay	S. aureus	None	Easy	30 min	93	108
BinaxNOW PBP2a	Immunoassay	S. aureus	mecA	Easy	30 min	95	109
Keypath MRSA/MSSA	Bacteriophage amplification	S. aureus	mecA	Easy	5.5 h	82–93	111,112
PNA FISH/QuickFISH	Hybridization	S. aureus/coagulase-negative staphylococci Enterococcus spp Candida spp Escherichia coli/ Klebsiella pneumoniae/ Pseudomonas aeruginosa	None	Moderate	30–90 min	98–100	76,116,151–154
BACcel	Microscopy	Unknown, potentially numerous	mecA bla_{KPC}	Unknown	4–6 h	Unknown	
MALDI-TOF	Mass spectrometry	Numerous	None	Moderate	30 min–2 h	37–99	123,126,128–132,134,135

Abbreviations: AST, antimicrobial susceptibility testing; ID, identification.

reduced by 1.6 days. However, these outcomes were in the context of an antimicrobial stewardship program, whereby an infectious disease pharmacist was contacted directly about the PCR results, who provided follow-up consultation. A subsequent study evaluating the GeneXpert MRSA/SA assay found that using the assay reduced unnecessary antimicrobial therapy by halting the use of antistaphylococcal therapy in patients without *S. aureus* bacteremia and also greatly improved time to initiation of appropriate therapy for those patients with MSSA.[142] It has been demonstrated that appropriate antibiotic therapy influences the outcome in patients with *S. aureus* bacteremia.[143,144]

Another study evaluating the clinical impact or a real-time PCR assay for *S. aureus* and methicillin resistance detection from positive blood cultures is less compelling[145]; however, this study was conducted in France, where the prevalence of MRSA is much less than what is typically observed in the United States. The study evaluated 250 instances of bacteremia with Gram-positive cocci in clusters during a 12 month period and compared standard phenotypic methods for organism identification and susceptibility testing to a rapid, real-time PCR assay for identification of *S. aureus* and methicillin resistance. This study found that although the assay was accurate, no difference in clinical outcome was observed postimplementation. The rate of clinical cure and absence of relapse was similar in both groups. In addition to a lower MRSA prevalence (24% of *S. aureus* were methicillin resistant in this study), another difference in this study is that the testing was not performed in conjunction with a specific antimicrobial stewardship program.[145]

The major theme that emerges from the studies is that if these assays are performed but passively reported, the results are less likely to have a major impact on patient care. However, if the results are actively reported, especially in conjunction with an antimicrobial stewardship program, they have the potential to improve patient outcomes and reduce health care costs. Although this might be limited to a small subset of pathogens/resistance mechanisms at present, detection of *S. aureus* and methicillin resistance accounts for a large proportion of clinically actionable results at many medical centers. As these testing methods have expanded menus and become more readily available, it is possible that the impact and cost-benefit ratio of rapid diagnostics for blood cultures will become more completely understood.

SUMMARY

The detection of blood stream infections is often considered one of the most important functions of the clinical microbiology laboratory. Sepsis is a clinical emergency, and mortality increases if commencement of appropriate antimicrobial therapy is delayed. To date, automated blood culture systems are the most sensitive approach for detection of the causative agent of sepsis. Using conventional techniques, once an automated blood culture system signals positive, the blood culture broth is Gram stained and subcultured to solid media. Once isolated colonies are growing, organism identification and susceptibility testing will proceed. In this review, we have described a number of laboratory methods that have been developed to expedite identification of organisms directly from positive blood culture broth.

REFERENCES

1. Dellinger RP, Levy MM, Carlet JM, et al. Surviving Sepsis Campaign: international guidelines for management of severe sepsis and septic shock. Intensive Care Med 2008;34(1):17–60.

2. Weinstein MP, Murphy JR, Reller LB, et al. The clinical significance of positive blood cultures: a comprehensive analysis of 500 episodes of bacteremia and fungemia in adults. II. Clinical observations, with special reference to factors influencing prognosis. Rev Infect Dis 1983;5(1):54–70.

3. Weinstein MP, Doern GV. A critical appraisal of the role of the clinical microbiology laboratory in the diagnosis of bloodstream infections. J Clin Microbiol 2011;49(9S):S26–9.

4. Beekmann SE, Diekema DJ, Chapin KC, et al. Effects of rapid detection of bloodstream infections on length of hospitalization and hospital charges. J Clin Microbiol 2003;41(7):3119–25.

5. Washington JA 2nd. Blood cultures: principles and techniques. Mayo Clin Proc 1975;50(2):91–8.

6. Brown DR, Kutler D, Rai B, et al. Bacterial concentration and blood volume required for a positive blood culture. J Perinatol 1995;15(2):157–9.

7. Connell TG, Rele M, Cowley D, et al. How reliable is a negative blood culture result? Volume of blood submitted for culture in routine practice in a children's hospital. Pediatrics 2007;119(5):891–6.

8. Sarkar S, Bhagat I, DeCristofaro JD, et al. A study of the role of multiple site blood cultures in the evaluation of neonatal sepsis. J Perinatol 2006;26(1):18–22.

9. Schelonka RL, Chai MK, Yoder BA, et al. Volume of blood required to detect common neonatal pathogens. J Pediatr 1996;129(2):275–8.

10. Lin HH, Liu YF, Tien N, et al. Evaluation of the blood volume effect on the diagnosis of bacteremia in automated blood culture systems. J Microbiol Immunol Infect 2013;46(1):48–52.

11. Cockerill FR 3rd, Wilson JW, Vetter EA, et al. Optimal testing parameters for blood cultures. Clin Infect Dis 2004;38(12):1724–30.

12. Ziegler R, Johnscher I, Martus P, et al. Controlled clinical laboratory comparison of two supplemented aerobic and anaerobic media used in automated blood culture systems to detect bloodstream infections. J Clin Microbiol 1998;36(3): 657–61.

13. Lee A, Mirrett S, Reller LB, et al. Detection of bloodstream infections in adults: how many blood cultures are needed? J Clin Microbiol 2007;45(11): 3546–8.

14. Richter SS, Beekmann SE, Croco JL, et al. Minimizing the workup of blood culture contaminants: implementation and evaluation of a laboratory-based algorithm. J Clin Microbiol 2002;40(7):2437–44.

15. Weinstein MP. Blood culture contamination: persisting problems and partial progress. J Clin Microbiol 2003;41(6):2275–8.

16. Wisplinghoff H, Bischoff T, Tallent SM, et al. Nosocomial bloodstream infections in US hospitals: analysis of 24,179 cases from a prospective nationwide surveillance study. Clin Infect Dis 2004;39(3):309–17.

17. Munson EL, Diekema DJ, Beekmann SE, et al. Detection and treatment of bloodstream infection: laboratory reporting and antimicrobial management. J Clin Microbiol 2003;41(1):495–7.

18. Wolk DM, Dunne WM. New technologies in clinical microbiology. J Clin Microbiol 2011;49(9S):S62–7.

19. Parta M, Goebel M, Matloobi M, et al. Identification of methicillin-resistant or methicillin-susceptible Staphylococcus aureus in blood cultures and wound swabs by GeneXpert. J Clin Microbiol 2009;47(5):1609–10.

20. Wolk DM, Struelens MJ, Pancholi P, et al. Rapid detection of Staphylococcus aureus and methicillin-resistant S. aureus (MRSA) in wound specimens and

blood cultures: multicenter preclinical evaluation of the Cepheid Xpert MRSA/ SA skin and soft tissue and blood culture assays. J Clin Microbiol 2009;47(3): 823–6.

21. Spencer DH, Sellenriek P, Burnham CA. Validation and implementation of the GeneXpert MRSA/SA blood culture assay in a pediatric setting. Am J Clin Pathol 2011;136(5):690–4.

22. Kelley PG, Grabsch EA, Farrell J, et al. Evaluation of the Xpert MRSA/SA Blood Culture assay for the detection of Staphylococcus aureus including strains with reduced vancomycin susceptibility from blood culture specimens. Diagn Microbiol Infect Dis 2011;70(3):404–7.

23. FDA. Corrective action notice for Cepheid MRSA/SA blood culture assay. 2010. Available at: http://www.fda.gov/MedicalDevices/Safety/ListofRecalls/ucm218002. htm. Accessed December 31, 2012.

24. Vincent M, Xu Y, Kong H. Helicase-dependent isothermal DNA amplification. EMBO Rep 2004;5(8):795–800.

25. Pasko C, Hicke B, Dunn J, et al. Staph ID/R: a rapid method for determining Staphylococcus species identity and detecting the mecA gene directly from positive blood culture. J Clin Microbiol 2012;50(3):810–7.

26. BD. GeneOhm StaphSR Assay. 2012. Available at: http://www.bd.com/geneohm/ english/products/idi_staphsr.asp. Accessed December 31, 2012.

27. BD. BD MAX System. 2012. Available at: http://www.bd.com/geneohm/english/ products/max/. Accessed December 31, 2012.

28. Stamper PD, Cai M, Howard T, et al. Clinical validation of the molecular BD GeneOhm StaphSR assay for direct detection of Staphylococcus aureus and methicillin-resistant Staphylococcus aureus in positive blood cultures. J Clin Microbiol 2007;45(7):2191–6.

29. Grobner S, Dion M, Plante M, et al. Evaluation of the BD GeneOhm StaphSR assay for detection of methicillin-resistant and methicillin-susceptible Staphylococcus aureus isolates from spiked positive blood culture bottles. J Clin Microbiol 2009;47(6):1689–94.

30. Huletsky A, Giroux R, Rossbach V, et al. New real-time PCR assay for rapid detection of methicillin-resistant Staphylococcus aureus directly from specimens containing a mixture of staphylococci. J Clin Microbiol 2004;42(5):1875–84.

31. Oberdorfer K, Pohl S, Frey M, et al. Evaluation of a single-locus real-time polymerase chain reaction as a screening test for specific detection of methicillin-resistant Staphylococcus aureus in ICU patients. Eur J Clin Microbiol Infect Dis 2006;25(10):657–63.

32. Stamper PD, Louie L, Wong H, et al. Genotypic and phenotypic characterization of methicillin-susceptible Staphylococcus aureus isolates misidentified as methicillin-resistant Staphylococcus aureus by the BD GeneOhm MRSA assay. J Clin Microbiol 2011;49(4):1240–4.

33. Snyder JW, Munier GK, Heckman SA, et al. Failure of the BD GeneOhm StaphSR assay for direct detection of methicillin-resistant and methicillin-susceptible Staphylococcus aureus isolates in positive blood cultures collected in the United States. J Clin Microbiol 2009;47(11):3747–8.

34. Thomas L, van Hal S, O'Sullivan M, et al. Failure of the BD GeneOhm StaphS/R assay for identification of Australian methicillin-resistant Staphylococcus aureus strains: duplex assays as the "gold standard" in settings of unknown SCCmec epidemiology. J Clin Microbiol 2008;46(12):4116–7.

35. Bartels MD, Boye K, Rohde SM, et al. A common variant of staphylococcal cassette chromosome mec type IVa in isolates from Copenhagen, Denmark,

is not detected by the BD GeneOhm methicillin-resistant *Staphylococcus aureus* assay. J Clin Microbiol 2009;47(5):1524–7.

36. Boyle-Vavra S, Daum RS. Reliability of the BD GeneOhm methicillin-resistant *Staphylococcus aureus* (MRSA) assay in detecting MRSA isolates with a variety of genotypes from the United States and Taiwan. J Clin Microbiol 2010;48(12): 4546–51.

37. Nanosphere. Gold Nanoparticle Technology. 2012. Available at: http://www.nanosphere.us/page/gold-nanoparticle-technology. Accessed December 31, 2012.

38. Buchan BW, Peterson JF, Cogbill CH, et al. Evaluation of a microarray-based genotyping assay for the rapid detection of cytochrome P450 2C19 *2 and *3 polymorphisms from whole blood using nanoparticle probes. Am J Clin Pathol 2011;136(4):604–8.

39. Tormo N, Medina R, Ocete MD, et al. Performance of the Nanosphere's Verigene BC-GP test for rapid detection of Gram-positive bacteria and resistance determinants directly from positive blood cultures (poster). London (UK): ECCMID; 2012.

40. Nanosphere. Gram-negative blood culture. 2012. Available at: http://www.nanosphere.us/product/gram-negative-blood-culture. Accessed December 31, 2012.

41. Anderson C, Kaul K, Voss B, et al. Evaluation of the Verigene Gram-Positive Blood Culture Test (BC-GP) (poster). San Francisco (CA): ASM; 2012.

42. Buchan BW, Mackey TL, Cahak C, et al. Rapid detection of Gram-positive bacteria and resistance determinants directly from positive blood cultures using the microarray-based sample-to-result Verigene BC-GP assay (poster). London (UK): ECCMID; 2012.

43. BioFire. FilmArray Blood Culture ID Panel. 2012. Available at: http://www.biofiredx.com/FilmArray/FutureApplications.html. Accessed December 31, 2012.

44. Blaschke AJ, Heyrend C, Byington CL, et al. Rapid identification of pathogens from positive blood cultures by multiplex polymerase chain reaction using the FilmArray system. Diagn Microbiol Infect Dis 2012;74(4):349–55.

45. Jordan JA, Butchko AR, Durso MB. Use of pyrosequencing of 16S rRNA fragments to differentiate between bacteria responsible for neonatal sepsis. J Mol Diagn 2005;7(1):105–10.

46. Haanpera M, Jalava J, Huovinen P, et al. Identification of alpha-hemolytic streptococci by pyrosequencing the 16S rRNA gene and by use of VITEK 2. J Clin Microbiol 2007;45(3):762–70.

47. Motoshima M, Yanagihara K, Morinaga Y, et al. Identification of bacteria directly from positive blood culture samples by DNA pyrosequencing of the 16S rRNA gene. J Med Microbiol 2012;61(Pt 11):1556–62.

48. Innings A, Krabbe M, Ullberg M, et al. Identification of 43 *Streptococcus* species by pyrosequencing analysis of the rnpB gene. J Clin Microbiol 2005; 43(12):5983–91.

49. Jordan JA, Jones-Laughner J, Durso MB. Utility of pyrosequencing in identifying bacteria directly from positive blood culture bottles. J Clin Microbiol 2009;47(2): 368–72.

50. Quiles-Melero I, Garcia-Rodriguez J, Romero-Gomez MP, et al. Rapid identification of yeasts from positive blood culture bottles by pyrosequencing. Eur J Clin Microbiol Infect Dis 2011;30(1):21–4.

51. Kaleta EJ, Clark AE, Johnson DR, et al. Use of PCR coupled with electrospray ionization mass spectrometry for rapid identification of bacterial and yeast

bloodstream pathogens from blood culture bottles. J Clin Microbiol 2011;49(1): 345–53.

52. Jeng K, Gaydos CA, Blyn LB, et al. Comparative analysis of two broad-range PCR assays for pathogen detection in positive-blood-culture bottles: PCR-high-resolution melting analysis versus PCR-mass spectrometry. J Clin Microbiol 2012;50(10):3287–92.

53. Endimiani A, Hujer KM, Hujer AM, et al. Rapid identification of bla KPC-possessing Enterobacteriaceae by PCR/electrospray ionization-mass spectrometry. J Antimicrob Chemother 2010;65(8):1833–4.

54. Wolk DM, Blyn LB, Hall TA, et al. Pathogen profiling: rapid molecular characterization of Staphylococcus aureus by PCR/electrospray ionization-mass spectrometry and correlation with phenotype. J Clin Microbiol 2009;47(10):3129–37.

55. Hujer KM, Hujer AM, Endimiani A, et al. Rapid determination of quinolone resistance in Acinetobacter spp. J Clin Microbiol 2009;47(5):1436–42.

56. Roche. LightCycler SeptiFast MGRADE Test 2012. Available at: http://molecular. roche.com/assays/Pages/LightCyclerSeptiFastTestMGRADE.aspx. Accessed December 31, 2012.

57. Lehmann LE, Hunfeld KP, Emrich T, et al. A multiplex real-time PCR assay for rapid detection and differentiation of 25 bacterial and fungal pathogens from whole blood samples. Med Microbiol Immunol 2008;197(3):313–24.

58. Arpi M, Bentzon MW, Jensen J, et al. Importance of blood volume cultured in the detection of bacteremia. Eur J Clin Microbiol Infect Dis 1989;8(9):838–42.

59. Ilstrup DM, Washington JA 2nd. The importance of volume of blood cultured in the detection of bacteremia and fungemia. Diagn Microbiol Infect Dis 1983;1(2): 107–10.

60. Kreger BE, Craven DE, Carling PC, et al. Gram-negative bacteremia. III. Reassessment of etiology, epidemiology and ecology in 612 patients. Am J Med 1980;68(3):332–43.

61. Kellogg JA, Manzella JP, Bankert DA. Frequency of low-level bacteremia in children from birth to fifteen years of age. J Clin Microbiol 2000;38(6):2181–5.

62. Rath PM, Saner F, Paul A, et al. Multiplex PCR for rapid and improved diagnosis of bloodstream infections in liver transplant recipients. J Clin Microbiol 2012; 50(6):2069–71.

63. Josefson P, Stralin K, Ohlin A, et al. Evaluation of a commercial multiplex PCR test (SeptiFast) in the etiological diagnosis of community-onset bloodstream infections. Eur J Clin Microbiol Infect Dis 2011;30(9):1127–34.

64. Mencacci A, Leli C, Montagna P, et al. Diagnosis of infective endocarditis: comparison of the LightCycler SeptiFast real-time PCR with blood culture. J Med Microbiol 2012;61(Pt 6):881–3.

65. Lucignano B, Ranno S, Liesenfeld O, et al. Multiplex PCR allows rapid and accurate diagnosis of bloodstream infections in newborns and children with suspected sepsis. J Clin Microbiol 2011;49(6):2252–8.

66. Dubska L, Vyskocilova M, Minarikova D, et al. LightCycler SeptiFast technology in patients with solid malignancies: clinical utility for rapid etiologic diagnosis of sepsis. Crit Care 2012;16(1):404.

67. Mauro MV, Cavalcanti P, Perugini D, et al. Diagnostic utility of LightCycler SeptiFast and procalcitonin assays in the diagnosis of bloodstream infection in immunocompromised patients. Diagn Microbiol Infect Dis 2012;73(4):308–11.

68. Casalta JP, Gouriet F, Roux V, et al. Evaluation of the LightCycler SeptiFast test in the rapid etiologic diagnostic of infectious endocarditis. Eur J Clin Microbiol Infect Dis 2009;28(6):569–73.

69. Varani S, Stanzani M, Paolucci M, et al. Diagnosis of bloodstream infections in immunocompromised patients by real-time PCR. J Infect 2009;58(5):346–51.

70. Mobidiag. Prove-it Sepsis bacterial and fungal targets. 2012. Available at: http://www.mobidiag.com/Products/ProveittradeSepsis/ProveittradeSepsisStripArray/tabid/242/Default.aspx. Accessed December 31, 2012.

71. Tissari P, Zumla A, Tarkka E, et al. Accurate and rapid identification of bacterial species from positive blood cultures with a DNA-based microarray platform: an observational study. Lancet 2010;375(9710):224–30.

72. Wellinghausen N, Wirths B, Essig A, et al. Evaluation of the Hyplex BloodScreen Multiplex PCR-enzyme-linked immunosorbent assay system for direct identification of gram-positive cocci and gram-negative bacilli from positive blood cultures. J Clin Microbiol 2004;42(7):3147–52.

73. Molzym. SepsiTest. 2012. Available at: http://www.sepsitest.com/lab-diagnostics.html. Accessed December 31, 2012.

74. Wellinghausen N, Kochem AJ, Disque C, et al. Diagnosis of bacteremia in whole-blood samples by use of a commercial universal 16S rRNA gene-based PCR and sequence analysis. J Clin Microbiol 2009;47(9):2759–65.

75. Kuhn C, Disque C, Muhl H, et al. Evaluation of commercial universal rRNA gene PCR plus sequencing tests for identification of bacteria and fungi associated with infectious endocarditis. J Clin Microbiol 2011;49(8):2919–23.

76. Carretto E, Bardaro M, Russello G, et al. Comparison of the Staphylococcus QuickFISH BC test with the tube coagulase test performed on positive blood cultures for evaluation and application in a clinical routine setting. J Clin Microbiol 2013;51(1):131–5.

77. Chapin K, Musgnug M. Evaluation of three rapid methods for the direct identification of Staphylococcus aureus from positive blood cultures. J Clin Microbiol 2003;41(9):4324–7.

78. Goldstein J, Roberts JW. Microtube coagulase test for detection of coagulase-positive staphylococci. J Clin Microbiol 1982;15(5):848–51.

79. McDonald CL, Chapin K. Rapid identification of Staphylococcus aureus from blood culture bottles by a classic 2-hour tube coagulase test. J Clin Microbiol 1995;33(1):50–2.

80. Speers DJ, Olma TR, Gilbert GL. Evaluation of four methods for rapid identification of Staphylococcus aureus from blood cultures. J Clin Microbiol 1998;36(4):1032–4.

81. Sturm PD, Kwa D, Vos FJ, et al. Performance of two tube coagulase methods for rapid identification of Staphylococcus aureus from blood cultures and their impact on antimicrobial management. Clin Microbiol Infect 2008;14(5):510–3.

82. Qian Q, Eichelberger K, Kirby JE. Rapid identification of Staphylococcus aureus in blood cultures by use of the direct tube coagulase test. J Clin Microbiol 2007;45(7):2267–9.

83. Varettas K, Mukerjee C, Taylor PC. Anticoagulant carryover may influence clot formation in direct tube coagulase tests from blood cultures. J Clin Microbiol 2005;43(9):4613–5.

84. Madison BM, Baselski VS. Rapid identification of Staphylococcus aureus in blood cultures by thermonuclease testing. J Clin Microbiol 1983;18(3):722–4.

85. Ratner HB, Stratton CW. Thermonuclease test for same-day identification of Staphylococcus aureus in blood cultures. J Clin Microbiol 1985;21(6):995–6.

86. Bergh K, Maeland JA. Same-day confirmation of Staphylococcus aureus bacteraemia by a thermonuclease test. Acta Pathol Microbiol Immunol Scand B 1986;94(4):291–2.

87. Skulnick M, Simor AE, Patel MP, et al. Evaluation of three methods for the rapid identification of *Staphylococcus aureus* in blood cultures. Diagn Microbiol Infect Dis 1994;19(1):5–8.

88. Lagace-Wiens PR, Alfa MJ, Manickam K, et al. Thermostable DNase is superior to tube coagulase for direct detection of *Staphylococcus aureus* in positive blood cultures. J Clin Microbiol 2007;45(10):3478–9.

89. Murray PR. Modification of the bile solubility test for rapid identification of *Streptococcus pneumoniae*. J Clin Microbiol 1979;9(2):290–1.

90. Wetkowski MA, Peterson EM, de la Maza LM. Direct testing of blood cultures for detection of streptococcal antigens. J Clin Microbiol 1982;16(1):86–91.

91. Shlaes DM, Toossi Z, Patel A. Comparison of latex agglutination and immunofluorescence for direct Lancefield grouping of streptococci from blood cultures. J Clin Microbiol 1984;20(2):195–8.

92. Lupetti A, Barnini S, Castagna B, et al. Rapid identification and antimicrobial susceptibility profiling of Gram-positive cocci in blood cultures with the Vitek 2 system. Eur J Clin Microbiol Infect Dis 2010;29(1):89–95.

93. Lupetti A, Barnini S, Castagna B, et al. Rapid identification and antimicrobial susceptibility testing of Gram-positive cocci in blood cultures by direct inoculation into the BD Phoenix system. Clin Microbiol Infect 2010;16(7):986–91.

94. Lupetti A, Barnini S, Morici P, et al. Saponin promotes rapid identification and antimicrobial susceptibility profiling of Gram-positive and Gram-negative bacteria in blood cultures with the Vitek 2 system. Eur J Clin Microbiol Infect Dis 2013; 32(4):493–502.

95. Bruins MJ, Bloembergen P, Ruijs GJ, et al. Identification and susceptibility testing of *Enterobacteriaceae* and *Pseudomonas aeruginosa* by direct inoculation from positive BACTEC blood culture bottles into Vitek 2. J Clin Microbiol 2004;42(1):7–11.

96. Chen JR, Lee SY, Yang BH, et al. Rapid identification and susceptibility testing using the VITEK 2 system using culture fluids from positive BacT/ALERT blood cultures. J Microbiol Immunol Infect 2008;41(3):259–64.

97. de Cueto M, Ceballos E, Martinez-Martinez L, et al. Use of positive blood cultures for direct identification and susceptibility testing with the Vitek 2 system. J Clin Microbiol 2004;42(8):3734–8.

98. Gherardi G, Angeletti S, Panitti M, et al. Comparative evaluation of the Vitek-2 Compact and Phoenix systems for rapid identification and antibiotic susceptibility testing directly from blood cultures of Gram-negative and Gram-positive isolates. Diagn Microbiol Infect Dis 2012;72(1):20–31.

99. Ling TK, Liu ZK, Cheng AF. Evaluation of the VITEK 2 system for rapid direct identification and susceptibility testing of Gram-negative bacilli from positive blood cultures. J Clin Microbiol 2003;41(10):4705–7.

100. Munoz-Davila MJ, Yague G, Albert M, et al. Comparative evaluation of Vitek 2 identification and susceptibility testing of Gram-negative rods directly and isolated from BacT/ALERT-positive blood culture bottles. Eur J Clin Microbiol Infect Dis 2012;31(5):663–9.

101. Yonetani S, Okazaki M, Araki K, et al. Direct inoculation method using BacT/ALERT 3D and BD Phoenix System allows rapid and accurate identification and susceptibility testing for both Gram-positive cocci and Gram-negative rods in aerobic blood cultures. Diagn Microbiol Infect Dis 2012;73(2):129–34.

102. Beuving J, van der Donk CF, Linssen CF, et al. Evaluation of direct inoculation of the BD PHOENIX system from positive BACTEC blood cultures for both Gram-positive cocci and Gram-negative rods. BMC Microbiol 2011;11:156.

103. Funke G, Funke-Kissling P. Use of the BD PHOENIX Automated Microbiology System for direct identification and susceptibility testing of Gram-negative rods from positive blood cultures in a three-phase trial. J Clin Microbiol 2004; 42(4):1466–70.

104. Colakoglu S, Aliskan H, Senger SS, et al. Performance of MRSA ID chromogenic medium for detection of methicillin-resistant *Staphylococcus aureus* directly from blood cultures and clinical specimens. Diagn Microbiol Infect Dis 2007; 59(3):319–23.

105. Murray CK, Beckius ML, Green JA, et al. Use of chromogenic medium in the isolation of yeasts from clinical specimens. J Med Microbiol 2005;54(Pt 10):981–5.

106. Tan GL, Peterson EM. CHROMagar Candida medium for direct susceptibility testing of yeast from blood cultures. J Clin Microbiol 2005;43(4):1727–31.

107. Ghelardi E, Pichierri G, Castagna B, et al. Efficacy of Chromogenic Candida Agar for isolation and presumptive identification of pathogenic yeast species. Clin Microbiol Infect 2008;14(2):141–7.

108. Alere. BinaxNOW *Staphylococcus aureus* card product insert. 2012. Available at: http://www.alere.com/us/en/product-details/binaxnow-s-aureus.html. Accessed December 31, 2012.

109. Romero-Gomez MP, Quiles-Melero I, Navarro C, et al. Evaluation of the Binax-NOW PBP2a assay for the direct detection of methicillin resistance in *Staphylococcus aureus* from positive blood culture bottles. Diagn Microbiol Infect Dis 2012;72(3):282–4.

110. Study of the performance of the KeyPath MRSA/MSSA blood culture test - BTA. Available at: http://clinicaltrials.gov/ct2/show/NCT01640886. Accessed November 20, 2012.

111. Bhowmick T, Mirrett S, Reller L, et al. Controlled multicenter evaluation of a bacteriophage based method for the rapid detection of *Staphylococcus aureus* in positive blood cultures (poster). New Orleans (LA): ASM; 2011.

112. Kingery J, Stamper P, Peterson L, et al. A novel phage technology for the detection of *S. aureus* and differentiation of MSSA and MRSA in positive blood culture bottles (poster). Philadelphia (PA): ASM; 2009.

113. Dreiling B, Reed K, Steinmark T, et al. The Keypath MRSA/MSSA blood culture test - BT accurately identifies S. aureus isolates that carry incomplete SCC elements (mecA dropouts) as MSSA (poster). Boston (MA): IDSA; 2011.

114. Nielsen PE, Egholm M. An introduction to peptide nucleic acid. Curr Issues Mol Biol 1999;1(1–2):89–104.

115. Stender H, Fiandaca M, Hyldig-Nielsen JJ, et al. PNA for rapid microbiology. J Microbiol Methods 2002;48(1):1–17.

116. Deck MK, Anderson ES, Buckner RJ, et al. Multicenter evaluation of the *Staphylococcus Quick*FISH method for simultaneous identification of *Staphylococcus aureus* and coagulase-negative staphylococci directly from blood culture bottles in less than 30 minutes. J Clin Microbiol 2012;50(6):1994–8.

117. Alexander BD, Ashley ED, Reller LB, et al. Cost savings with implementation of PNA FISH testing for identification of *Candida albicans* in blood cultures. Diagn Microbiol Infect Dis 2006;54(4):277–82.

118. Forrest GN, Mehta S, Weekes E, et al. Impact of rapid in situ hybridization testing on coagulase-negative staphylococci positive blood cultures. J Antimicrob Chemother 2006;58(1):154–8.

119. Heil EL, Daniels LM, Long DM, et al. Impact of a rapid peptide nucleic acid fluorescence in situ hybridization assay on treatment of *Candida* infections. Am J Health Syst Pharm 2012;69(21):1910–4.

120. Ly T, Gulia J, Pyrgos V, et al. Impact upon clinical outcomes of translation of PNA FISH-generated laboratory data from the clinical microbiology bench to bedside in real time. Ther Clin Risk Manag 2008;4(3):637–40.

121. Forrest GN, Roghmann MC, Toombs LS, et al. Peptide nucleic acid fluorescent in situ hybridization for hospital-acquired enterococcal bacteremia: delivering earlier effective antimicrobial therapy. Antimicrob Agents Chemother 2008; 52(10):3558–63.

122. Metzger S, Price CS, Hance K, et al. Same-day blood culture with digital microscopy (poster). San Francisco (CA): ICAAC; 2012.

123. Loonen AJ, Jansz AR, Stalpers J, et al. An evaluation of three processing methods and the effect of reduced culture times for faster direct identification of pathogens from BacT/ALERT blood cultures by MALDI-TOF MS. Eur J Clin Microbiol Infect Dis 2012;31(7):1575–83.

124. Juiz PM, Almela M, Melcion C, et al. A comparative study of two different methods of sample preparation for positive blood cultures for the rapid identification of bacteria using MALDI-TOF MS. Eur J Clin Microbiol Infect Dis 2012; 31(7):1353–8.

125. Meex C, Neuville F, Descy J, et al. Direct identification of bacteria from BacT/ALERT anaerobic positive blood cultures by MALDI-TOF MS: MALDI Sepsityper kit versus an in-house saponin method for bacterial extraction. J Med Microbiol 2012;61(Pt 11):1511–6.

126. Klein S, Zimmermann S, Kohler C, et al. Integration of matrix-assisted laser desorption/ionization time-of-flight mass spectrometry in blood culture diagnostics: a fast and effective approach. J Med Microbiol 2012;61(Pt 3):323–31.

127. Buchan BW, Riebe KM, Ledeboer NA. Comparison of the MALDI Biotyper system using Sepsityper specimen processing to routine microbiological methods for identification of bacteria from positive blood culture bottles. J Clin Microbiol 2012;50(2):346–52.

128. Moussaoui W, Jaulhac B, Hoffmann AM, et al. Matrix-assisted laser desorption ionization time-of-flight mass spectrometry identifies 90% of bacteria directly from blood culture vials. Clin Microbiol Infect 2010;16(11):1631–8.

129. La Scola B, Raoult D. Direct identification of bacteria in positive blood culture bottles by matrix-assisted laser desorption ionisation time-of-flight mass spectrometry. PLoS One 2009;4(11):e8041.

130. Romero-Gomez MP, Mingorance J. The effect of the blood culture bottle type in the rate of direct identification from positive cultures by matrix-assisted laser desorption/ionisation time-of-flight (MALDI-TOF) mass spectrometry. J Infect 2011;62(3):251–3.

131. Wimmer JL, Long SW, Cernoch P, et al. Strategy for rapid identification and antibiotic susceptibility testing of Gram-negative bacteria directly recovered from positive blood cultures using the Bruker MALDI Biotyper and the BD Phoenix system. J Clin Microbiol 2012;50(7):2452–4.

132. Ferreira L, Sanchez-Juanes F, Porras-Guerra I, et al. Microorganisms direct identification from blood culture by matrix-assisted laser desorption/ionization time-of-flight mass spectrometry. Clin Microbiol Infect 2011;17(4): 546–51.

133. Stevenson LG, Drake SK, Murray PR. Rapid identification of bacteria in positive blood culture broths by matrix-assisted laser desorption ionization-time of flight mass spectrometry. J Clin Microbiol 2010;48(2):444–7.

134. Spanu T, Posteraro B, Fiori B, et al. Direct MALDI-TOF mass spectrometry assay of blood culture broths for rapid identification of *Candida* species causing

bloodstream infections: an observational study in two large microbiology laboratories. J Clin Microbiol 2012;50(1):176–9.

135. Fothergill A, Kasinathan V, Hyman J, et al. Rapid identification of bacteria and yeasts from positive BacT/ALERT blood culture bottles by using a lysis-filtration method and MALDI-TOF mass spectrum analysis with SARAMIS database. J Clin Microbiol 2013;51(3):805–9.

136. Schmidt V, Jarosch A, Marz P, et al. Rapid identification of bacteria in positive blood culture by matrix-assisted laser desorption ionization time-of-flight mass spectrometry. Eur J Clin Microbiol Infect Dis 2012;31(3):311–7.

137. Kaleta EJ, Clark AE, Cherkaoui A, et al. Comparative analysis of PCR-electrospray ionization/mass spectrometry (MS) and MALDI-TOF/MS for the identification of bacteria and yeast from positive blood culture bottles. Clin Chem 2011;57(7):1057–67.

138. Prod'hom G, Bizzini A, Durussel C, et al. Matrix-assisted laser desorption ionization-time of flight mass spectrometry for direct bacterial identification from positive blood culture pellets. J Clin Microbiol 2010;48(4):1481–3.

139. Pletz MW, Wellinghausen N, Welte T. Will polymerase chain reaction (PCR)-based diagnostics improve outcome in septic patients? A clinical view. Intensive Care Med 2011;37(7):1069–76.

140. Forrest GN, Mankes K, Jabra-Rizk MA, et al. Peptide nucleic acid fluorescence in situ hybridization-based identification of *Candida albicans* and its impact on mortality and antifungal therapy costs. J Clin Microbiol 2006; 44(9):3381–3.

141. Bauer KA, West JE, Balada-Llasat JM, et al. An antimicrobial stewardship program's impact with rapid polymerase chain reaction methicillin-resistant *Staphylococcus aureus*/*S. aureus* blood culture test in patients with *S. aureus* bacteremia. Clin Infect Dis 2010;51(9):1074–80.

142. Parta M, Goebel M, Thomas J, et al. Impact of an assay that enables rapid determination of *Staphylococcus* species and their drug susceptibility on the treatment of patients with positive blood culture results. Infect Control Hosp Epidemiol 2010;31(10):1043–8.

143. Blot SI, Vandewoude KH, Hoste EA, et al. Outcome and attributable mortality in critically ill patients with bacteremia involving methicillin-susceptible and methicillin-resistant *Staphylococcus aureus*. Arch Intern Med 2002;162(19): 2229–35.

144. McHugh CG, Riley LW. Risk factors and costs associated with methicillin-resistant *Staphylococcus aureus* bloodstream infections. Infect Control Hosp Epidemiol 2004;25(5):425–30.

145. Cattoir V, Merabet L, Djibo N, et al. Clinical impact of a real-time PCR assay for rapid identification of *Staphylococcus aureus* and determination of methicillin resistance from positive blood cultures. Clin Microbiol Infect 2011;17(3): 425–31.

146. Chihara S, Hayden MK, Minogue-Corbett E, et al. Shortened time to identify *Staphylococcus* species from blood cultures and methicillin resistance testing using CHROMagar. Int J Microbiol 2009;2009:636502.

147. Pape J, Wadlin J, Nachamkin I. Use of BBL CHROMagar MRSA medium for identification of methicillin-resistant *Staphylococcus aureus* directly from blood cultures. J Clin Microbiol 2006;44(7):2575–6.

148. Wendt C, Havill NL, Chapin KC, et al. Evaluation of a new selective medium, BD BBL CHROMagar MRSA II, for detection of methicillin-resistant *Staphylococcus aureus* in different specimens. J Clin Microbiol 2010;48(6):2223–7.

149. Riedel S, Dam L, Stamper PD, et al. Evaluation of Bio-Rad MRSASelect agar for detection of methicillin-resistant *Staphylococcus aureus* directly from blood cultures. J Clin Microbiol 2010;48(6):2285–8.
150. Peterson JF, Dionisio AA, Riebe KM, et al. Alternative use for Spectra MRSA chromogenic agar in detection of methicillin-resistant *Staphylococcus aureus* from positive blood cultures. J Clin Microbiol 2010;48(6):2265–7.
151. Hensley DM, Tapia R, Encina Y. An evaluation of the AdvanDx *Staphylococcus aureus*/CNS PNA FISH assay. Clin Lab Sci 2009;22(1):30–3.
152. Morgan MA, Marlowe E, Novak-Weekly S, et al. A 1.5 hour procedure for identification of *Enterococcus* species directly from blood cultures. J Vis Exp 2011;(48). pii:2616.
153. Della-Latta P, Salimnia H, Painter T, et al. Identification of *Escherichia coli, Klebsiella pneumoniae*, and *Pseudomonas aeruginosa* in blood cultures: a multicenter performance evaluation of a three-color peptide nucleic acid fluorescence in situ hybridization assay. J Clin Microbiol 2011;49(6):2259–61.
154. Hall L, Le Febre KM, Deml SM, et al. Evaluation of the Yeast Traffic Light PNA FISH probes for identification of *Candida* species from positive blood cultures. J Clin Microbiol 2012;50(4):1446–8.

Future-Generation Sequencing and Clinical Microbiology

Benjamin C. Kirkup, PhD[a], Steven Mahlen, PhD[b],
George Kallstrom, PhD[c],*

KEYWORDS

- Sequencing • Clinical microbiology • Genomics

KEY POINTS

- Emerging nucleic acid sequencing technologies will augment and replace traditional clinical microbiology services as detection, characterization and computing technologies mature.
- Sequencing technology is outpacing software support and data storage solutions that are required for functional analysis and incorporation into patients' records.
- There are few clinical professionals trained in interpreting sequence data.
- Current reference databases are far from perfect.
- Physicians must be made aware of the limitations and unanticipated consequences associated with sequencing for clinical diagnosis.

NUCLEIC ACID SEQUENCING

Nucleic acid (NA) sequencing has evolved over the past few decades to allow the generation of vast amounts of sequences at a relatively low cost. In **Fig. 1**, the authors show an approximate cost of sequencing a base of DNA over time. DNA sequencing has progressed from reading Sanger sequencing via films exposed to radiolabeled gels, through fluorescent di-deoxyNTPs on gels and in capillaries, to pyrosequencing, ion detection sequencing, single polymerase sequencing, pore sequencing, and other future-generation methods. Unique benefits and limitations have emerged with each generation of sequencing technology such as sequencing biases, error rates, cost

Disclaimer: The views expressed in this article are those of the authors and do not reflect the official policy or position of the Department of the Army, Department of Defense, or the US Government.

[a] Department of Wound Infections, Walter Reed Army Institute of Research, Room 3A24, 503 Robert Grant Avenue, Silver Spring, MD 20910, USA; [b] Bacterial Diseases Branch, Walter Reed Army Institute of Research, Room 3A16, 503 Robert Grant Avenue, Silver Spring, MD 20910, USA; [c] Department of Pathology, Tripler Army Medical Center, 1 Jarrett White Road, Honolulu, HI 96859, USA
* Corresponding author. Department of Pathology, Tripler Army Medical Center, 1 Jarrett White Road, Honolulu, HI 96859.
E-mail address: george.kallstrom@us.army.mil

Clin Lab Med 33 (2013) 685–704
http://dx.doi.org/10.1016/j.cll.2013.03.011
0272-2712/13/$ – see front matter Published by Elsevier Inc.

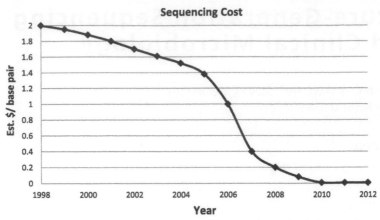

Fig. 1. This figure shows the approximate cost of sequencing a single base pair over time. The dramatic reduction in cost during 2006 to 2008 coincided with the release and increased use of the next-generation sequencing technologies. Est, estimated.

per base pair, and read length. As a result differing methods currently coexist in distinct niches. Examples of these varied methods include continued use of Sanger sequencing for difficult repetitive regions and the ability for Pacific Biosciences SMRT-cell sequencing (Pacific Biosciences, Menlo Park, CA) to reach beyond Watson-Crick base pairing and distinguish modified bases. A large knowledge gap exists between the true technical expert and the naïve. Because the different sequencing technologies have variable technical specifications and performance characteristics, very few people are proven experts in more than one sequencing method at any given time. Sequencing is only used selectively in clinical microbiology at the time of publication of this article, rather than the broad applicability that might have been suggested in an era of scientific claims of imminent personal genomes and real-time molecular epidemiology studies.

CLINICAL MICROBIOLOGY

The clinical microbiology laboratory is chiefly responsible for the diagnosis of individual patient infections, distinguishing between infections and other diseases, identifying the pathogens present in patient specimens, and providing therapeutic recommendations (such as antibiotic susceptibility). In addition to the primary mission of diagnosis, the clinical laboratory frequently assists in outbreak detection and epidemiologic investigations, including the processing of surveillance and carriage samples, which can be used to implement more stringent isolation precautions.

The incorporation of microbial NA sequencing into various aspects of clinical microbiology has begun and will play an increasing role in the future as technology improves and data analysis solutions are uncovered. Increasingly, microbial identification is tied to molecular phylogeny (genomics) rather than biochemical tests. Early bacterial taxonomy began by noting physical similarities and differences between bacteria. Bacterial taxonomy evolved over the decades to include biochemical profiling and some genetic information, but the determination of bacterial taxonomy has largely remained intuitive until very recently with the advent of complete genomic sequencing.[1–4] However, even without taxonomy, phylogeny always had a clear application in epidemiology.[5] Tracing the parentage of patient isolates among a background of commensal and environmental microbes is a key epidemiologic task, and the historical record of semiconservative replication phylogeny is physically tied to the NA sequence.[6-13]

Because of the moderate mutation rates in bacteria and higher mutation rates in many viruses, many outbreaks can be tracked patient to patient via sequencing of specific areas of bacterial genomes without resorting to more creative methods (like measurements of epigenetics,[14] phenotypic noise, or intracellular NA diversity) to gain additional resolution. Microbial molecular epidemiology, originally practiced without NA sequencing,[15] was one of the early applications of sequence-based phylogeny.[16] The increasing speed and throughput of NA sequencing may soon allow for near real-time detection and characterization of ongoing outbreaks.[8,17] Finally, the genetic capabilities of bacteria, fungi, viruses, and communities[18,19] are increasingly available through genetic inference, including extensive databases of known drug-resistance mutations for viruses (hivdb.stanford.edu) and resistance (www.tdbreamdb.com; ardb.cbcb.umd.edu) and virulence factors of pathogenic bacteria (www.mgc.ac.ca/VFS/).

CLINICAL PRACTICE AND SEQUENCING

Most clinicians are understandably naïve of the technical details of NA sequencing, particularly because technology keeps changing. The physicians' chief difficulties are in asking useful questions of the scientists sequencing microbial NA, having realistic expectations of the results the laboratory will return, and having the appropriate medical knowledge to integrate the answers into diagnosis and treatment. Currently, the data provided to promote and evaluate new sequencing technologies do not help the physicians answer these questions about clinical utility. The advertised, requested, and anticipated benefits of new sequencing technologies are typically increases in the volume of sequences generated, reduced cost per base, and increased speed with which results are returned. Certainly, each is important to bringing research technologies into the clinical enterprise. However, the details of newer methods that are required to attain a higher volume at a lower cost typically undermine some intended uses and open alternative applications. Thus, the new technologies do not readily substitute for the earlier technologies, such as Sanger sequencing.

As a result, more sophisticated users focus on nonobvious technological parameters, such as increased base-calling accuracy, lower bias in sequencing from diverse libraries, and longer read lengths[20,21]; the first is important for accurately identifying single nucleotide mutations, the second for evenly sequencing large libraries, and the third for constructing accurate assemblies and, thus, identifying gene content and genome structure mutations. Downstream, improved accuracy, and increased length of reads will provide increases in the precision of isolate identifications, the resolution and accuracy of phylogeny reconstruction, and the specificity of resistance gene identifications—all core elements of the clinical microbiology mission.

UNCOVERING MOLECULAR PHYLOGENY

In addition to the benefits of sequencing described earlier, several unexpected benefits are also becoming available to the clinician. One positive byproduct of ready genome sequencing is that now many closely related genomes have been sequenced. This development has allowed for the creation of robust databases, such as Pathos-Systems Resource Integration Center, Integrated Microbial Genomes, Metagenomics analysis server, and the Human Microbiome Project. These efforts begin to comprehend the phylogeny of pathogenic organisms.

When single genes were all that could be generated by Sanger sequencing, linkage disequilibrium suggested a degree of clonal structure interrupted by homologous recombination to create something of a phylogenetic network within each species or genus,[22] which often confused the pool of the pathogens or symbionts, depending on the species. This view is rapidly being overturned, first in the environmental organisms and now in known pathogenic organisms, by the impact of large-scale sequencing. The pan-genome has proven much larger and more variable than originally expected.[23] Further, a relatively few core genes are closely correlated with ecological roles like *pathogen*, and they can be largely independent of the recombinational processes shuffling the housekeeping genes, be they shuffled slowly or quickly.[24–28]

The new understanding of genomic microdiversity permitted by large databases undermines the failing vision of ready microbiological diagnosis via several extant characterization schemes, such as multilocus sequence typing, multiple-locus variable number tandem repeat analysis, 16S ribosomal DNA sequencing, and more traditional techniques like restriction fragment length polymorphism and pulsed field gel electrophoresis (PFGE). Delineating pathogen from nonpathogen requires careful pathology to study DNA from both pathogenic- and nonpathogenic-type organisms and identify the specific and discrete genetic elements determinative of ecological partitioning. Genomic data and ecological data can be linked via informatics[29–31] to define the loci that define the ecology. Linking data together will be useful when evaluating complex specimens using shotgun metagenomics (discussed later).

Reference sequences for each locus, additional isolates, or samples can be readily typed by a range of molecular methods, including but not limited to standard sequencing. At the same time, all of those other recombining housekeeping genes and mobile genetic elements that compose most of the microbial genome have important parts to play in microbiology and can provide critical information to clinicians. Some of the information is diagnostic, including antibiotic resistance genes.[32] Other information is epidemiologic[33,34] in nature; the network of housekeeping genes, more than was previously imagined, is a rich historical tapestry.[35–37] Many elementary textbooks demonstrate the tree of life as something clearly rooted with neatly bifurcating branches to demonstrate taxonomy, and the original phylogenetic methods were predicated on this assumption. The absence of a bifurcating tree may frustrate older analytical techniques, but mathematics and computing are quickly stepping in to fill in gaps and provide sound interpretations tied to sociology,[38] biogeography,[39] and time.[40,41]

Without the explosion in sequencing, the possibility to understand the genome network was infeasible. Finding the appropriate ecological markers requires sequencing hundreds of strains on an ongoing basis. Even with the current technologies, discovering genomic microdiversity is a significant challenge. More than one technology will be required to address each and every genome; simply to confirm single-nucleotide polymorphisms (SNPs) and major genomic arrangements requires the simultaneous application of 2 or more technologies, one for high accuracy and another for structural determination.[42–45]

The process of characterizing genomic microdiversity in bacterial species has barely begun; its impact will not be fully realized for a decade or more. Major pathogen types have emerged in as little as a decade, so any lasting technology will require continual database development as new pathogens arise and must provide the ability to capture emerging, previously uncharacterized pathogens in real time[46]; identifying novel and emerging pathogens will not be a single completed project. Pathogen definitions are not a series of successive approximations, refinements toward the truth, as much as active tracking in a dynamic social network. The definitions will require indefinite maintenance and attention as novel organisms and variant strains emerge.

METAGENOMICS IN THE CLINICAL SETTING

An additional nascent sequencing strategy is shotgun metagenomics,[47–52] which is sequencing the genomes of a community of bacteria simultaneously, prepared from a single sample. This strategy naturally has the possibility to capture all of the genomic data from all of the community members; but because the distribution of membership can be radically skewed (ie, some members are 80% and others are 0.0001%),[53,54] the depth of sequencing required to effectively capture and assemble all the genes in all the minority members can be radically disproportionate. Still, this may also enter the clinical laboratory in the future, although its future is being hotly debated at this moment. It provides an entry point to visualize certain constants that underlie phylogenetic diversity, such as the abundance of key metabolic pathways,[55] and may be the only way to reconstruct complex systems because genomic microdiversity and community diversity act simultaneously.

Freed from the confines of classic culture methods, sequencing has revealed a vast new diversity associated with all body sites, including some that are thought to be aseptic, like the lower respiratory tract.[56] In addition, relevant microbial diversity has been characterized in a range of pathogenic conditions, some that are thought to be nonmicrobial[57] and others that are thought to be monomicrobial.[58] Neurologic,[59,60] immunologic,[61,62] metabolic,[63] and putatively genetic diseases have all been identified with microbial components, impacts, and associations. Many of the published associations are simply observed differences between the microbiome of one or more body sites in patients with and without some clinical presentation. However, there are a growing number of cases in which the evidence is much stronger, either through animal models or other experimental studies. In chronic wound care, the use of sequencing to guide antibiotic selection already results in vastly improved healing times.[64–66] Brain abscesses, including those that are culture negative, can be classified by their often polymicrobial infections; more importantly, when comorbidities are analyzed, the mechanism of infection and the source communities for the abscesses are mechanistically readily explained (ie, dental vs sinus).[67,68]

One of the significant challenges faced by proponents of molecular methods is that culture overall can be much more sensitive to the detection of bacteria than molecular methods, even polymerase chain reaction (PCR); this complicates the idea of replacing culture with molecular methods because the new methods are not simply better culture. However, sequencing reveals diversity that culture simply does not reveal. The debate about sensitivity has been very lively in the area of prosthetic joint infections; many physicians are primarily concerned about the presence or absence of bacteria and not their identity. The discordance between molecular methods and culture-based methods creates challenges (sometimes one or the other is the more sensitive).[69–71] This issue might be conceivably resolved by using even more sensitive molecular methods,[72] but culture has a great advantage of auto-amplification when detecting culture-friendly organisms.

Where there is a single-culturable organism, there are often others that cannot be cultured, in pyogenic infections,[58] in pleural infections,[73] and in urinary catheter infections.[74]

Where there is no culturable organism, the results are more striking. These results include some newly discovered brain infections validated through dramatic animal studies,[75] culture-negative eye infections,[76] and amniotic fluid.[77] Another key application for sequencing is during asymptomatic spells in chronic infections; only information-rich methods can demonstrate conclusively that the infection has continued rather than simply recurred. Periods of quiescent infection occur in chronic otitis media[78,79] but also between frank sepsis and later infections.[80]

In addition to the previously mentioned cases of undetected or misidentified infectious agents, although Koch's postulates are still valuable as one possible standard of evidence to which infectious disease research must aspire, the mindset they have reinforced (one pathogen, one disease) is being eroded on all sides. The most extreme cases are the diseases in which there is no pathogen per se[81,82]; the absence of a microbe[83] or simply a change in community structure,[63,84] such as an increase or decrease in effective diversity, is central to the illness. This already seems to be the case in chronic sinusitis.[85] A hybrid model has been demonstrated for *Clostridium difficile* infection, with the depleted flora opening patients to infection[86-88] and restoration treating the disease.[89] It is beginning to become clear that sequencing, although maybe not the ultimate universal diagnostic tool, will be used in many cases in determining the diseased state, whether by definitive identification of the pathogen or a marked imbalance in the normal microbiota of the host. Sequencing technology is advancing faster than other diagnostic methods.

DIVERSITY AND THE OPEN NATURE OF SEQUENCING

Sequencing will continue to be used clinically in part because it can be open, that is, finding diversity not described before the collection of the data and able to be interpreted without a reference database. The theory that underpins this capability was developed by Pace,[90] which is that in semiconservative replication with mutation, DNA is effectively a historical document. A broad set of mutational classes can be represented by the matrix of a Markov process, with transitions, transversions, insertions of various sizes, rearrangements, and other kinds of mutations occurring at different rates.[91] In specific molecules, such as 16S rRNA, mutation rates can be specified with even greater detail based on the stem-loop secondary and functional tertiary structure required for ribosomal function.[92,93] This allows an entirely novel 16S rRNA sequence (or protein sequence or genome sequence) to be interpreted into the context of the known diversity in a way that a PFGE profile or matrix-assisted laser desorption/ionization–time of flight mass spectrometry peak pattern fundamentally cannot.

Further, sequencing in some of its current implementations is necessarily massively parallel. The method is performing the same assay in multiplicate to derive a highly precise value for a single measurement; it is sequencing many different molecules independently and incidentally simultaneously. The biggest change in sequencing technologies has occurred over the past decade from Sanger sequencing in which a single sequence present in numerous copies is analyzed in a lane to nanopore[94,95] or captive enzyme sequencing[96] whereby a single copy of each target is used to generate NA sequence data. Other molecular methods have not made the leap from precision to diversity. Real-time PCR can be multiplexed, for example, to detect a few dozen to a few hundred targets at a time; but newer sequencing technologies detect a few million to a few billion separate entities in a single run. The only technologies that compete with sequencing for the characterization of diversity may be some of the modern imaging technologies, such as flow cytometry and automated microscopy, but they are typically limited by the division of the spectrum into measuring a few dozen parameters about each target at any given time. The processivity of sequencing provides an additional dimension to the physical entity studied, the secret to its high throughput.

CHALLENGES TO INTEGRATING SEQUENCING INTO CLINICAL DIAGNOSTICS

Applying sequencing to the clinic has long been anticipated to create several challenges for the clinician and clinical laboratory. Not the least of these is the cost of implementing the method, the length of time required to process a sample, and the number of samples required to use a full lane of sequencing. These problems are important; but advances in technology are making unmistakable progress against each one, in a variety of combinations. Turn-around times are now dependent more on library construction and data analysis than on sequencing itself.[97] Sequencing technology is rapidly being automated, the data analyses are the limiting factor requiring processing power and algorithmic optimization, not physical limitations on the system. As sequencers are being marketed to the clinical and diagnostic laboratory, they are appearing at a variety of scales and a range of price points competitive with the diagnostic instruments of prior eras (MiSeq Personal Sequencer [Illumina, San Diego, CA], 454 GSJr [454Life Sciences, Brandford, CT], Ion Proton Sequencer [Ion Torrent, San Francisco, CA]). The cost of sequencing is currently decreasing more rapidly than the cost of computing[98]; frankly, this decline in cost itself begins to present a significant and well-anticipated problem.[99–101]

DATA STORAGE PROBLEMS

Sequence data was once the object of intense, intelligent scrutiny. Every gene that was sequenced was a topic of conversation, publication, and experimentation. Now, entire microbial genomes are submitted into databases half annotated by automated pipelines.[102,103] The information storage challenges alone are massive, and sequencing has become so inexpensive that some individuals have proposed storing information on DNA directly and reading it off via sequencing as a form of computer data rather than reading DNA and storing the sequence in computers as a form of biologic data.[104] The short-read archive at the National Center for Biotechnology Information was threatened with insufficient funding because of the high volumes of data being stored.[105] The analysis of vast quantities of data requires substantial computing power; as of yet, using that power effectively requires expertise that is rare. Software exists to make prior analyses ubiquitous, but the scale and scope of the available data is running ahead of the analytical methods.

These problems will not entirely be resolved in the foreseeable future. As usual, the expected problems are not ultimately the ones that are most troubling. Cloud computing facilities have grown into a substantial industry, with clusters that are HIPPA (Health Insurance Portability and Accountability Act) compliant [106,107] and massive storage capabilities. Holography for static data structures has been on the horizon for a long time now; perhaps sequencing will push it into general use. Institutions are developing user-friendly analysis that are already being adapted for the clinical laboratory in standard configurations.[108,109] Many of the problems encountered applying existing sequence interpretation methods to the clinical laboratory grow out of the poor programing practices of professional biologists and software designed for ultimate flexibility instead of efficiency, which is a balance struck in the research laboratory but ill-suited to the clinic.

ESTABLISHING STANDARDS

There are other issues that have resulted because much of the sequencing has grown out of the creative and minimally coordinated world of academic biology. Various academic groups are currently wrestling with issues such as the standardization of skin sampling for the purposes of sequencing the microbial diversity or the standardization of population genetic analyses from microbial population; once clinical microbiologists enter the arena in numbers, Standard Operating Procedures (SOPs) will quickly be drafted, compared, translated, reconciled in committee, and published. Forensic scientists have been wrestling with the equivalent problems in their own sequencing endeavors over the past decade; the clinical laboratories will make short work of developing standards, confirmatory tests, quality analysis/quality control, and sensitivity and specificity bounds. The Clinical Laboratory Standards Institute (CLSI) has already issued numerous CLSI standards regarding sequencing.[110–112]

REFERENCE DATABASE QUALITY AND SEQUENCING ERRORS

A much more significant issue is the present condition of the reference databases. In an environment of continual contribution and accretion with relatively little curation, it is unsurprising that there are major problems in the reference sequence databases. What has been surprising to almost everyone is the scope and scale of the problems, even in curated 16S rRNA databases. This problem was first brought to light during the crisis of chimeric 16S rRNA sequences when it was discovered that there was a significant amount of chimeras generated with newer sequencing technologies. Now, professional 16s rRNA sequence analysis pipelines have chimera checks in place to clean the sequences; but at one time this was not yet a known problem, and a large number of chimeric sequences entered the databases unfiltered.[113–115] Scrutiny has intensified on the use of 16s rRNA to classify organisms at the species level[116]; but in doing so, substantial problems with the quality of the curated databases have been brought to light, including misclassification of organisms from other genera, families, and so on.

The reflexive solutions to some data quality problems, such as discarding singleton sequences in a study, may lead to inaccuracies. It has been demonstrated that many of the singletons are actually accurate,[53] an important tail to the frequency distribution, and, worst yet, ecologically relevant even when dormant[117–120] but often disproportionately metabolically active.[121,122] Discarding them may not be *conservative* unless one proposes that the scientific claim is a one-tailed test of rare diversity, in which case understating the diversity might be conceivably considered *conservative*. The good news is that as more data enters the reference sets and can be quality controlled, better software solutions can be implemented to provide accurate operational taxonomic units and enzyme function measures. In the same fashion that human genome sequencing is progressing with the validation of SNPs, copy number variants, and other known variants, microbes sequenced in the medical context are just barely becoming known; it will be some time before those recognized only from sequence are as familiar to a trained microbiologist as reading the growth from a culture plate.

INTERPRETING GENOMIC DATA

This issue raises the other major class of well-anticipated problems: difficulties with the clinical interpretation and use of both genome and community composition data.[123] The problem is hardly a new one; already, medical microbiologists and clinicians know all the caveats that accompany automated identification and susceptibility testing. The diagnostics and therapeutics that compose our present system of medical care are complex and include such variables as the clinical picture, the culture conditions, microscopy, empiric therapy, the drugs to be tested, drug-testing cutoffs and minimal inhibitory concentrations and the treatment that will be used.[124–128] These rules are not as straightforward as measuring the response of the organisms to a set concentration of an antibiotic and titrating to that concentration in the patient's bloodstream; a hosts of factors,[129] many uncharacterized, complicate the scenario and are corrected for in the context of clinical experience. Without comparative effectiveness testing, clinical microbiology and infectious disease practice would not work as well as it does today.

Integrating sequencing data into the system does not somehow break the elegant simplicity of the existing model, based on phenotypic testing of axenic cultures. It also does not introduce mathematically simple answers based on digital genotype data, allowing drug concentrations to be calculated to treat any arbitrary organism. The vast number of potential genotypes and their complex relationship to phenotype is a well-known challenge. This challenge has been made substantially more difficult than previously anticipated by the significant microdiversity of genomes and the community effects of host and microbiome.[130] Novel mutations and rare taxa both present hard problems for interpretation. Clinical microbiology previously reached for machine learning solutions to a set of problems.[131–134] Although instruments have automated some of the manual testing performed in the clinical microbiology laboratory, the algorithms used by the machines often provide erroneous results that need to be interpreted in context with the laboratory technologist, infectious disease physician, and clinical microbiologist to troubleshoot conflicting or very unlikely results.

LIMITATIONS OF PATTERN RECOGNITION IN COMPUTER SYSTEMS

The discussion of prior machine learning and expert systems attempts raises an issue very much pertinent to the interpretation of microbial community data in the context of clinical care. That is, why have automated systems performed so poorly in clinical microbiology to date? With all of the technology innovation, many providers prefer to consult with a microbiologist with 20 years bench experience over the fast computers provided with automated systems to interpret a complex clinical sample. It seems that technologists are commonly underestimating the power of the human mind to do certain kinds of tasks, particularly pattern recognition. The gamification of several complex calculations, including protein folding[135] and other optimizations[136] or computationally hard problems,[137–140] has demonstrated repeatedly that a focused human effort can exceed the collective computing power of a massively distributed computer system, itself much more powerful than any given computer dedicated to a single task.[141] Appropriate systems to visualize microbial data are already being built.[142–144]

Human computing systems tend to focus on the novice, perhaps mistakenly ignoring the significantly enhanced capabilities of the human expert. Underestimating the power of the alternative they sought to replace with computers, technologists imagined the problem of clinical microbiology to be easier than it was and failed to achieve the baseline level of accuracy they had advertised to exceed. This trap is a very easy trap to fall into again, particularly when interpreting the vast flood of data present in genomes and microbial communities. In some sense, the current technologists are playing against a straw man because very few, if any, clinical microbiologists have sat with this new class of data for the amount of time that they have sat with culture data.

There are no well-trained humans to compete against the computers. The vast amount of genomic data generated exceeds the computing capacity of the relatively unaided human brain. A valuable question is whether technology should be developed primarily to interpret the data for the clinician or primarily to provide intuitive interfaces and visualizations to the clinical microbiologists for sophisticated interpretation via the human expert. Trained clinical microbiologists will likely exist in the foreseeable future, but technology may replace some of the traditional microbiology technologists. The microbiology laboratory of the future will require a different set of competency skills, such as mechanical technicians and bioinformatics experts. Clinical microbiologists will need to work on bridging the gap as they currently do between test result and what that means to the clinician, but they must first understand and embrace the coming sequencing technologies.

PRIVACY ISSUES

As complex as these anticipated problems of interpretation are, there are other problems that sequencing will introduce into the clinical laboratory that are less well anticipated. One problem raised recently is the problem of privacy.[145,146] Clinical sequencing of human genomes has been anticipated to raise a host of concerns; but now it is becoming obvious that the microbiome is just as much a part of a person as his or her eukaryotic genome, that it is distinctive and traceable. Recent research has demonstrated tracing individual fingertips to keyboard keys via the microflora; bite marks can be identified by the oral flora[147]; tooth surfaces are similarly distinctive; and the face can be mapped in a manner that identifies where a person touches his face with his hands, via the microbial communities. An additional layer of privacy invasion exists with the potential for source tracking,[148,149] that is, the potential ability to backtrack through experiences, locations, and behaviors by sampling the microbiome.

What may be a boon for epidemiology becomes a problem for privacy. Currently, one can determine whether people use their shoes to flush the toilet in a public restroom.[150] It is not a large leap to determine that a person has visited a public restroom from their shoes and hands. As this ability to track sources emerges, so do potential threats to privacy. Dealing with privacy issues was not as much a problem with classic microbiology. As microbiological sequencing becomes more common, issues with personal information will likely become more closely entwined with microbiology.

INCIDENTAL FINDINGS

Another problem that has challenged microbiology previously is that of incidental findings.[65,151] In fact, Koch's postulates were in essence a response to the medical community's inability to deal with incidental findings of culturable pathogens in many different contexts. Koch was attempting to construct a strong evidentiary basis for infectious disease at a time when charlatans would use every culturable microorganism as an excuse to sell snake oil–type remedies. Legitimate scientists were questioning the basis of infectious disease in practice. Eventually the boundaries of legitimate medical inference from culture became fixed; every new microbiology student learns at some point that skin may be colonized with *Staphylococcus aureus* and that there is no need to panic. However, sequencing upsets that equilibrium. For chronic wounds, it has already raised questions because it has been found that ulcers are colonized by cyanobacteria, algae, various fungi,[152] predatory bacteria, and other unexpected organisms. Questions will be raised as to what should be done about this abnormal community or colonization or virulence factor.[153]

In a current analogy, medical imaging is facing challenges with regard to incidental findings[154,155]; similarly, microbiology via sequencing is likely to turn up a host of incidental findings for patients, depending on the depth of the sequencing. One solution in medical imaging is to narrow the scope of inspection; this is analogous to taking fewer samples or reducing the sequencing depth. Each of these has an internal logic, and each might have an impact both on patient care and epidemiology. But this is when the analogy with medical imaging breaks down. The greater the inspection is of the individual patient's microbiologically, the greater the potential contribution is to public health and infectious disease epidemiology. Narrowing the scope of observation for the purposes of avoiding incidental findings may relieve physicians of the difficult task of deciding what to treat, at the cost of losing insight at the population level. The potential impact for incidental findings in clinical microbiology will require significant forethought as sequencing is implemented.

ANTIMICROBIAL SUSCEPTIBILITY RESULTS AND CLINICAL OUTCOMES

The selection of which antibiotic susceptibility testing to perform in the laboratory has been an area of debate between the physicians and clinical microbiologists. The introduction of sequencing will potentially create a new area of debate as different areas and specialties jockey over the border between laboratory work, data interpretation, and therapy selection. Addressing the promise and difficulty of integrating sequencing into clinical microbiology or, as some may have it, remaking clinical microbiology around it, will require research, development, advanced development, and the active participation of the clinical laboratorians and clinicians. The interface where this struggle will likely play out is in part in the development of new software in which laboratorians and clinicians must come together.

It currently makes sense to integrate data cleaning, interpretation, and therapeutic selection into a single engine that draws on electronic health records and laboratory results; however, as stated earlier, computers are not necessarily well suited to the kinds of pattern recognition required for the interpretation of very complex data, although they may be invaluable in storing, retrieving, and presenting it. In addition, the travails of telemedicine present an ample warning against overestimating the possibility of diagnosis directly from electronic health records. Physicians do not necessarily enter the data well[156,157]; further, there are many nuances to the patient interaction, which must enter into diagnosis and therapeutic selection. As a result, software that draws on sequencing from the clinical microbiology laboratory and patients' records will probably also require an asynchronous collaborative capacity to allow the physician and microbiologist to each contribute to patient care in the same way that some do today, with electronic communication, telephonic consults, and in-person consultations.

THE ROAD AHEAD FROM GENOME TO MICROBIOME

The shaping of clinical microbiology around sequencing will require a massive quantity of clinical research, including the development of new reference databases to define the associations between microbiology and health or disease and comparative effectiveness research determining the impact of diverse interventions framed with an awareness of the entire microbiome. These studies have been initiated by the National Institutes of Health under the auspices of the Human Microbiome Project.[158] The creation and ongoing maintenance of these enormous resources is a monumental challenge, which is certainly an unforeseen cost of clinical sequencing beyond the cost per base sequenced.

Currently, most sequencing technologies have been driven by the requirements of sequencing human genomes; as sequencing becomes a major component of microbiology, it will be increasingly important to include microbiologists in the development of sequencing technologies. As discussed earlier, many of the limitations of sequencing technologies appear in the context of optimizing particular parameters, such as throughput or cost per base. As microbiology becomes an increasingly defined and routinized application of sequencing, the opportunity to produce specialized platforms that are optimized to specific clinical microbiology tasks will appear. Microbiologists can capitalize on this opportunity by being dissatisfied with current technologies and not making arbitrary concessions to the platforms that are presented to market.

INCORPORATING GENOMICS INTO MEDICAL EDUCATION

Finally, new educational materials, programs, and strategies are required for both laboratory professionals and physicians. Effective education will be a major requirement for the effective transformation of not only infectious diseases but also every medical specialty that will be impacted by the coming revolutions in microbiology. Laboratory professionals practicing over the past 30 years have seen the fragmented and inadequate impact of both information technology and molecular biology on the clinical laboratory. In each case, adoption has been inevitable but uneven. Difficulties with adoption are related to substantial investment costs, standardization, and education. As microbiology responds to its newfound awareness of microbial diversity and population dynamics, its increased ability to characterize both individual strains and communities, both accepting change and leading change require enhanced and accelerated education.

Clinical laboratories will require professionals versed in genomics and professionals versed in microbial ecology. They will also require a new wave of information technology, particularly in places that had difficulty adopting information technology in the past. The integration of these educational requirements into present certifications may be difficult because of the glacial pace at which certifying bodies move. As a result, savvy laboratory directors will require alternative methods for identifying capable and appropriately educated technicians. These methods may include college minors that provide a needed subspecialty or alternative educational opportunities, such as online course completion and certificates.

For sequencing to recognize its full potential impact on medicine, sequencing cannot be isolated in the clinical laboratory; physician education will also need to adapt. Currently, the flood of publications is too turbulent for a practicing physician to keep up with findings in the human microbiome or the news in microbial genomics. This material demands presentation in a condensed form for continuing education and inclusion in the current medical curricula. The development of these educational materials must start quickly because education on sequencing technology and its applications and limitations is currently lagging.

SUMMARY

Every level of health care management will have a role in organizing the enterprise to absorb and support the introduction of sequencing to clinical microbiology. The implementation of sequencing capabilities, research and collaboration requirements, educational opportunities, and regulatory atmosphere will be a large enterprise within medicine for decades to come. Anticipation of the challenges inherent in future waves of sequencing technology is critical. Sequencing technologies bring not only the intended benefits of the improvements around which they were designed but also the challenges of the unforeseen weaknesses that are closely linked to their underlying mechanisms. In addition, anticipation of the disruption that microbial sequencing will cause in medicine, public health, and related fields should lead to the early, almost premature development of educational materials, collaborative software, and a regulatory environment designed to deal with the inevitable disruptions.

REFERENCES

1. Cowan ST. Heretical taxonomy for bacteriologists. J Gen Microbiol 1970;61(2): 145–54.
2. Staley TE, Colwell RR. Application of molecular genetics and numerical taxonomy to the classification of bacteria. Annu Rev Ecol Syst 1973;4:273–300.
3. Wayne LG, Brenner DJ, Clowell RR, et al. Report of the ad hoc committee on reconciliation of approaches to bacterial systematics. Int J Syst Bacteriol 1987;37(4):463–4.
4. Stackebrandt E. Phylogenetic relationships vs. phenotypic diversity: how to achieve a phylogenetic classification system of the eubacteria. Can J Microbiol 1988;34(4):552–6.
5. Ou CY, Ciesielski CA, Myers G, et al. Molecular epidemiology of HIV transmission in a dental practice. Science 1992;256:1165–71.
6. Woese CR, Fox GE. Phylogenetic structure of the prokaryotic domain: the primary kingdoms. Proc Natl Acad Sci U S A 1977;74(11):5088–90.
7. Köser CU, Holden MT, Ellington MJ, et al. Rapid whole-genome sequencing for investigation of a neonatal MRSA outbreak. N Engl J Med 2012;366(24): 2267–75.
8. Harris SR, Cartwright EJ, Török ME, et al. Whole-genome sequencing for analysis of an outbreak of methicillin-resistant Staphylococcus aureus: a descriptive study. Lancet Infect Dis 2013;13(2):130–6.
9. Snitkin ES, Zelazny AM, Thomas PJ, et al. Tracking a hospital outbreak of carbapenem-resistant Klebsiella pneumoniae with whole-genome sequencing. Sci Transl Med 2012;4(148):148ra116.
10. Sandora TJ, Goldmann DA. Preventing lethal hospital outbreaks of antibiotic-resistant bacteria. N Engl J Med 2012;367(23):2168–70.
11. Holden MT, Hsu LY, Kurt K, et al. A genomic portrait of the emergence, evolution and global spread of a methicillin resistant Staphylococcus aureus pandemic. Genome Res 2013;23(4):653–64.
12. Reuter S, Harrison TG, Köser CU, et al. A pilot study of rapid whole-genome sequencing for the investigation of a Legionella outbreak. BMJ Open 2013; 3(1). pii: e002175.
13. Lipkin WI. The changing face of pathogen discovery and surveillance. Nat Rev Microbiol 2013;11(2):133–41.
14. Flusberg BA, Webster DR, Lee JH, et al. Direct detection of DNA methylation during single-molecule, real-time sequencing. Nat Methods 2010;7(6):461–5.
15. Stull TL, LiPuma JJ, Edlind TD. A broad-spectrum probe for molecular epidemiology of bacteria: ribosomal RNA. J Infect Dis 1988;157(2):280–6.
16. Li WH, Tanimura M, Sharp PM. Rates and dates of divergence between AIDS virus nucleotide sequences. Mol Biol Evol 1988;5(4):313–30.
17. Jolley KA, Hill DM, Bratcher HB, et al. Resolution of a meningococcal disease outbreak from whole-genome sequence data with rapid web-based analysis methods. J Clin Microbiol 2012;50(9):3046–53.
18. Flores R, Shi J, Gail MH, et al. Association of fecal microbial diversity and taxonomy with selected enzymatic functions. PLoS One 2012;7(6):e39745.
19. Gifford SM, Sharma S, Booth M, et al. Expression patterns reveal niche diversification in a marine microbial assemblage. ISME J 2013;7(2):281–98.
20. Loman NJ, Constantinidou C, Chan JZ, et al. High-throughput bacterial genome sequencing: an embarrassment of choice, a world of opportunity. Nat Rev Microbiol 2012;10(9):599–606.

21. Loman NJ, Misra RV, Dallman TJ, et al. Performance comparison of benchtop high-throughput sequencing platforms. Nat Biotechnol 2012;30(5):434–9.
22. Spratt BG, Hanage WP, Feil EJ. The relative contributions of recombination and point mutation to the diversification of bacterial clones. Curr Opin Microbiol 2001;4(5):602–6.
23. Medini D, Donati C, Tettelin H, et al. The microbial pan-genome. Curr Opin Genet Dev 2005;15(6):589–94.
24. Hunt DE, David LA, Gevers D, et al. Resource partitioning and sympatric differentiation among closely related bacterioplankton. Science 2008;320(5879): 1081–5.
25. Szabo G, Preheim SP, Kauffman KM, et al. Reproducibility of Vibrionaceae population structure in coastal bacterioplankton. ISME J 2013;7(3):509–19.
26. Connor N, Sikorski J, Rooney AP, et al. Ecology of speciation in the genus Bacillus. Appl Environ Microbiol 2010;76(5):1349–58.
27. Weissman SJ, Johnson JR, Tchesnokova V, et al. High-resolution two-locus clonal typing of extraintestinal pathogenic Escherichia coli. Appl Environ Microbiol 2012;78(5):1353–60.
28. Paul S, Linardopoulou EV, Billig M, et al. Role of homologous recombination in adaptive diversification of extra-intestinal Escherichia coli. J Bacteriol 2012; 195(2):231–42.
29. Kopac S, Cohan FM. A theory-based pragmatism for discovering and classifying newly divergent bacterial species. London: Division III Faculty Publications; 2011 [Paper 214].
30. Preheim SP, Timberlake S, Polz MF. Merging taxonomy with ecological population prediction in a case study of Vibrionaceae. Appl Environ Microbiol 2011; 77(20):7195–206.
31. Francisco JC, Cohan FM, Krizanc D. Demarcation of bacterial ecotypes from DNA sequence data: a comparative analysis of four algorithms. 2nd IEEE International Conference on Computational Advances in Bio and Medical Sciences (ICCABS). February 23, 2012, Las Vegas, NV. p. 1–6.
32. Poirel L, Bonnin RA, Nordmann P. Analysis of the resistome of a multidrug-resistant NDM-1-producing Escherichia coli strain by high-throughput genome sequencing. Antimicrob Agents Chemother 2011;55(9):4224–9.
33. Price JR, Didelot X, Crook DW, et al. Whole genome sequencing in the prevention and control of Staphylococcus aureus infection. J Hosp Infect 2013;83(1): 14–21.
34. Cho YJ, Yi H, Lee JH, et al. Genomic evolution of Vibrio cholerae. Curr Opin Microbiol 2010;13(5):646–51.
35. Marttinen P, Hanage WP, Croucher NJ, et al. Detection of recombination events in bacterial genomes from large population samples. Nucleic Acids Res 2012; 40(1):e6.
36. Blount ZD, Barrick JE, Davidson CJ, et al. Genomic analysis of a key innovation in an experimental Escherichia coli population. Nature 2012;489(7417):513–8.
37. Ford C, Yusim K, Loerger T, et al. Mycobacterium tuberculosis–heterogeneity revealed through whole genome sequencing. Tuberculosis 2012;92(3):194–201.
38. Gardy JL, Johnston JC, Ho Sui SJ, et al. Whole-genome sequencing and social-network analysis of a tuberculosis outbreak. N Engl J Med 2011; 364(8):730–9.
39. Chaffron S, Rehrauer H, Pernthaler J, et al. A global network of coexisting microbes from environmental and whole-genome sequence data. Genome Res 2010;20(7):947–59.

40. Grad YH, Lipsitch M, Feldgarden M, et al. Genomic epidemiology of the Escherichia coli O104: H4 outbreaks in Europe, 2011. Proc Natl Acad Sci U S A 2012; 109(8):3065–70.

41. Makkoch J, Suwannakarn K, Payungporn S, et al. Whole genome characterization, phylogenetic and genome signature analysis of human pandemic H1N1 virus in Thailand, 2009–2012. PLoS One 2012;7(12):e51275.

42. Nagarajan N, Cook C, Di Bonaventura M, et al. Finishing genomes with limited resources: lessons from an ensemble of microbial genomes. BMC Genomics 2010;11(1):242.

43. English AC, Richards S, Han Y, et al. Mind the gap: upgrading genomes with pacific biosciences RS long-read sequencing technology. PLoS One 2012; 7(11):e47768.

44. Au KF, Underwood JG, Lee L, et al. Improving PacBio long read accuracy by short read alignment. PLoS One 2012;7(10):e46679.

45. Turner PC, Yomano LP, Jarboe LR, et al. Optical mapping and sequencing of the Escherichia coli KO11 genome reveal extensive chromosomal rearrangements, and multiple tandem copies of the Zymomonas mobilispdc and adhB genes. J Ind Microbiol Biotechnol 2012;39(4):629–39.

46. Peirano G, Pitout JD. Molecular epidemiology of Escherichia coli producing CTX-M β-lactamases: the worldwide emergence of clone ST131 O25: H4. Int J Antimicrob Agents 2010;35(4):316–21.

47. DeLong EF, Pace NR. Environmental diversity of bacteria and archaea. Syst Biol 2001;50(4):470–8.

48. Schloss PD, Handelsman J. Biotechnological prospects from metagenomics. Curr Opin Biotechnol 2003;14(3):303–10.

49. Tringe SG, Rubin EM. Metagenomics: DNA sequencing of environmental samples. Nat Rev Genet 2005;6(11):805–14.

50. Tyson GW, Chapman J, Hugenholtz P, et al. Community structure and metabolism through reconstruction of microbial genomes from the environment. Nature 2004;428(6978):37–43.

51. Woyke T, Xie G, Copeland A, et al. Assembling the marine metagenome, one cell at a time. PLoS One 2009;4(4):e5299.

52. Iverson V, Morris RM, Frazar CD, et al. Untangling genomes from metagenomes: revealing an uncultured class of marine Euryarchaeota. Science 2012; 335(6068):587–90.

53. Sogin ML, Morrison HG, Huber JA, et al. Microbial diversity in the deep sea and the underexplored "rare biosphere". Proc Natl Acad Sci U S A 2006;103(32): 12115–20.

54. Elshahed MS, Youssef NH, Spain AM, et al. Novelty and uniqueness patterns of rare members of the soil biosphere. Appl Environ Microbiol 2008;74(17):5422–8.

55. Abubucker S, Segata N, Goll J, et al. Metabolic reconstruction for metagenomic data and its application to the human microbiome. PLoS Comput Biol 2012;8(6): e1002358.

56. Beck JM, Young VB, Huffnagle GB. The microbiome of the lung. Transl Res 2012;160(4):258–66.

57. Grif K, Heller I, Prodinger WM, et al. Improvement of detection of bacterial pathogens in normally sterile body sites with a focus on orthopedic samples by use of a commercial 16S rRNA broad-range PCR and sequence analysis. J Clin Microbiol 2012;50(7):2250–4.

58. Sibley CD, Church DL, Surette MG, et al. Pyrosequencing reveals the complex polymicrobial nature of invasive pyogenic infections: microbial constituents of

empyema, liver abscess, and intracerebral abscess. Eur J Clin Microbiol Infect Dis 2012;31(10):2679–91.

59. Finegold SM, Dowd SE, Gontcharova V, et al. Pyrosequencing study of fecal microflora of autistic and control children. Anaerobe 2010;16(4):444–53.

60. Benach JL, Li E, McGovern MM. A microbial association with autism. MBio 2012;3(1). pii: e00019–12.

61. Larsen N, Vogensen FK, van den Berg FW, et al. Gut microbiota in human adults with type 2 diabetes differs from non-diabetic adults. PLoS One 2010;5(2): e9085.

62. Giongo A, Gano KA, Crabb DB, et al. Toward defining the autoimmune micro-biome for type 1 diabetes. ISME J 2010;5(1):82–91.

63. Huang YJ, Lynch SV, Wiener-Kronish JP. From microbe to microbiota: consid-ering microbial community composition in infections and airway diseases. Am J Respir Crit Care Med 2012;185(7):691–2.

64. Dowd SE, Wolcott RD, Kennedy J, et al. Molecular diagnostics and personalised medicine in wound care: assessment of outcomes. J Wound Care 2011;20(5): 232–9.

65. Rhoads DD, Wolcott RD, Sun Y, et al. Comparison of culture and molecular iden-tification of bacteria in chronic wounds. Int J Mol Sci 2012;13(3):2535–50.

66. Dowd SE, Delton Hanson J, Rees E, et al. Survey of fungi and yeast in polymi-crobial infections in chronic wounds. J Wound Care 2011;20(1):40–7.

67. Al Masalma M, Armougom F, Scheld WM, et al. The expansion of the microbio-logical spectrum of brain abscesses with use of multiple 16S ribosomal DNA sequencing. Clin Infect Dis 2009;48(9):1169–78.

68. Al Masalma M, Lonjon M, Richet H, et al. Metagenomic analysis of brain ab-scesses identifies specific bacterial associations. Clin Infect Dis 2012;54(2): 202–10.

69. Moojen DJ, van Hellemondt G, Vogely HC, et al. A prospective multicenter study investigating the incidence of low-grade infection in aseptic loosening of total hip arthroplasty. Acta Orthop 2010;81(6):667–73.

70. Bjerkan G, Witsø E, Nor A, et al. A comprehensive microbiological evaluation of fifty-four patients undergoing revision surgery due to prosthetic joint loosening. J Med Microbiol 2012;61(Pt 4):572–81.

71. Xu Y, Rudkjøbing VB, Simonsen O, et al. Bacterial diversity in suspected pros-thetic joint infections: an exploratory study using 16S rRNA gene analysis. FEMS Immunol Med Microbiol 2012;65(2):291–304.

72. Motoshima M, Yanagihara K, Morinaga Y, et al. Identification of bacteria directly from positive blood culture samples by DNA pyrosequencing of the 16S rRNA gene. J Med Microbiol 2012;61(Pt 11):1556–62.

73. Insa R, Marín M, Martín A, et al. Systematic use of universal 16S rRNA gene poly-merase chain reaction (PCR) and sequencing for processing pleural effusions im-proves conventional culture techniques. Medicine (Baltimore) 2012;91(2):103–10.

74. Xu Y, Moser C, Al-Soud WA, et al. Culture-dependent and -independent inves-tigations of microbial diversity on urinary catheters. J Clin Microbiol 2012;50(12): 3901–8.

75. Branton WG, Ellestad KK, Maingat F, et al. Brain microbial populations in HIV/ AIDS: α-proteobacteria predominate independent of host immune status. PLoS One 2013;8(1):e54673.

76. Aarthi P, Harini R, Sowmiya M, et al. Identification of bacteria in culture negative and polymerase chain reaction (PCR) positive intraocular specimen from pa-tients with infectious endophthalmitis. J Microbiol Methods 2011;85(1):47–52.

77. DiGiulio DB, Romero R, Kusanovic JP, et al. Prevalence and diversity of microbes in the amniotic fluid, the fetal inflammatory response, and pregnancy outcome in women with preterm pre-labor rupture of membranes. Am J Reprod Immunol 2010;64(1):38–57.

78. Foreman A, Boase S, Psaltis A, et al. Role of bacterial and fungal biofilms in chronic rhinosinusitis. Curr Allergy Asthma Rep 2012;12(2):127–35.

79. Liu CM, Cosetti MK, Aziz M, et al. The otologic microbiome: a study of the bacterial microbiota in a pediatric patient with chronic serous otitis media using 16SrRNA gene-based pyrosequencing. Arch Otolaryngol Head Neck Surg 2011;137(7):664–8.

80. Wang T, Derhovanessian A, DeCruz S, et al. Subsequent infections in survivors of sepsis epidemiology and outcomes. J Intensive Care Med 2013;28(2). in press.

81. Leid JG, Cope E. Population level virulence in polymicrobial communities associated with chronic disease. Front Biol 2011;6(6):435–45.

82. Nelson A, De Soyza A, Perry JD, et al. Polymicrobial challenges to Koch's postulates: ecological lessons from the bacterial vaginosis and cystic fibrosis microbiomes. Innate Immun 2012;18(5):774–83.

83. Ren T, Glatt DU, Nguyen TN, et al. 16S rRNA survey revealed complex bacterial communities and evidence of bacterial interference on human adenoids. Environ Microbiol 2013;15(2):535–47.

84. Jeraldo P, Sipos M, Chia N, et al. Quantification of the relative roles of niche and neutral processes in structuring gastrointestinal microbiomes. Proc Natl Acad Sci U S A 2012;109(25):9692–8.

85. Abreu NA, Nagalingam NA, Song Y, et al. Sinus microbiome diversity depletion and Corynebacterium tuberculostearicum enrichment mediates rhinosinusitis. Sci Transl Med 2012;4(151):151ra124.

86. Khoruts A, Dicksved J, Jansson JK, et al. Changes in the composition of the human fecal microbiome after bacteriotherapy for recurrent Clostridium difficile-associated diarrhea. J Clin Gastroenterol 2010;44(5):354–60.

87. Reeves AE, Theriot CM, Bergin IL, et al. The interplay between microbiome dynamics and pathogen dynamics in a murine model of Clostridium difficile Infection. Gut Microbes 2011;2(3):145–58.

88. Im GY, Modayil RJ, Lin CT, et al. The appendix may protect against clostridium difficile recurrence. Clin Gastroenterol Hepatol 2011;9(12):1072–7.

89. Lawley TD, Clare S, Walker AW, et al. Targeted restoration of the intestinal microbiota with a simple, defined bacteriotherapy resolves relapsing Clostridium difficile disease in mice. PLoS Pathog 2012;8(10):e1002995.

90. Pace NR. Mapping the tree of life: progress and prospects. Microbiol Mol Biol Rev 2009;73(4):565–76.

91. Kimura M. Estimation of evolutionary distances between homologous nucleotide sequences. Proc Natl Acad Sci U S A 1981;78(1):454–8.

92. Cole JR, Chai B, Marsh TL, et al. The Ribosomal Database Project (RDP-II): previewing a new autoaligner that allows regular updates and the new prokaryotic taxonomy. Nucleic Acids Res 2003;31(1):442–3.

93. Schloss PD. Secondary structure improves OTU assignments of 16S rRNA gene sequences. ISME J 2013;7(3):457–60.

94. Clarke J, Wu HC, Jayasinghe L, et al. Continuous base identification for single-molecule nanopore DNA sequencing. Nat Nanotechnol 2009;4(4):265–70.

95. Korlach J, Bjornson KP, Chaudhuri BP, et al. Real-time DNA sequencing from single polymerase molecules. Meth Enzymol 2010;472:431–55.

96. Eid J, Fehr A, Gray J, et al. Real-time DNA sequencing from single polymerase molecules. Science 2009;323(5910):133–8.

97. Eyre DW, Golubchik T, Gordon NC, et al. A pilot study of rapid benchtop sequencing of Staphylococcus aureus and Clostridium difficile for outbreak detection and surveillance. BMJ Open 2012;2(3):e0011224.

98. Angiuoli SV, White JR, Matalka M, et al. Resources and costs for microbial sequence analysis evaluated using virtual machines and cloud computing. PLoS One 2011;6(10):e26624.

99. Rogers YH, Venter JC. Genomics: massively parallel sequencing. Nature 2005; 437(7057):326–7.

100. Mardis ER. Anticipating the $1,000 genome. Genome Biol 2006;7(7):112.

101. Gullapalli RR, Desai KV, Santana-Santos L, et al. Next generation sequencing in clinical medicine: challenges and lessons for pathology and biomedical informatics. J Pathol Inform 2012;3(1):40.

102. Mavromatis K, Land ML, Brettin TS, et al. The fast changing landscape of sequencing technologies and their impact on microbial genome assemblies and annotation. PLoS One 2012;7(12):e48837.

103. Klassen JL, Currie CR. Gene fragmentation in bacterial draft genomes: extent, consequences and mitigation. BMC Genomics 2012;13(1):14.

104. Church GM, Gao Y, Kosuri S. Next-generation digital information storage in DNA. Science 2012;337(6102):1628.

105. Wiecek AS. NCBI database shut down averted. Biotechniques 2011;50:4.

106. Schweitzer EJ. Reconciliation of the cloud computing model with US federal electronic health record regulations. J Am Med Inform Assoc 2012;19(2): 161–5.

107. Ahuja SP, Mani S, Zambrano J. A survey of the state of cloud computing in healthcare. Netw Comm Tech 2012;1(2):12.

108. Torri F, Dinov ID, Zamanyan A, et al. Next generation sequence analysis and computational genomics using graphical pipeline workflows. Genes (Basel) 2012;3(3):545–75.

109. Zhang Y, Erdmann J, Chilton J, et al. CLIA-certified next-generation sequencing analysis in the cloud. BMC Proc 2012;6(Suppl 6):54.

110. Clinical and Laboratory Standards Institute (CLSI). Nucleic acid sequencing methods in diagnostic laboratory medicine; approved guideline. CLSI document MM9-A (ISBN 1-56238-558-3). Wayne (PA): Clinical and Laboratory Standards Institute; 2004.

111. Clinical and Laboratory Standards Institute (CLSI). Genotyping for infectious diseases: identification and characterization; approved guideline (MM10-A). Wayne (PA): Clinical and Laboratory Standards Institute; 2004.

112. Clinical and Laboratory Standards Institute (CLSI). Interpretive criteria for identification of bacteria and fungi by DNA target sequencing; approved guideline (MM18-A). Wayne (PA): Clinical and Laboratory Standards Institute; 2004.

113. Ashelford KE, Chuzhanova NA, Fry JC, et al. At least 1 in 20 16S rRNA sequence records currently held in public repositories is estimated to contain substantial anomalies. Appl Environ Microbiol 2005;71(12):7724–36.

114. Schloss PD, Gevers D, Westcott SL. Reducing the effects of PCR amplification and sequencing artifacts on 16S rRNA-based studies. PLoS One 2011;6(12): e27310.

115. Haas BJ, Gevers D, Earl AM, et al. Chimeric 16S rRNA sequence formation and detection in Sanger and 454-pyrosequenced PCR amplicons. Genome Res 2011;21(3):494–504.

116. Conlan S, Kong HH, Segre JA. Species-level analysis of DNA sequence data from the NIH human microbiome project. PLoS One 2012;7(10):e47075.

117. Campbell BJ, Kirchman DL. Bacterial diversity, community structure and potential growth rates along an estuarine salinity gradient. ISME J 2012;7(1): 210–20.

118. Gilbert JA, Field D, Swift P, et al. The seasonal structure of microbial communities in the Western English Channel. Environ Microbiol 2009;11(12):3132–9.

119. Gilbert JA, Field D, Swift P, et al. Defining seasonal marine microbial community dynamics. ISME J 2011;6(2):298–308.

120. Caporaso JG, Paszkiewicz K, Field D, et al. The Western English Channel contains a persistent microbial seed bank. ISME J 2011;6(6):1089–93.

121. Campbell BJ, Yu L, Heidelberg JF, et al. Activity of abundant and rare bacteria in a coastal ocean. Proc Natl Acad Sci U S A 2011;108(31):12776–81.

122. Hunt DE, Lin Y, Church MJ, et al. The relationship between abundance and specific activity of bacterioplankton in open ocean surface waters. Appl Environ Microbiol 2012;79(1):177–84.

123. Gilbert KJ, Andrew RL, Bock DG, et al. Recommendations for utilizing and reporting population genetic analyses: the reproducibility of genetic clustering using the program STRUCTURE. Mol Ecol 2012;21(20):4925–30.

124. MacGowan AP, Wise R. Establishing MIC breakpoints and the interpretation of in vitro susceptibility tests. J Antimicrob Chemother 2001;48(Suppl 1):17–28.

125. Phillips I. Reevaluation of antibiotic breakpoints. Clin Infect Dis 2001;33(Suppl 3): S230–2.

126. Kahlmeter G, Brown DF, Goldstein FW, et al. European harmonization of MIC breakpoints for antimicrobial susceptibility testing of bacteria. J Antimicrob Chemother 2003;52(2):145–8.

127. Turnidge J, Paterson DL. Setting and revising antibacterial susceptibility breakpoints. Clin Microbiol Rev 2007;20(3):391–408.

128. Mitka M. Antibiotic breakpoints. JAMA 2012;307(10):1015.

129. Frei CR, Wiederhold NP, Burgess DS. Antimicrobial breakpoints for Gram-negative aerobic bacteria based on pharmacokinetic–pharmacodynamic models with Monte Carlo simulation. J Antimicrob Chemother 2008;61(3):621–8.

130. Benfey PN, Mitchell-Olds T. From genotype to phenotype: systems biology meets natural variation. Science 2008;320(5875):495–7.

131. Shortliffe EH, Axline SG, Buchanan BG, et al. An artificial intelligence program to advise physicians regarding antimicrobial therapy. Comput Biomed Res 1973; 6(6):544–60.

132. Sielaff BH, Johnson EA, Matsen JM. Computer-assisted bacterial identification utilizing antimicrobial susceptibility profiles generated by autobac 1. J Clin Microbiol 1976;3(2):105–9.

133. Williams KN, Davidson JM, Lynn R, et al. A computer system for clinical microbiology. J Clin Pathol 1978;31(12):1193–201.

134. Kricheysky MI. Coping with computers and computer evangelists. Annu Rev Microbiol 1982;36(1):311–41.

135. Khatib F, Cooper S, Tyka MD, et al. Algorithm discovery by protein folding game players. Proc Natl Acad Sci U S A 2011;108(47):18949–53.

136. Carruthers S, Masson ME, Stege U. Human performance on hard non-Euclidean graph problems: vertex cover. J Problem Solving 2012;5(1) [article 5].

137. Von Ahn L. Games with a purpose. Computer 2006;39(6):92–4.

138. Quinn A, Bederson B. Human computation: charting the growth of a burgeoning field. Computer 2010;1(3):10–37.

139. Nov O, Ofer A, Anderson D. Dusting for science: motivation and participation of digital citizen science volunteers. Proc of the 2011 iConference. February 8–11, 2011, Seattle WA. p. 68–74.

140. Barrington L, Turnbull D, Lanckriet G. Game-powered machine learning. Proc Natl Acad Sci U S A 2012;109(17):6411–6.

141. Korpela EJ. SETI@ home, BOINC, and volunteer distributed computing. Annu Rev Earth Planet Sci 2012;40:69–87.

142. Moore JH, Lari RC, Hill D, et al. Human microbiome visualization using 3d technology. Pac Symp Biocomput 2011;154–64.

143. Zhu Z, Niu B, Chen J, et al. MGAviewer: a desktop visualization tool for analysis of metagenomics alignment data. Bioinformatics 2013;29(1):122–3.

144. Ondov BD, Bergman NH, Phillippy AM. Interactive metagenomic visualization in a Web browser. BMC Bioinformatics 2011;12(1):385.

145. Hawkins AK, O'Doherty KC. "Who owns your poop?": insights regarding the intersection of human microbiome research and the ELSI aspects of biobanking and related studies. BMC Med Genomics 2011;4:72.

146. Fierer N, Lauber CL, Zhou N, et al. Forensic identification using skin bacterial communities. Proc Natl Acad Sci U S A 2010;107(14):6477–81.

147. Kennedy DM, Stanton JA, García JA, et al. Microbial analysis of bite marks by sequence comparison of streptococcal DNA. PLoS One 2012;7(12):e51757.

148. Knights D, Kuczynski J, Charlson ES, et al. Bayesian community-wide culture-independent microbial source tracking. Nat Methods 2011;8(9):761–3.

149. Flores GE, Bates ST, Caporaso JG, et al. Diversity, distribution and sources of bacteria in residential kitchens. Environ Microbiol 2013;15(2):588–96.

150. Flores GE, Bates ST, Knights D, et al. Microbial biogeography of public restroom surfaces. PLoS One 2011;6(11):e28132.

151. Biesecker LG, Burke W, Kohane I, et al. Next-generation sequencing in the clinic: are we ready? Nat Rev Genet 2012;13(11):818–24.

152. Dowd SE, Delton Hanson J, Rees E, et al. Research survey of fungi and yeast in polymicrobial infections in chronic wounds. J Wound Care 2011;20(1):40–7.

153. Wolcott R, Dowd S. The role of biofilms: are we hitting the right target? Plast Reconstr Surg 2011;127(Suppl 1):36S–7S.

154. Berland LL, Silverman SG, Gore RM, et al. Managing incidental findings on abdominal CT: white paper of the ACR incidental findings committee. J Am Coll Radiol 2010;7(10):754–73.

155. Morris Z, Whiteley WN, Longstreth WT Jr, et al. Incidental findings on brain magnetic resonance imaging: systematic review and meta-analysis. BMJ 2009;339:b3016.

156. Wagner MM, Hogan WR. The accuracy of medication data in an outpatient electronic medical record. J Am Med Inform Assoc 1996;3(3):234–44.

157. Peabody JW, Luck J, Jain S, et al. Assessing the accuracy of administrative data in health information systems. Med Care 2004;42(11):1066–72.

158. Gevers D, Knight R, Petrosino JF, et al. The human microbiome project: a community resource for the healthy human microbiome. PLoS Biol 2012;10(8):e1001377.

Integration of Technology Into Clinical Practice

Christopher D. Doern, PhD

KEYWORDS

- MALDI-TOF MS • Walk away PCR • Clinical outcome(s) • Respiratory virus panel
- Immunocompromised • Decision support • Electronic medical record
- Polymerase chain reaction

KEY POINTS

- The first step in optimizing the clinical impact of new technology begins with selecting the right product for the laboratory environment.
- New technology can improve laboratory work flow but may not have the desired clinical impact if not properly implemented.
- MALDI-TOF MS promises to revolutionize the diagnosis of bacterial and fungal disease by identifying organisms faster, cheaper, and more accurately than conventional methods.
- New technological developments in molecular biology will allow laboratories without experienced molecular biologists to perform testing they previously could not.
- Passive reporting using an electronic medical record has greatly improved the transmission of laboratory information to physicians but also represents a barrier to optimal uptake of new technology.

INTRODUCTION

Historically, the diagnosis of most bacterial, fungal, and even viral infections has relied on growth and isolation of the causative pathogen in culture-based systems; only once a pathogen had been isolated could identification be attempted. This process was originally very labor intensive but, with advances in technology, it has become more automated, and as a result faster and more reliable. The purpose of this review is to discuss the implementation of several different technologies that are revolutionizing all aspects of microbiology. This article discusses subjects such as organism identification and multiplex diagnostic systems as well as reporting programs with a focus on implementation and maximizing the impact of these technologies on patient care.

Disclosures: C.D. Doern has received research funds and speaker's honoraria from bioMerieux, Siemens, and Becton Dickinson and consulting fees from Thermo Fisher.
Department of Pathology, Children's Medical Center Dallas, University of Texas Southwestern Medical Center, 1935 Medical District Drive, Mailcode B1.06, Dallas, TX 75235, USA
E-mail address: christopher.doern@utsouthwestern.edu

Clin Lab Med 33 (2013) 705–729
http://dx.doi.org/10.1016/j.cll.2013.03.004
0272-2712/13/$ – see front matter © 2013 Elsevier Inc. All rights reserved.

RAPID BACTERIAL IDENTIFICATION AND SUSCEPTIBILITY SYSTEMS

In 1982 Doern and colleagues[1] published a study assessing the clinical impact of rapid disk diffusion susceptibility testing from bacterial blood cultures. Of the 173 patients enrolled in this study, greater than 25% were found to be in need of a modification to their antibiotic regimen according to the rapid susceptibility result. Doern and colleagues found that rapid susceptibility testing led to a change in antibiotic therapy 24 hours earlier than conventional testing in two-thirds of the patients in which a change was warranted.

Although this study used low-technology disk diffusion, it illustrates a central theme for laboratories looking to implement technology: faster results improve patient care. Since that time, several other studies have evaluated the impact of rapid automated systems on patient care. Most of these studies have focused on blood culture identification because patients with bloodstream infection are often very ill and stand to derive the most benefit from improved turnaround times.[2–4]

One of the first studies assessing the impact of automated bacterial identification and susceptibility systems on patient care was published by Trenholme and colleagues[5] in the *Journal of Clinical Microbiology* in 1989. They used the Vitek AutoMicrobic system (bioMeriéux, Marcy l'Étoile, France) to generate identifications and susceptibilities directly from positive blood culture isolates. They found that the direct method generated results nearly 40 hours earlier than conventional methods and was significantly more likely to result in a change in patient care. This method suggests that rapid technologies will allow physicians to manage their patients more efficiently. Although Trenholme and coworkers did not assess clinical outcomes such as rate of mortality, they did find rapid test methods to result in less antibiotic usage through de-escalating or switching to effective but less expensive therapies. Other studies investigating different rapid methodologies from all specimens[6,7] or from normally sterile body sites[8] have come to similar conclusions.

These studies all come to the obvious conclusion that faster is better. Trenholme and colleagues[5] offer some unique data to explain this phenomenon. In their study they found that not only did rapid results improve parameters surrounding antibiotic use and hospital charges, but in addition, infectious disease recommendations were more likely to be accepted when presented from the rapid method. The reasons for this finding are unclear, but it seems likely that when recommendations are made 48 hours or more after specimen collection, patients have already declared themselves by responding or not responding to therapy. Physicians are less likely to change therapy in patients who are improving and have already changed in those patients who are worsening, thus minimizing the impact of advice given at later time points.

A less obvious component of these studies is the manner in which reporting of results occurred. The Doern (1982), Trenholme, Kerremans, and Doern (1994) studies all relied on actively reporting of laboratory results via a telephone call to either an infectious disease fellow or the patient's provider.[1,5,6,8] This observation is important because the current standard practice in most laboratories is to send results passively to an electronic medical record (EMR). A significant disadvantage of this reporting system is the gap in time between when a result is sent to the EMR and when a physician accesses that result. That gap may minimize or eliminate the benefits of implemented technologies designed to improve turnaround times. These studies all eliminated this lag and optimized the impact of their systems by actively reporting results.

Interestingly, one randomized controlled study in the Netherlands found that shortening turnaround times for microbial procedures had no effect on clinical outcomes.[9]

An important difference in this study, though, is that only those results deemed "clinically relevant" by technologists were communicated orally. The definition of "clinical significance" was not given in this study so it is unclear which results were actually communicated orally. The reasons for this observation are unclear. It may be that differences in the way health care is delivered in the Netherlands contributed to their findings.

Negative data are rarely published so it is difficult to make conclusions about what strategies fail to improve patient care. Nonetheless, the Bruins study, contrasted with others, seems to suggest that active reporting is critical to realizing the full benefit of implemented technologies.[9]

These studies also represent what has become the norm in clinical microbiology. Automated identification and susceptibility technology resulted in a significant improvement in microbiology result turnaround times. With the advent of matrix-assisted laser desorption ionization time-of-flight mass spectrometry (MALDI-TOF MS) for organism identification and rapid molecular techniques, microbiology turnaround times will again be accelerated. These studies suggest that this will improve patient care.

DIAGNOSTIC TESTS PERFORMED ON POSITIVE BLOOD CULTURE SPECIMENS

Episodes of bloodstream infection constitute medical emergencies and as a result numerous molecular assays have been designed to identify organisms from positive blood cultures rapidly. These assays have been shown to have excellent analytical performance.[10–13]

Given the emergent nature of bloodstream infections, rapid blood culture diagnostic methods may be one of the most important tests a clinical microbiology laboratory could implement. Indeed, several studies have shown that the use of these assays can improve patient care.[14–17] It is important to note, however, that all of these studies, like those mentioned earlier in this review, used antimicrobial stewardship programs and active reporting. The reader is referred to the article on rapid diagnostics from positive blood culture broth in this monograph for the specific details and performance characteristics of these assays. **Table 1** lists studies that investigated the impact of implementing rapid diagnostics.

In addition to communicating critical results directly, laboratories must also carefully craft electronic reports so that they are clearly understood. Implementation of rapid blood culture diagnostics will constitute a significant change for the practice of most providers. In the initial phases of implementation this could lead to confusion and misuse of information if results are not clearly communicated. Another important aspect of implementation is educating the medical staff as to the pending changes. It is vital that infectious disease specialists, pharmacists, and antimicrobial stewardship programs (if they exist) be involved in the implementation process.

Last, these tests are expensive and do not supplant traditional culture-based techniques for confirmatory identification and susceptibility. In light of the fact that conventional testing is not eliminated, laboratories will need to implement policies addressing the frequency of repeat testing as a cost-containment measure. As an example, Spencer and colleagues[10] limited molecular testing of positive blood cultures to every 3 days for patients with previously positive cultures for methicillin-resistant *Staphylococcus aureus*. Laboratories can also argue that, although their budget will increase with the use of these tests, the hospital can expect to save money overall as demonstrated by these studies.[14–16]

Table 1
List of select studies evaluating the clinical impact of implementing different technology platforms

Technology	Intervention/Application	Study Type	Number of Patients	Reporting Method	Findings	Reference
Disk diffusion SUS	Rapid SUS performed directly from pos bid cx bottle	Retrospective review	173	Active (telephone)	Antibiotic regimen altered within 24 h of rapid result in 66.7% of patients in which a change was warranted	Doern et al,[1] 1982
Vitek AutoMicrobic ID and SUS	Rapid ID and SUS performed directly from pos bid cx bottle	Prospective randomized	226	Active (telephone)	Results available 40 h earlier with direct method. Recommendations from direct method more likely to be followed. Significant cost savings to patient.	Trenholme et al,[5] 1989
Baxter-Microscan WALKAWAY-96 ID and SUS	Rapid ID and SUS performed on all bacterial cultures	Prospective randomized	573	Active (telephone)	Results available ~12 h earlier with rapid method. Mortality rate lower in rapid method group (8.8% vs 15.3%). Lower hospital resource utilitization and cost in rapid method group.	Doern et al,[6] 1994
Vitek AutoMicrobic ID and SUS	Rapid verification of ID and SUS	Prospective intervention group with retrospective controls	765	Passive (EMR)	SUS results available 5 h earlier rapid verification group. Mortality was lowered but not statistically significant. Length of stay shorter by 1.9 d. Patient cost reduced by $1750.	Barenfanger et al,[7] 1999

bioMerieux Vitek 2 ID and SUS	Rapid ID and SUS performed on all bacterial cultures	Prospective randomized	597	Only results considered to be clinically significant were actively reported (telephone)	Turnaround time shorter in the rapid group. No difference in mortality, morbidity, or hospital cost observed.	Bruins et al,[9] 2005
Cepheid GeneXpert MRSA/SA rPCR blood culture test	Rapid ID of S. aureus and detection of mecA	Prospective intervention group with retrospective controls	156	Active (telephone)	Faster de-escalation from vancomycin to cefazolin/nafcillin by 1.7 d. Length of stay shortened by 6.2 d. Hospital costs decreased by >$20,000.	Bauer et al,[14] 2010
AdvanDx PNA FISH	Rapid ID of Candida albicans from pos bld cx bottle	Prospective intervention group with retrospective controls	72	Active (telephone)	Reduction in caspofungin usage. Hospital costs reduced by $1729.	Forrest et al,[16] 2006
AdvanDx PNA FISH	Rapid ID of Enterococcus faecium and E faecium from pos bld cx bottle	Prospective intervention group with retrospective controls	224	Active (telephone)	ID results available 2.3–3 d earlier. Time to initiating effective therapy was reduced. 30-d mortality reduced.	Forrest et al,[17] 2008
Bruker MALDI-TOF MS and BD Phoenix	Rapid ID (MALDI-TOF MS) and SUS (Phoenix) performed on all bacterial cultures	Prospective intervention group with retrospective controls	317	Active (telephone)	Length of stay shortened by 2.6 d. Hospital costs reduced by >$19,000.	Perez et al,[36] 2012

Abbreviations: EMR, electronic medical record; ID, identification; MRSA, methicillin-resistant *Staphylococcus aureus*; Pos bld cx, positive blood culture; SUS, susceptibility.

MALDI-TOF MS FOR ORGANISM IDENTIFICATION
Introduction

MALDI-TOF MS for microorganism identification is a technology that is rapidly gaining traction in the clinical microbiology laboratory and promises to revolutionize the way bacterial and fungal diseases are diagnosed. In contrast to conventional methods that rely on biochemical reactivity patterns for organism identification, MALDI-TOF MS generates identifications through analysis of whole cell protein fingerprints. The resulting identifications are produced much more rapidly and in many cases more accurately than with conventional methods. Another advantage of MALDI-TOF MS is that consumable costs on a per-test basis are generally much cheaper than conventional methods.[18] Last, because MALDI-TOF MS assesses preexisting protein components of an organism, it is capable of identifying fastidious or biochemically inert organisms that could not be reliably identified with conventional biochemical methods.

Given these improvements over conventional methods, MALDI-TOF MS is likely to replace conventional methods as the primary identification system in the very near future. As laboratories move to implement this technology, they will be faced with several decisions regarding how to maximize its potential. The following discussion provides some perspective on the critical issues surrounding implementation of MALDI-TOF MS.

Economics of MALDI-TOF MS

Unfortunately, one of the most important factors in deciding whether to implement any technology is cost. Like most technologies, MALDI-TOF MS comes with a steep price tag and laboratories can expect to pay several hundred thousand dollars for the instrument, easily making it one of the most expensive instruments in the microbiology laboratory. In addition, the service contracts can be very expensive but are typically considered to be essential.

Fortunately though, the consumable cost for MALDI-TOF MS analysis is quite low and much less than what laboratories are likely paying for existing conventional methods. Cherkaoui and colleagues[19] determined that on a per-test basis MALDI-TOF MS costs $0.50. They went on to do a comparison study to assess the savings generated by implementation of MALDI-TOF MS. They estimated that conventional methods cost about $10 for non-*Escherichia coli*, non-*S. aureus* identifications. Like many laboratories, they used a limited identification scheme for *E. coli* and *S. aureus* and estimated their cost to be $0.20 and $1.50, respectively. Even when they accounted for isolates requiring additional identifications (ie, isolates where MALDI-TOF MS failed) and factoring in the cost of the limited identifications, they found that it cost them ~$3,400 less to identify 720 consecutively collected clinical isolates over 21 days. The findings published by Cherkaoui can be extrapolated to estimate the expected return on investment for a MALDI-TOF MS. For example, a return on investment for a laboratory in a 600-bed hospital with an average of 10,000 annual organism identifications would be less than 3 years (unpublished data).

MALDI-TOF MS Work Flow

Given the simplicity and broad applicability of MALDI-TOF MS, it is tempting to conclude that implementation will decrease labor demands. Most laboratories have not found this to be the case. Many laboratories use combination panels or automated systems that allow them to process both a phenotypic identification and a susceptibility profile on the same instrument. MALDI-TOF MS requires that the identification be performed on a separate platform, which increases workload. One area where laboratories may see a decreased workload is in the workup of complicated, biochemically unreactive and unusual organisms. In particular, laboratories working with cultures from cystic fibrosis patients will likely find a simplified work flow.[20] In the author's laboratory, 6 months following implementation of MALDI they had essentially eliminated the use of auxiliary test methodologies. A few examples of tests that were no longer necessary were the API test strips (bioMeriéux, Marcy l'Etoile, France), Lancefield antigen testing, *Haemophilus* ID Triplate (Thermo Scientific, Waltham, MA, USA), and the Rapid Yeast ID (Siemens, Erlangen, Germany). If the experience is extrapolated out to a full year of using MALDI approximately $20,000 in API reagent costs alone will be saved. If an API takes on average 10 minutes of hands-on time to perform, 150 annual man-hours just in reduced API strip testing will also be saved (author's unpublished observation).

In analyzing cystic fibrosis cultures specifically, it was found before implementing MALDI-TOF MS that gram-negative isolates required on average 2.4 methods to generate a correct identification (spot or rapid biochemical tests, such as Gram-stain and oxidase were not counted as an "identification method" in this analysis). Following MALDI-TOF MS implementation, that number dropped to exactly 1. Importantly, this yielded a much improved turnaround time. Following implementation of MALDI-TOF MS, identifications were reported an average of 6 days earlier, which had the collateral benefit of improving reporting of susceptibility test results by 4.9 days as well. If and how this will impact patient care is yet unstudied.

Clinical Utility of MALDI-TOF MS

Dangers of MALDI-TOF MS

There is no question that MALDI-TOF MS will produce organism identifications more rapidly than conventional methods, which should translate into improved patient care.[20,21] Many investigators are starting studies to evaluate the benefit of MALDI beyond the laboratory, but laboratories must also be aware of the ways in which MALDI-TOF MS may have a negative impact on patient care.

Protocol deviation seems to be a natural part of the process of adopting MALDI-TOF MS technologies. Laboratories have strict protocols and procedures to guide culture workups. These protocols and procedures guide not only what types of organisms are identified but how they are reported. For example, most laboratory protocols state that single positive blood cultures growing non-*anthracis Bacillus* should be reported as "*Bacillus* spp." Before MALDI-TOF MS was used, many laboratories would not have attempted to identify these organisms to species level. In fact most laboratories would not have the ability to do so, requiring that the isolate be sent to a reference laboratory for identification. MALDI-TOF MS now gives laboratories the ability to identify *Bacillus* to the species level.

There are several potential pitfalls here. For laboratories using the Bruker instrument, unless they purchase a special database, *Bacillus anthracis* will not be present in the MALDI-TOF MS database and could therefore be misidentified as some other *Bacillus* spp. A second problem is that these *Bacillus* spp can now be easily sent to MALDI for definitive identifications and are subsequently reported to the species level, which is problematic because definitively identifying such an organism may suggest that it is of greater clinical significance than was intended. Laboratories should be sure to review protocols to ensure that technologists are familiar with proper resulting practice so that procedural drift does not occur.

The negative aspect of speed and ease

The ease with which MALDI-TOF MS can be performed is a blessing, but it can also be a curse. Due to the fact that MALDI-TOF MS identifications only require a single isolated colony and because a relatively small amount of growth is needed, technologists can obtain identifications earlier in the workup process than ever before. This speed makes a big difference for critical sterile cultures where physicians need information as quickly as possible.[2–4] However, in nonsterile cultures where the interpretation of a culture depends on the relative proportions of different organisms, this can prove problematic. In the past, these mixed cultures required subculturing to isolate pure colonies before conducting definitive identification testing. Although slow, this method had the benefit of allowing the culture to mature before reporting of organism identification and susceptibility results. Because MALDI-TOF MS does not ordinarily require such subcultures, definitive identifications can be obtained a full day earlier. In some cases slower growing organisms may not be apparent at the time of initial testing, leading to misinterpretation of culture results. This manifests itself most commonly in urine cultures where faster growing gram-negative bacilli are identified on the first day of analysis but, on reincubation, recovery of more slowly growing organisms may change the interpretation of the culture result (From Children's Medical Center Dallas, Microbiology Laboratory, unpublished observations). What initially appeared to be a culture consistent with urinary tract infection becomes a mixed specimen suggestive of urogenital flora colonization. One recommendation for avoiding this problem might be to set minimum incubation periods before reporting identifications. Although this strategy will extend turnaround times, it will help to minimize interpretation errors. It is also important for technologists to correlate specimen Gram-stain findings (when available) with those of their culture results.

Laboratory reporting of unusual organisms

A major limitation of MALDI-TOF MS is that currently it only produces organism identifications and does not provided susceptibility information. As a result, physicians will receive identifications in the absence of any kind of guidance as to what an organism can be treated with. Susceptibility information in most cases will follow at best 24 hours later, necessitating that physicians understand the appropriate empiric treatment of a given organism. In these cases the laboratory director can plan an important role in clarifying the interpretation of the culture result. Directors may want to conduct literature reviews and directly consult with providers to help guide the management of patients infected with unusual organisms.

In some cases, MALDI-TOF MS results may be confusing to physicians if they are not reported clearly. As an example, many organisms are actually part of large complexes that previously had only been reported to the complex level of resolution. Even most microbiologists would struggle to identify all members of the *Pseudomonas aeruginosa* group, of which there are over 40. **Table 2** lists some commonly reported organisms that are part of larger groups or complexes.[22,23]

In many cases MALDI-TOF MS is capable of producing identifications to a higher degree of resolution than the complex-level identification that is delivered using conventional phenotypic identification schemes.[20,24] However, this may lead to confusion about appropriate antibiotic selection. *Enterobacter cloacae*, for example, encodes a chromosomal, inducible *ampC* gene. The presence of this inducible mechanism is important because a high percentage of isolates will develop resistance when treated with third-generation cephalosporins.[25,26] *E. cloacae* is also a complex of organisms and reporting an identification of a species within that complex could be unfamiliar

Table 2
List of commonly encountered organisms that are part of groups or complexes

Enterobacter cloacae Complex	Citrobacter freundii Complex	Burkholderia cepacia Complex	Pseudomonas putida Group	Pseudomonas fluorescens Group	Pseudomonas aeruginosa Group
E. asburiae	C. braakii	B. multivorans	P. cremoricolorata	[a]	P. citronellolis
E. cancerogenus	C. freundii	B. cepacia	P. fulva		P. jinjuensis
E. dissolvens	C. gillenii	B. cenocepacia	P. mosselii		P. nitroreducens
E. hormaechei	C. murliniae	B. ambifaria	P. monteilii		P. panipatensis
E. kobei	C. rodenticum	B. anthina	P. parafulva		P. knackmussii
E. nimipressuralis	C. sedlakii	B. arboris	P. plecoglossicida		P. resinovorans
	C. wekmanii	B. contaminans			P. otitidis
	C. youngae	B. diffusa			P. indica
		B. dolosa			P. thermotolerans
		B. lata			P. alcaligenes
		B. lateens			
		B. metallica			
		B. pyrrocina			
		B. seminalis			
		B. stabiliz			
		B. vietnamiensis			

[a] There are currently >40 members of the P. fluorescens group.

or misleading. The same could be said about reporting within the *Citrobacter freundii* complex.

Strategies for implementing MALDI-TOF MS into clinical practice

Given the hurdles mentioned earlier, implementation of MALDI-TOF MS presents challenges that other technologies do not. Microbiology laboratories will need to manage implementation from several levels; in this section two are focused on: (1) the technologist and (2) the physician.

Most microbiologists will say that their initial reaction to using mass spectrometry for bacterial identification was skepticism. Microbiologists have been using traditional biochemical methods to identify organisms for decades. Using a methodology such as MALDI-TOF MS constitutes a departure from those methods and results in initial lack of trust in the results. The distrust is short-lived and quickly replaced by enthusiasm as technologists begin to experience the power and robustness of the results (personal observation and communication with laboratory directors). Nonetheless, the process of bringing in such a foreign technology requires education and time to become familiar with the new method. Verification studies provide an ideal opportunity for laboratory staff to familiarize themselves with MALDI-TOF MS before using it for clinical specimens.

Generally speaking, physicians do not care how organism identifications are derived, provided that the results they receive are accurate and actionable. MALDI-TOF MS will be no exception, but what MALDI-TOF MS may allow laboratories to do is report results on a more predictable schedule, allowing physicians to understand better when to expect results.

Nearly all reporting in microbiology is passive and as a result there is often a large gap in the time between when a result is ready for review and when it is actually acted on. If laboratories can produce results on a more regular schedule, physicians can know when to look for, and hopefully act on, those results. In a 2009 French study by Seng and colleagues,[27] a process is described by which results are available consistently by 9:30 AM. They claim that this has greatly improved physician uptake of the information and their ability to act on the results because most decision-making and follow-up orders are placed by 1 PM.

MALDI-TOF MS has a positive impact on laboratory/physician relations (personal observation and communication with laboratory directors). Technologists are regularly contacted by physicians requesting additional workup of organisms from nonsterile cultures, generally isolates that were originally deemed to be clinically insignificant by laboratory protocols. In most cases, response to these requests takes several days. The ability to provide near-immediate answers makes for an exciting and rewarding interaction with health care providers.

Making MALDI-TOF MS count for the patient

Thus far, no study has evaluated the impact of MALDI-TOF MS organism identification (from routine cultures) on patient outcomes. Several studies, discussed later, have assessed outcomes when MALDI-TOF MS is used to identify organisms directly from positive blood culture bottles. It remains to be seen if patient management will change when MALDI-TOF MS is applied as the primary system for routine organism identification. All studies that have been performed to date have focused on the improvements achieved in laboratory work flow, budget, result quality, and turnaround time.[27] One can reasonably infer from these findings that patient care will be positively impacted but to date no studies have measured the effect.

MALDI-TOF MS and blood cultures

It is now well-documented that MALDI-TOF MS is capable of identifying organisms directly out of positive blood culture bottles.[28–33] These methods are now being increasingly applied in clinical practice and studies are demonstrating the clinical benefit.

It seems intuitive that faster organism identification from positive blood cultures would improve the accuracy with which antibiotics are prescribed. However a high percentage of patients have antibiotic decisions made at the time of phlebotomy. These antibiotics decisions are empiric and generally include broad gram-positive and gram-negative coverage,[34] so it would seem that in most cases any change in antibiotic management would come in the form of narrowing or de-escalating therapy.

One interesting finding from the Munson study was that a larger percentage of patients had antibiotic changes made following the Gram-stain report than with the release of definitive antimicrobial susceptibility testing (AST).[34] The most likely interpretation of this finding is that definitive AST results are merely confirming the empiric decisions that physicians have been making based on patient information and Gram-stain results, suggesting that MALDI-TOF MS identifications applied to positive blood cultures bottles would have a significant impact on patient care because it would provide more definitive information at an important decision point for antimicrobial management.

Indeed, when Clerc and colleagues[35] conducted a prospective observational study looking at the impact of using MALDI-TOF MS on positive blood cultures, they found that Gram-stain had an impact on the care of approximately 21% of cases and MALDI-TOF MS impacted 35% of cases. This study focused on gram-negative organisms exclusively, and patients who were not being seen by infectious disease physicians were excluded. When the authors analyzed the changes in antibiotic use that were made, they found that most interventions based on MALDI-TOF MS results were broadening of antibiotic coverage, which is not surprising considering that most gram-negative bloodstream infections are due to the *Enterobacteriaceae* and nonfermenting gram-negative bacilli. These categories of organisms are not considered to be predictably susceptible to narrow spectrum antibiotics so physicians usually wait for AST results before de-escalating therapy.

If the primary impact of MALDI-TOF MS identification on gram-negative bacteremia is broadening of coverage, then its usefulness will be impacted directly by the institutions' most commonly used empiric therapy. Institutions with very broad empiric choices such as a carbapenems will probably find MALDI-TOF MS identification of gram-negative isolates less useful than that an institution that relies on third-generation cephalosporins. This, of course, will also be impacted directly by local resistance patterns.

A recent study published by Perez and colleagues[36] demonstrated a more profound effect on the care of patients with gram-negative bacteremia. In this study MALDI-TOF MS was used to identify organisms directly from positive blood culture bottles, and in addition, a susceptibility panel was directly inoculated from the blood culture broth. This study found that time to identification and susceptibility improved by 25 and 23 hours, respectively. In addition they found that the time to an antibiotic adjustment improved by 31 hours. All findings were statistically significant. The study also assessed parameters such as length of stay and hospital charges. Overall hospital charges were reduced by approximately $19,000 and length of stay following the positive culture was 1.8 days shorter in the invention group.

In contrast to bloodstream infections caused by gram-negative bacteria, it is much easier to envision scenarios involving gram-positive bacteria in which organism identification directly from blood culture bottles would provide information that would allow a physician to de-escalate antibiotic therapy. A common dilemma faced by clinicians is deciding whether a gram-positive coccus isolate constitutes real infection or is a blood culture contaminant.[37] MALDI-TOF MS could be used to establish the difference rapidly between coagulase-negative Staphylococci and *S. aureus* or between a viridans group streptococci and group A *Streptococcus*, Group B *Streptococcus, Streptococcus pneumoniae*, or even *Enterococcus*. Armed with these more rapid identifications, physicians would better be able to decide whether aggressive treatment was warranted, to decide if antibiotics could be discontinued, or even to prevent a patient being readmitted for antimicrobial therapy (as in the case of a contaminant).

Indeed, several publications are starting to show that MALDI-TOF MS can be used effectively in this way.[28–31,33,38] The Clerc study is one of the only studies conducted to date to look at the impact of MALDI-TOF MS results on antibiotic use. However, Romero-Gomez and colleagues[32] developed an interesting technique in which they combined a MALDI-TOF MS identification with a rapid susceptibility test. In their study they performed direct identifications with MALDI-TOF MS as well as a susceptibility test inoculated directly from the positive blood culture bottle. Of over 300 positive monomicrobic blood cultures, 97.7% of the *Enterobacteriaceae*, 75.8% of *S. aureus*, and 63.3% of coagulase-negative Staphylococci were identified correctly. This method did not produce any incorrect identification results. However, the study did not include any isolates of *S. pneumoniae* or viridans group streptococci, organisms that MALDI-TOF MS cannot reliably differentiate.[30] The correlation of the rapid susceptibility method with standardized methods was between 92% and 98%. Despite relatively high agreement, there were a significant number of very major errors (VME), or false susceptibility. Of critical importance are errors made for drugs likely to be used empirically, such as cefotaxime (3 VME), ceftazidime (1 VME), cefepime (1 VME), and piperacillin-tazobactam (4 VME). Given the extent of VMEs, laboratories may be slow to adopt such an approach. These errors also necessitate that the results be confirmed with standardized susceptibility testing, resulting in a duplication of effort. In addition, these processes require significant amounts of hands-on time and are technically demanding, which may make it difficult to accommodate on shifts where staff is minimal.

That said, determination of methicillin susceptibility for *S. aureus* is one of the most important and time-sensitive susceptibility results that can be provided for a blood culture. The Romero-Gomez study tested 18 *S. aureus* isolates and found no errors with methicillin testing.[32] This susceptibility method involved inoculating Vitek 2 susceptibility cards based on the identification provided by MALDI-TOF MS. A standard inoculum was prepared and organism collected by centrifuging blood culture broth.

Another critical result for physician decision-making is *Enterococcus* vancomycin susceptibility. In this study all 22 Enterococci were accurately categorized with the direct susceptibility method.[32]

As laboratories consider implementing MALDI-TOF MS testing from positive blood cultures, the lack of a corresponding susceptibility result could significantly diminish its clinical impact. Although direct susceptibility testing has its limitations, it may be that it performs accurately for the bug/drug combinations that matter most. Thus a combination approach could augment the utility of MALDI-TOF MS identifications and improve clinical impact.

In the absence of providing susceptibility testing for individual isolates, laboratories may take other approaches to guide therapeutic decisions. One strategy might be to include antibiogram information along with organism identification. Laboratories may even choose to develop unit-specific or patient-specific information in institutions providing care for diverse patient populations.

MOLECULAR TECHNOLOGY
Introduction

Molecular biology has revolutionized the way viral infections are diagnosed and emerging assays promise to do the same for bacterial infections. In virology, what used to be slow (culture) and insensitive (direct fluorescence antigen [DFA], rapid antigen) has become fast, highly sensitive, and specific with molecular techniques. The power of a polymerase chain reaction (PCR) assay is that it can be designed to detect a wide variety of pathogens and in many cases can provide quantitative values.

The objective of this review is to discuss implementing these technologies so as to maximize clinical impact. There are far too many different platform/analyte combinations to discuss them all in detail. Rather, the following paragraphs analyze the pertinent characteristics that one would want to consider when adopting a given platform. Also discussed is what has been learned about the clinical impact of implementing a few of the more commonly ordered molecular tests, namely respiratory viral panels and quantitative Epstein-Barr virus (EBV). Last the future of molecular diagnostics and gastroenteritis is discussed.

Product Selection

Many laboratories now find that send-out test volumes are increasing and account for a disproportionate percentage of laboratory costs.[39] In some laboratories, molecular diagnostics for infectious diseases may constitute a high percentage of the microbiology send-out volume. Due to the high price and slow turnaround time of this testing, there are both financial and clinical incentives to perform these tests on site. A good first step when assessing what tests to target for development is to simply look at volumes, costs, and turnaround times of send-out testing. As an example, the author's institution provides care for a complex pediatric population that includes active solid organ and bone marrow transplant programs. Consequently, the physicians order high volumes of quantitative EBV (n = 3700/y), adenovirus (n = 550/y), and BK (n = 360/y) PCRs, all of which were being sent out. By bringing these tests in-house, it is estimated that the laboratory would save well over $100,000 annually.

Once the decision has been made to perform molecular testing in the clinical laboratory, a testing platform must be selected. There are several factors a laboratory must consider when selecting a molecular platform. What is driving the implementation of most technologies is clinical necessity and a surprisingly large number of clinically important tests are *not* FDA cleared. The Association for Molecular Pathology provides an updated document that tracks FDA-cleared assays (www.amp.org/FDATable/FDATable.doc; accessed February 2013). This information can also be obtained on the FDA's Web site itself (http://www.accessdata.fda.gov/scripts/cdrh/devicesatfda/index.cfm; accessed February 2013). The decision to bring on a non-FDA-cleared assay is not a trivial one, as these tests require more rigorous verification studies than FDA-cleared assays. Cumitech 31A[40] provides guidance on verifying the performance of laboratory tests. In addition, depending on whether the assay contains research use only reagents, the laboratory may choose not to bill for testing.

Laboratories opting to bring non-FDA-cleared tests in-house will need an open platform on which to develop their test. There are many traditional real-time PCR instrument options but very few that offer the ability to develop what is referred to as "walk-away" assays. Walk-away assays are performed on an instrument that completes the nucleic acid extraction, purification, amplification, and detection all on one instrument. These instruments are generally self-contained and require very little specimen and reagent manipulation and, in most cases, minimal technologist time.

One of the first such instruments to come to market was the Cepheid GeneXpert (Sunnyvale, CA, USA). Originally this instrument was an open platform allowing for test development, but it has since been closed and only assays produced by Cepheid can be performed on the instrument. Other variations of walk-away technology include the Tigris (Gen-Probe, San Diego, CA, USA), FilmArray (BioFire Diagnostics, Inc, Salt Lake City, UT, USA), Verigene (Nanosphere, Northbrook, IL, USA), and Integrated Cycler (Focus Diagnostics, Cypress, CA, USA). None of these technologies would be considered open platforms, although Focus sells a variety of analyte-specific reagents produced for use with the Integrated Cycler.

Becton Dickinson (Franklin Lakes, NJ, USA) has recently acquired the BD MAX system, which offers consumers an open "walk-away" platform on which they can develop their own assays. Becton Dickinson has developed a series of extraction products made specifically for the instrument, leaving only the analyte-specific portion of the assay open for development. The instrument is capable of running up to 24 samples simultaneously.

Laboratories seeking to develop molecular tests where amplification is performed separately from nucleic acid purification have a large number of options. A few of the more common platforms for real-time PCR test development are the LighCycler (Roche, Indianapolis, IN, USA), Cepheid SmartCycler, and Applied Biosystems ABI 7500 (Melbourne, Australia).

Quantitative Tests

Laboratories that provide testing for immunocompromised patients have a high demand for several important molecular tests for which no FDA-approved assays are available. Such tests include quantitative assays for EBV, BK virus, and adenovirus. Herpes simplex virus PCR from blood is also a commonly ordered quantitative assay.

The central problem surrounding quantitative tests is that the results are highly variable from laboratory to laboratory and there is no standardized interpretation for the values provided.[41] Although there are numerous articles assessing their clinical relevance, it is difficult to extrapolate findings into another institution's clinical practice because of the variability in test methodologies.[42] The first step in developing interpretive criteria for these assays is establishing a standard by which all assays can be compared, which has recently been accomplished with the development of the World Health Organization CMV standard. Using this standard, Hirsch and colleagues[43] were able to demonstrate high interlaboratory agreement for quantitative CMV viral loads over 4 orders of magnitude.

The following sections discuss some specific assays and look at the steps that laboratories may want to take to integrate each assay properly into clinical practice.

EBV PCR

Quantitative EBV PCR is used as a marker of B-cell expansion in post-transplant lymphoproliferative disease (PTLD). The diagnosis of PTLD can be very challenging and having a noninvasive marker of the disease, such as EBV PCR, can be extremely valuable. The problem is that there is no one value that is diagnostic for PTLD and, although EBV PCR positivity is very sensitive for PTLD associated with EBV, it lacks specificity.[44] Although rare, there are also forms of PTLD that are not associated with EBV.[45]

A significant problem when a laboratory brings in or decides to change quantitative EBV assays is that the values of the new test will be different from the old test. These changes in interpretive value can significantly impact the way the physicians manage their patients. At Children's Medical Center in Dallas, TX, their assay was found to produce values that were roughly 10-fold higher than that of their reference laboratory (data not shown). Implementing a test that produced significantly different values required extensive collaboration with physicians so they could adjust their clinical practice. They learned through this collaboration that despite the lack of interpretive guidance for EBV PCR values, their physicians had adopted a rough viral load cutoff value, above which they began to consider enacting their PTLD protocols. These protocols involved nontrivial interventions like increased imaging frequency and adjustments in immunosuppression. A critical part to implementing the new test methodology successfully was working with the physicians to establish new clinically actionable values.

To facilitate the transition between old and new tests, laboratories may want to conduct parallel testing to compare the old and new methods for the first phase of implementation. This implementation is a costly practice but goes a long way toward improving physician comfort with the new testing and helps to transition previously positive patients onto the new assay. It was found that with this approach parallel testing is only required for a very short time before physicians become comfortable with the new results.

It is not uncommon for EBV PCR to be ordered to make the diagnosis of infectious mononucleosis. The test is not intended for this purpose and should not be ordered in this capacity. If resources are available, it can be beneficial financially and for patient care if EBV PCR's for nontransplant patients are approved by a pathologist, which allows the pathologist to get involved before test results have been obtained. It also provides a valuable opportunity to educate providers on the proper use and interpretation of the test. Because a high percentage of the population has been exposed and is therefore latently infected, the PCR has poor specificity for diagnosing active EBV disease.[46] At best, the assay might be reasonably used as an adjunct to ambiguous serologic results.[47] However, in most cases EBV PCR adds nothing but cost and confusion to the diagnosis of infectious mononucleosis.

Multiplex Testing

Multiplex molecular panels are becoming commonplace in the laboratory. Any test that detects greater than one analyte is a multiplex test. However, for the purposes of this review the implementation of multiplexed panels with 4 or more analytes is focused on.

Respiratory Virus Testing

These assays are all capable of detecting multiple pathogens simultaneously and offer significant advantages in sensitivity and specificity when compared with DFA, viral culture, and rapid antigen detection. Superior sensitivity and specificity notwithstanding, there is significant debate about whether the high price tag is justified by clinical utility.

Clinical Utility of Respiratory Viral Testing

Of all the viruses detected from respiratory specimens, only influenza is routinely treated with antiviral agents. This begs the question, why test for respiratory viral infection? Beyond guiding use of antiviral drugs, there are many important reasons to test for respiratory viral infection. It is well documented that undetected viral infections are a significant driver of antibiotic use, which almost certainly contributes to emerging antimicrobial resistance in bacteria.[48] Likewise, undetected viral infection drives unnecessary laboratory and radiologic investigations to rule out alternative causes of disease. It stands to reason then that identifying these viral pathogens would eliminate diagnostic uncertainty and result in reduced use of health care resources, including antibiotics.

Several studies have looked at the impact of rapid respiratory viral testing on the medical management of patients. Most investigate the impact of rapid antigen, DFA, or viral culture methodologies and only a relatively small number look at how molecular methods affect patient care. A modeling study from Mahony and colleagues[49] suggested that when compared with DFA and/or shell vial culture, the xTAG RVP by Luminex (Austin, TX) resulted in lower patient charges.[50] Interestingly though, the primary cost savings were derived from decreased length of stay and not a reduction in antibiotic usage or other diagnostic testing. The findings of the Mahony study conflict with those of Wishaupt and colleagues,[51] who found that real-time-PCR and rapid reporting of the results had no impact on length of stay, antibiotic use, or hospital admission. A similar study conducted in the Netherlands also concluded that real-time PCR testing had no impact on antibiotic usage in children with respiratory viral infection.[52] All studies were from single centers, which may limit their applicability to other institutions and the practice of their physicians.

A limitation of PCR testing methodologies is that they are often batched and suffer from slow turnaround times (TAT). Given the acute course of respiratory viral illness, it is possible that their clinical utility is limited by slow TAT. Rapid antigen tests have poor sensitivity and specificity but are simple to perform and can yield results in 15 to 30 minutes. With multiplex PCR methods such as the FilmArray (TAT = 1 h) entering the market, patients may be able to have the best of both worlds. There are no studies looking at the impact of rapid molecular tests on patient care but some insight can be gained into their possible impact by reviewing the rapid antigen detection literature.

A recent Cochrane Database review identified 4 randomized controlled studies looking at rapid antigen testing and their impact on patient care.[53] Taken together, these 4 studies demonstrated a minor reduction in antibiotic use in pediatric patients seen in the emergency department (ED), but this finding was not statistically significant. However, when taken individually, 2 of the 4 studies did find rapid antigen testing to have a statistically significant change on patient care. Bonner and colleagues[54] found that when rapid results were available fewer antibiotic prescriptions written, there were lower rates of chest X rays and ED length of stay was shorter. All findings were statistically significant. Doan and colleagues[55] did not find a difference in length of ED visit, chest X ray, blood tests, urine analysis, or initial antibiotic prescription with the use of a rapid antigen test. Interestingly though, they did find that rapid antigen test results significantly reduced antibiotic prescription 1 week after discharge from the ED.

The aforementioned studies provide very little evidence that respiratory viral testing has any impact on patient care. However, the molecular methods assessed were slow and the rapid antigen tests suffer from poor quality. It remains to be seen if the newer generation of "walk-away" platforms, such as the FilmArray, the GeneXpert, or the Integrated Cycler, which combine rapid (<2-h turnaround time) results with high sensitivity and specificity, will have a significant impact on patient care. The clinical impact of these platforms has not yet been evaluated.

Regardless of what the clinical outcome studies show, laboratories are seeing increased demand for this type of testing. In many cases this demand comes from inpatient providers who are caring for immunocompromised patients whereby these viral infections have a more severe course.[56] It is in these complex patients that respiratory viral panel testing promises to be of maximal benefit.

Multiplex Detection of Gastrointestinal Pathogens

It is likely that diagnostic testing for acute gastroenteritis will change significantly in the very near future. Several companies are developing or have developed multiplex molecular assays that are capable of detecting multiple pathogens in one test. These assays will combine diagnostics for bacterial, viral, and parasitic pathogens and, in some cases, their toxins, into one panel and promise to do so with greater sensitivity than conventional methods. As of yet, only the Luminex xTAG panel is FDA cleared for use in the United States, but it is expected that many will become available in 2013.

Implementing molecular testing for gastrointestinal pathogens is appealing to clinical microbiology laboratories because it would replace the vast majority of stool cultures. These cultures use numerous plates and are laborious to process. Instead, laboratories would use molecular methods as their primary test and culture only those that required susceptibility testing or epidemiologic investigation. The negative aspect for the laboratory is that the culture is relatively inexpensive compared with molecular testing and budgets will have to expand to accommodate these new methods.

Given the likely increase in cost to the laboratory, the question of whether to implement molecular testing will amount to differences in performance, clinical impact, and overall institutional costs.

Assessing Multiplex Panels and Their Possible Impact on the Management of Gastroenteritis

Of the multiplex products about to enter the market, there are some similarities in panel design but also some important differences that laboratories may want to consider. One important difference is the presence of *Clostridium difficile* on the panels. It has been well documented that high percentages of young children are asymptomatically colonized with *C. difficile*.[57] By age 3, carriage rates are similar to that of nonhospitalized adults (less than 3%).[58,59] However, carriage rates in hospitalized patients may be 10% or more.[60] Given these high rates of asymptomatic carriage, it is likely that indiscriminant testing for *C. difficile* will result in a high number of misleading positive results and clinical confusion. It is unclear what the final versions of these products will look like but it may be possible to blind certain results or laboratories may choose a selective reporting strategy.

Laboratories will also want to consider how these panels are offered to providers. Currently, providers select tests for specific categories of pathogens. Although there is significant overlap in symptoms between these pathogens, ordering patterns would suggest that providers think they can differentiate between viral, bacterial, and parasitic gastrointestinal disease. Introducing multiplex panels as they are currently configured will significantly change the way laboratories and providers think about diagnosing gastroenteritis.

First, laboratories commonly reject stool specimens for bacterial culture and/or ova and parasite analysis that are obtained from patients who have been hospitalized for greater than 3 days. In fact, it is a College of American Pathologists requirement to do so. However, there is a growing body of evidence suggesting that nosocomial acquisition of rotavirus and norovirus does occur.[61,62] With the combination of viral and bacterial diagnostics, it may no longer be reasonable or even possible for laboratories to have such rejection policies.

Second, these assays will readily detect mixed infections, the significance of which may not be fully understood, which has proven to be the case with implementation of multiplex respiratory viral panels, which detect a high rate of mixed infection.[63] Despite coinfection rates as high as 30%, the significance of these infections remains unclear.[63,64] The US Acute Gastroenteritis Etiology Study Team recently surveyed the cause of acute gastroenteritis in adults and found that nearly 10% of patients had mixed infections, many of which were mixed viral/bacterial infections.[65]

Third, a high percentage of stool cultures submitted for diagnostic testing are not accompanied by orders for viral pathogens. Nevertheless, the Bresee study as well as others, has suggested that a high percentage of viral gastroenteritis is probably undiagnosed.[65] It is unclear how the implementation of multiplex gastrointestinal panels will impact clinical outcomes as the management of many of these diseases is supportive. However, one positive outcome might be a reduction in unnecessary diagnostic procedures in patients infected with previously undiagnosed infections. These assays will also lead to a better understanding of nosocomial acquisition of viral gastroenteritis and aid in more rapid outbreak investigation.

COMMUNICATION OF RESULTS

Whether it is a bacterial identification, a susceptibility test, or a quantitative value, the importance of effective reporting cannot be overstated. New technology can improve laboratory efficiency, quality of results, and perhaps even reduce costs, but unless results are effectively communicated to the provider, they will not have the intended impact on patient care.

Earlier, the impact of rapid blood culture diagnostics on patient care was reviewed and it was concluded that their benefit was maximized when combined with active reporting. Communicating results directly is an obvious way to decrease reporting time but this is not a practical option for all laboratory values. As a result, the vast majority of communication takes place through the EMR. Given that the ability of any technology to improve patient care depends on communicating its results, a brief review of EMRs and other information management systems is warranted.

Electronic Medical Records

EMR are now ubiquitous in health care and offer significant advantages to hardcopy reporting. EMR provide easy access to large amounts of information, eliminate the waste and inconvenience of hardcopied data, and improve the speed with which data can be communicated. In some ways though, EMR are less effective means of communicating results. All microbiology results, with the exception of a small list of critical results, are passively reported. That is to say, the laboratory completes a test and sends information to the EMR, where a provider may or may not view it at some later date.

A survey study conducted by Bruins and colleagues[66] found that most, but not all, physicians preferred electronic to hardcopy reporting. This study also found that implementation of an EMR greatly reduced telephone calls to the laboratory as well as time to reporting of results. It is therefore somewhat surprising that they did not observe any change in provider decision-making. A likely explanation for this finding is that only final results were communicated electronically. Preliminary reports in this study were only reported by hardcopy, thus delaying their uptake by physicians. There are surprisingly few studies investigating the impact of EMRs on patient management. Ferris and colleagues[67] documented the benefits of an EMR on clinician and nurse work flow, but no measurement of its impact on patient outcomes has been published.

One study looked at the rate of missed test results in an Australian ED and found some discouraging results. They found that 32% of microbiology results were not accessed on the day they were provided.[68] Similarly, Kilpatrick and Holding[69] found that 45% of laboratory results issued for patients seen in the ED were never accessed.

Laboratories should be aware of their own institution's practices as they consider adopting expensive technologies to improve turnaround times for providers in time-sensitive situations. Understanding the true provider needs will help resource-strapped laboratories to prioritize the performance of tests that are needed and will be acted on in a timely manner.

Prior discussion may have suggested that in order for laboratories to maximize their clinical impact, all laboratory results should be communicated by telephone. This solution is of course impractical and one that the laboratory could not reasonably accommodate, nor would physicians want to be burdened with a high volume of telephone calls. One alternative that may be acceptable to both parties is an automated pager system. The impact of such a system has not been studied for microbiology results, but Kuperman and colleagues[70] studied its impact on notification of critical chemistry values. In this system, an automatic pager alert was sent to physicians to notify them of abnormal results, which were defined by rule-based alerting criteria. They found this system to significantly reduce the time it took a physician to act on the critical laboratory value and put patients on appropriate therapy.

Decision Support and Selective Reporting

Within the EMR, laboratories can use other tools to maximize their impact on patient care. A common strategy for laboratories is to report antibiotics selectively so as to direct providers to select optimal therapies. Not only can this approach reduce the chance than an ineffective antibiotic will be used, but it can also limit the use of potent antibiotics that are reserved for infections by more resistant organisms. Selective reporting can therefore be an important part of a hospital's antibiotic stewardship program.

No studies have shown a direct link between selective reporting and reduced emergence of antimicrobial resistance. However, Coupat and colleagues[71] suggested through a case-vignette study that selective reporting increased compliance with current recommendations for treating urinary tract infection. They also showed less variation and reduced use of broad-spectrum antibiotics in the intervention group exposed to selective reporting, which is important because in the same study they found that nearly 40% of physicians declared that they were not comfortable interpreting susceptibility results. Given this finding, it is not surprising that most physicians preferred having fewer antibiotics reported to them.

Computerized decision support systems can also be implemented to help providers make better use of laboratory information. Numerous studies have shown their impact on antibiotic prescriptions.[72–76] There are many forms in which these support models can be presented to providers. The most obvious and readily accessible will be to generate applications for the now ubiquitous smartphone. Indeed, at least one study has shown this to be a very effective way of making information accessible to providers at the bedside.[77] However, clinical decision support can have many forms, all of which can be used to either passively or actively modify clinician behavior.[78]

SUMMARY

The microbiology laboratory and its processes are being revolutionized with the implementation of new technology. In the era of diagnosis-related groups, laboratories are no longer compensated for each test performed; thus, it is important to analyze carefully which technology to adopt and how to do so. Laboratories will be asked to justify expensive instrumentation in several ways, including cost, laboratory work flow, and, most importantly, impact on patient outcome. In the final analysis, the technologies discussed in this review will only improve patient care if they are implemented carefully and with consideration for the practice of the providers they serve. Nearly all of the technologies discussed in this review promise to change the results and how they are reported to the provider. In most cases the end result will be higher quality information that is provided in a more rapid timeframe. Of critical importance to realizing the full potential of these improvements will be educating those acting on the results. Last, laboratories should be mindful of the limitations in their reporting systems and look for ways to communicate results efficiently, such that they are easily understood and can be acted on for maximal patient benefit.

REFERENCES

1. Doern GV, Scott DR, Rashad AL. Clinical impact of rapid antimicrobial susceptibility testing of blood culture isolates. Antimicrob Agents Chemother 1982; 21(6):1023–4.
2. Dellinger RP, Levy MM, Carlet JM, et al. Surviving Sepsis Campaign: international guidelines for management of severe sepsis and septic shock: 2008. Crit Care Med 2008;36(1):296–327.
3. Weinstein MP, Murphy JR, Reller LB, et al. The clinical significance of positive blood cultures: a comprehensive analysis of 500 episodes of bacteremia and fungemia in adults. II. Clinical observations, with special reference to factors influencing prognosis. Rev Infect Dis 1983;5(1):54–70.
4. Beekmann SE, Diekema DJ, Chapin KC, et al. Effects of rapid detection of bloodstream infections on length of hospitalization and hospital charges. J Clin Microbiol 2003;41(7):3119–25.
5. Trenholme GM, Kaplan RL, Karakusis PH, et al. Clinical impact of rapid identification and susceptibility testing of bacterial blood culture isolates. J Clin Microbiol 1989;27(6):1342–5.
6. Doern GV, Vautour R, Gaudet M, et al. Clinical impact of rapid in vitro susceptibility testing and bacterial identification. J Clin Microbiol 1994;32(7):1757–62.
7. Barenfanger J, Drake C, Kacich G. Clinical and financial benefits of rapid bacterial identification and antimicrobial susceptibility testing. J Clin Microbiol 1999; 37(5):1415–8.
8. Kerremans JJ, Verboom P, Stijnen T, et al. Rapid identification and antimicrobial susceptibility testing reduce antibiotic use and accelerate pathogen-directed antibiotic use. J Antimicrob Chemother 2008;61(2):428–35.
9. Bruins M, Oord H, Bloembergen P, et al. Lack of effect of shorter turnaround time of microbiological procedures on clinical outcomes: a randomised controlled trial among hospitalised patients in the Netherlands. Eur J Clin Microbiol Infect Dis 2005;24(5):305–13.
10. Spencer DH, Sellenriek P, Burnham CA. Validation and implementation of the GeneXpert MRSA/SA blood culture assay in a pediatric setting. Am J Clin Pathol 2011;136(5):690–4.
11. Blaschke AJ, Heyrend C, Byington CL, et al. Rapid identification of pathogens from positive blood cultures by multiplex polymerase chain reaction using the FilmArray system. Diagn Microbiol Infect Dis 2012;74(4):349–55.
12. Harris DM, Hata DJ. Rapid identification of bacteria and candida using PNA-FISH from blood and peritoneal fluid cultures: a retrospective clinical study. Ann Clin Microbiol Antimicrob 2013;12(1):2.
13. Hensley DM, Tapia R, Encina Y. An evaluation of the advandx Staphylococcus aureus/CNS PNA FISH assay. Clin Lab Sci 2009;22(1):30–3.

14. Bauer KA, West JE, Balada-Llasat JM, et al. An antimicrobial stewardship program's impact with rapid polymerase chain reaction methicillin-resistant Staphylococcus aureus/S. aureus blood culture test in patients with S. aureus bacteremia. Clin Infect Dis 2010;51(9):1074–80.

15. Forrest GN, Mehta S, Weekes E, et al. Impact of rapid in situ hybridization testing on coagulase-negative staphylococci positive blood cultures. J Antimicrob Chemother 2006;58(1):154–8.

16. Forrest GN, Mankes K, Jabra-Rizk MA, et al. Peptide nucleic acid fluorescence in situ hybridization-based identification of Candida albicans and its impact on mortality and antifungal therapy costs. J Clin Microbiol 2006;44(9):3381–3.

17. Forrest GN, Roghmann MC, Toombs LS, et al. Peptide nucleic acid fluorescent in situ hybridization for hospital-acquired enterococcal bacteremia: delivering earlier effective antimicrobial therapy. Antimicrob Agents Chemother 2008; 52(10):3558–63.

18. Bizzini A, Greub G. Matrix-assisted laser desorption ionization time-of-flight mass spectrometry, a revolution in clinical microbial identification. Clin Microbiol Infect 2010;16(11):1614–9.

19. Cherkaoui A, Emonet S, Fernandez J, et al. Comparison of two matrix-assisted laser desorption ionization-time of flight mass spectrometry methods with conventional phenotypic identification for routine identification of bacteria to the species level. J Clin Microbiol 2010;48(4):1169–75.

20. Desai AP, Stanley T, Atuan M, et al. Use of matrix assisted laser desorption ionisation-time of flight mass spectrometry in a paediatric clinical laboratory for identification of bacteria commonly isolated from cystic fibrosis patients. J Clin Pathol 2012;65(9):835–8.

21. Tan KE, Ellis BC, Lee R, et al. Prospective evaluation of a matrix-assisted laser desorption ionization-time of flight mass spectrometry system in a hospital clinical microbiology laboratory for identification of bacteria and yeasts: a bench-by-bench study for assessing the impact on time to identification and cost-effectiveness. J Clin Microbiol 2012;50(10):3301–8.

22. Mulet M, Lalucat J, Garcia-Valdes E. DNA sequence-based analysis of the Pseudomonas species. Environ Microbiol 2010;12(6):1513–30.

23. Brenner DJ, Grimont PA, Steigerwalt AG, et al. Classification of citrobacteria by DNA hybridization: designation of Citrobacter farmeri sp. nov., Citrobacter youngae sp. nov., Citrobacter braakii sp. nov., Citrobacter werkmanii sp. nov., Citrobacter sedlakii sp. nov., and three unnamed Citrobacter genomospecies. Int J Syst Bacteriol 1993;43(4):645–58.

24. Lambiase A, Del Pezzo M, Cerbone D, et al. Rapid identification of Burkholderia cepacia complex species recovered from cystic fibrosis patients using matrix assisted laser desorption ionization time-of-flight mass spectrometry. J Microbiol Methods 2012;92(2):145–9.

25. Choi SH, Lee JE, Park SJ, et al. Emergence of antibiotic resistance during therapy for infections caused by Enterobacteriaceae producing AmpC beta-lactamase: implications for antibiotic use. Antimicrob Agents Chemother 2008; 52(3):995–1000.

26. Kaye KS, Cosgrove S, Harris A, et al. Risk factors for emergence of resistance to broad-spectrum cephalosporins among Enterobacter spp. Antimicrob Agents Chemother 2001;45(9):2628–30.

27. Seng P, Drancourt M, Gouriet F, et al. Ongoing revolution in bacteriology: routine identification of bacteria by matrix-assisted laser desorption ionization time-of-flight mass spectrometry. Clin Infect Dis 2009;49(4):543–51.

28. Ferroni A, Suarez S, Beretti JL, et al. Real-time identification of bacteria and Candida species in positive blood culture broths by matrix-assisted laser desorption ionization-time of flight mass spectrometry. J Clin Microbiol 2010; 48(5):1542–8.

29. Fothergill A, Kasinathan V, Hyman J, et al. Rapid identification of bacteria and yeasts from positive BacT/ALERT blood culture bottles by using a lysis-filtration method and MALDI-TOF Mass Spectrum Analysis with SARAMIS Database. J Clin Microbiol 2013;51:805–9.

30. Kok J, Thomas LC, Olma T, et al. Identification of bacteria in blood culture broths using matrix-assisted laser desorption-ionization Sepsityper and time of flight mass spectrometry. PLoS One 2011;6(8):e23285.

31. Loonen AJ, Jansz AR, Stalpers J, et al. An evaluation of three processing methods and the effect of reduced culture times for faster direct identification of pathogens from BacT/ALERT blood cultures by MALDI-TOF MS. Eur J Clin Microbiol Infect Dis 2012;31(7):1575–83.

32. Romero-Gomez MP, Gomez-Gil R, Pano-Pardo JR, et al. Identification and susceptibility testing of microorganism by direct inoculation from positive blood culture bottles by combining MALDI-TOF and Vitek-2 Compact is rapid and effective. J Infect 2012;65(6):513–20.

33. Schmidt V, Jarosch A, Marz P, et al. Rapid identification of bacteria in positive blood culture by matrix-assisted laser desorption ionization time-of-flight mass spectrometry. Eur J Clin Microbiol Infect Dis 2012;31(3):311–7.

34. Munson EL, Diekema DJ, Beekmann SE, et al. Detection and treatment of bloodstream infection: laboratory reporting and antimicrobial management. J Clin Microbiol 2003;41(1):495–7.

35. Clerc O, Prod'hom G, Vogne C, et al. Impact of Matrix-Assisted Laser Desorption Ionization Time-Of-Flight Mass Spectrometry (MALDI-TOF) on the clinical management of patients with Gram-negative bacteremia: a prospective observational study. Clin Infect Dis 2013. [Epub ahead of print].

36. Perez KK, Olsen RJ, Musick WL, et al. Integrating rapid pathogen identification and antimicrobial stewardship significantly decreases hospital costs. Arch Pathol Lab Med 2012. [Epub ahead of print].

37. Gander RM, Byrd L, DeCrescenzo M, et al. Impact of blood cultures drawn by phlebotomy on contamination rates and health care costs in a hospital emergency department. J Clin Microbiol 2009;47(4):1021–4.

38. Meex C, Neuville F, Descy J, et al. Direct identification of bacteria from BacT/ALERT anaerobic positive blood cultures by MALDI-TOF MS: MALDI Sepsityper kit versus an in-house saponin method for bacterial extraction. J Med Microbiol 2012;61(Pt 11):1511–6.

39. MacMillan D, Lewandrowski E, Lewandrowski K. An analysis of reference laboratory (send out) testing: an 8-year experience in a large academic medical center. Clin Leadersh Manag Rev 2004;18(4):216–9.

40. Clark BC, Lewinski MA, Loeffelholz MJ, et al. Verification and validation of procedures in the clinical microbiology laboratory. Cumitech 31A. Herndon, VA: ASM Press; 2009.

41. Hayden RT, Yan X, Wick MT, et al. Factors contributing to variability of quantitative viral PCR results in proficiency testing samples: a multivariate analysis. J Clin Microbiol 2012;50(2):337–45.

42. de Pagter PJ, Schuurman R, de Vos NM, et al. Multicenter external quality assessment of molecular methods for detection of human herpesvirus 6. J Clin Microbiol 2010;48(7):2536–40.

43. Hirsch HH, Lautenschlager I, Pinsky BA, et al. An international multicenter per-formance analysis of cytomegalovirus load tests. Clin Infect Dis 2013;56(3): 367–73.
44. Green M, Webber SA. EBV viral load monitoring: unanswered questions. Am J Transplant 2002;2(10):894–5.
45. Zimmermann H, Oschlies I, Fink S, et al. Plasmablastic posttransplant lym-phoma: cytogenetic aberrations and lack of Epstein-Barr virus association linked with poor outcome in the prospective German Posttransplant Lymphopro-liferative Disorder Registry. Transplantation 2012;93(5):543–50.
46. Sousa H, Silva J, Azevedo L, et al. Epstein-Barr virus in healthy individuals from Portugal. Acta Med Port 2011;24(5):707–12.
47. Vouloumanou EK, Rafailidis PI, Falagas ME. Current diagnosis and manage-ment of infectious mononucleosis. Curr Opin Hematol 2012;19(1):14–20.
48. Barenfanger J, Drake C, Leon N, et al. Clinical and financial benefits of rapid detection of respiratory viruses: an outcomes study. J Clin Microbiol 2000; 38(8):2824–8.
49. Mahony JB, Blackhouse G, Babwah J, et al. Cost analysis of multiplex PCR testing for diagnosing respiratory virus infections. J Clin Microbiol 2009;47(9): 2812–7.
50. Banerji A, Greenberg D, White LF, et al. Risk factors and viruses associated with hospitalization due to lower respiratory tract infections in Canadian Inuit chil-dren: a case-control study. Pediatr Infect Dis J 2009;28(8):697–701.
51. Wishaupt JO, Russcher A, Smeets LC, et al. Clinical impact of RT-PCR for pedi-atric acute respiratory infections: a controlled clinical trial. Pediatrics 2011; 128(5):e1113–20.
52. Huijskens EG, Biesmans RC, Buiting AG, et al. Diagnostic value of respiratory virus detection in symptomatic children using real-time PCR. Virol J 2012;9:276.
53. Doan Q, Enarson P, Kissoon N, et al. Rapid viral diagnosis for acute febrile respi-ratory illness in children in the Emergency Department. Cochrane Database Syst Rev 2012;(5):CD006452.
54. Bonner AB, Monroe KW, Talley LI, et al. Impact of the rapid diagnosis of influ-enza on physician decision-making and patient management in the pediatric emergency department: results of a randomized, prospective, controlled trial. Pediatrics 2003;112(2):363–7.
55. Doan QH, Kissoon N, Dobson S, et al. A randomized, controlled trial of the impact of early and rapid diagnosis of viral infections in children brought to an emergency department with febrile respiratory tract illnesses. J Pediatr 2009;154(1):91–5.
56. El Saleeby CM, Somes GW, DeVincenzo JP, et al. Risk factors for severe respi-ratory syncytial virus disease in children with cancer: the importance of lympho-penia and young age. Pediatrics 2008;121(2):235–43.
57. Jangi S, Lamont JT. Asymptomatic colonization by Clostridium difficile in in-fants: implications for disease in later life. J Pediatr Gastroenterol Nutr 2010; 51(1):2–7.
58. Sunenshine RH, McDonald LC. Clostridium difficile-associated disease: new challenges from an established pathogen. Cleve Clin J Med 2006;73(2):187–97.
59. Barbut F, Petit JC. Epidemiology of Clostridium difficile-associated infections. Clin Microbiol Infect 2001;7(8):405–10.
60. Katz DA, Lynch ME, Littenberg B. Clinical prediction rules to optimize cytotoxin testing for Clostridium difficile in hospitalized patients with diarrhea. Am J Med 1996;100(5):487–95.

61. Sidler JA, Haberthur C, Heininger U. A retrospective analysis of nosocomial viral gastrointestinal and respiratory tract infections. Pediatr Infect Dis J 2012;31(12): 1233–8.

62. Beersma MF, Sukhrie FH, Bogerman J, et al. Unrecognized norovirus infections in health care institutions and their clinical impact. J Clin Microbiol 2012;50(9): 3040–5.

63. Zhang G, Hu Y, Wang H, et al. High incidence of multiple viral infections identified in upper respiratory tract infected children under three years of age in Shanghai, China. PLoS One 2012;7(9):e44568.

64. De Schutter I, De Wachter E, Crokaert F, et al. Microbiology of bronchoalveolar lavage fluid in children with acute nonresponding or recurrent community-acquired pneumonia: identification of nontypeable Haemophilus influenzae as a major pathogen. Clin Infect Dis 2011;52(12):1437–44.

65. Bresee JS, Marcus R, Venezia RA, et al. The etiology of severe acute gastroenteritis among adults visiting emergency departments in the United States. J Infect Dis 2012;205(9):1374–81.

66. Bruins MJ, Ruijs GJ, Wolfhagen MJ, et al. Does electronic clinical microbiology results reporting influence medical decision making: a pre- and post-interview study of medical specialists. BMC Med Inform Decis Mak 2011;11:19.

67. Ferris TG, Johnson SA, Co JP, et al. Electronic results management in pediatric ambulatory care: qualitative assessment. Pediatrics 2009;123(Suppl 2): S85–91.

68. Callen JL, Westbrook JI, Georgiou A, et al. Failure to follow-up test results for ambulatory patients: a systematic review. J Gen Intern Med 2012;27(10): 1334–48.

69. Kilpatrick ES, Holding S. Use of computer terminals on wards to access emergency test results: a retrospective audit. BMJ 2001;322(7294):1101–3.

70. Kuperman GJ, Teich JM, Tanasijevic MJ, et al. Improving response to critical laboratory results with automation: results of a randomized controlled trial. J Am Med Inform Assoc 1999;6(6):512–22.

71. Coupat C, Pradier C, Degand N, et al. Selective reporting of antibiotic susceptibility data improves the appropriateness of intended antibiotic prescriptions in urinary tract infections: a case-vignette randomised study. Eur J Clin Microbiol Infect Dis 2012. [Epub ahead of print].

72. Gonzales R, Anderer T, McCulloch CE, et al. A cluster randomized trial of decision support strategies for reducing antibiotic use in acute bronchitis. JAMA Intern Med 2013;1–7.

73. Litvin CB, Ornstein SM, Wessell AM, et al. Use of an electronic health record clinical decision support tool to improve antibiotic prescribing for acute respiratory infections: the ABX-TRIP Study. J Gen Intern Med 2012. [Epub ahead of print].

74. Patel J, Esterly JS, Scheetz MH, et al. Effective use of a clinical decision-support system to advance antimicrobial stewardship. Am J Health Syst Pharm 2012; 69(18):1543–4.

75. Mainous AG 3rd, Lambourne CA, Nietert PJ. Impact of a clinical decision support system on antibiotic prescribing for acute respiratory infections in primary care: quasi-experimental trial. J Am Med Inform Assoc 2013;20: 317–24.

76. Litvin CB, Ornstein SM, Wessell AM, et al. Adoption of a clinical decision support system to promote judicious use of antibiotics for acute respiratory infections in primary care. Int J Med Inform 2012;81(8):521–6.

77. Charani E, Kyratsis Y, Lawson W, et al. An analysis of the development and implementation of a smartphone application for the delivery of antimicrobial prescribing policy: lessons learnt. J Antimicrob Chemother 2013;68:960–7.
78. Rothman B, Leonard JC, Vigoda MM. Future of electronic health records: implications for decision support. Mt Sinai J Med 2012;79(6):757–68.

Index

Note: Page numbers of article titles are in **boldface** type.

A

Clin Lab Med 33 (2013) 731–748

http://dx.doi.org/10.1016/S0272-2712(13)00056-5

0272-2712/13/$ – see front matter © 2013 Elsevier Inc. All rights reserved.

labmed.theclinics.com

Moving?

Make sure your subscription moves with you!

To notify us of your new address, find your **Clinics Account Number** (located on your mailing label above your name), and contact customer service at:

Email: journalscustomerservice-usa@elsevier.com

800-654-2452 (subscribers in the U.S. & Canada)
314-447-8871 (subscribers outside of the U.S. & Canada)

Fax number: 314-447-8029

Elsevier Health Sciences Division
Subscription Customer Service
3251 Riverport Lane
Maryland Heights, MO 63043

*To ensure uninterrupted delivery of your subscription, please notify us at least 4 weeks in advance of move.

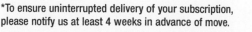

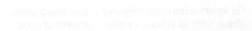

Printed and bound by CPI Group (UK) Ltd, Croydon, CR0 4YY

03/10/2024

01040478-0013